Perspectives on Adolescent Health Care

Perspectives on Adolescent Health Care

Ramona T. Mercer, R.N., Ph.D.

Associate Professor, Department of Family Health Care Nursing
University of California, San Francisco

J. B. LIPPINCOTT COMPANY

PHILADELPHIA   NEW YORK   TORONTO

Library of Congress Catalog Card Number 79-11274
ISBN   0-397-54314-X
PRINTED IN THE UNITED STATES OF AMERICA

1   3   5   7   9   8   6   4   2

Library of Congress Cataloging in Publication Data

Mercer, Ramona Thieme.
   Perspectives on adolescent health care.

   Includes bibliographies and index.
   1. Youth—Health and hygiene. 2. Youth—Diseases. I. Title.
RJ550.M47   613'.04'33   79-11274
ISBN 0-397-54314-X

Contributors

TERESA A. BELLO, R.N., M.S.
  Assistant Clinical Professor
  Department of Mental Health and Community Nursing
  University of California, San Francisco

ROBERT T. BROWN, M.D.
  Assistant Professor of Pediatrics
  Division of Adolescent Medicine
  Assistant Director, Interdisciplinary Training
  Program for Adolescent Health
  University of Alabama Medical Center
  Birmingham, Alabama

WILLIAM A. DANIEL, JR., M.D.
  Professor of Pediatrics
  Division of Adolescent Medicine
  Director, Interdisciplinary Training Program for Adolescent Health
  University of Alabama Medical Center
  Birmingham, Alabama

CAROLYN M. FONG, R.N., M.S.
  Pediatric Instructor
  Merritt College
  Oakland, California

CAROL L. GARRISON, R.N., M.S.N., P.N.P.
  Assistant Professor, School of Nursing
  Core Faculty, Interdisciplinary Training Program for Adolescent Health
  University of Alabama Medical Center
  Birmingham, Alabama

YOLANDA GUTIERREZ, M.S.

Assistant Clinical Professor
Department of Family Health Care Nursing
University of California, San Francisco

CARNIE A. HAYES, JR., R.N., M.S.

University of Mississippi Medical Center
Jackson, Mississippi

RAMONA T. MERCER, R.N., PH.D.

Associate Professor, Department of Family Health Care Nursing
University of California, San Francisco

FREDERICK H. MEYERS, M.D.

Professor of Pharmacology
Department of Pharmacology and the Toxicology Research Laboratory
University of California, San Francisco

SISTER PENNY PROPHIT, R.N., D.N.SC.

Assistant Professor, Psychiatric-Mental Health Nursing
The Catholic University of America
Washington, D.C.

MARILYN SAVEDRA, R.N., D.N.S.

Assistant Professor, Department of Family Health Care Nursing
University of California, San Francisco

DIANA TAYLOR, R.N., M.S.

Obstetric-Gynecological Clinical Specialist
Multnomah County Division of Health
5848 SE Milwaukie Avenue
Portland, Oregon

EUGENIA H. WAECHTER, R.N., PH.D., F.A.A.N.

Associate Professor, Department of Family Health Care Nursing
University of California, San Francisco

LOIS J. WELCHES, R.N., D.N.S.

Assistant Professor, Department of Family Health Care Nursing
Nursing Coordinator, Interdisciplinary Training Program for Adolescent Health
University of California, San Francisco

To my parents, NELL *and* WILLIAM THIEME, *who lovingly supported me through my adolescence; my daughter* CAMILLE, *who gave me many happy, and sobering, glimpses back into my adolescence; and my husband,* LEWIS, *for his infinite patience and understanding in my middlescence.*

Contents

SECTION 4: The Adolescent, the Health Professional, and the Health Care System

Foreword

Only in recent times has there been general recognition and acceptance by members of different health professions that adolescence is a distinctive developmental stage meriting close attention. In some situations adolescents were viewed as older children who, when hospitalized, naturally shared rooms with other children, many times with five- and six-year-olds. Often this resulted in chaos and occasionally it was disastrous. Equally unfitting was viewing adolescents as immature adults.

Even as the incongruities of treating adolescents as members of either of these other two developmental groups became apparent, other much more difficult problems arose. Firstly, while we have gained in our understanding of what adolescence is not, our knowledge of what it *is* has remained limited. For example, we know that beginning to develop a healthy body image is one of the tasks of adolescent development. But while we can readily identify behaviors which tell us that the toddler is learning to talk or walk, we do not know how to measure concretely whether the adolescent has accepted and achieved comfort with his or her own body image. We know that coming to terms with this image is a dynamic phenomenon continuing throughout the adult years. What, then, constitutes the range of normal body image attainment for the adolescent? What indicates abnormality? We just don't know. Finally we are uncertain as to the interrelationships among the various developmental tasks which occur during adolescence. How do they interfere with or augment one another?

The indefiniteness of our knowledge about these developmental tasks creates the second major problem of working with adolescents: provision of effective care. Even though our knowledge of the developmental tasks specific to this stage is elementary, we do understand that adolescence is a period of transition and that, like any transitional time, it is characterized by turbulence. This turbulence is reflected in the adolescent's extremely labile moods, behaviors, and needs. The adolescent may change drastically from day to day. Not only must the health care provider change the tone of approach to meet these changing moods but often the very content of the intervention as well. What alleviated an adolescent's emotional pain yesterday may no longer do so today. The words and explanations he or she comprehended previously may no longer have meaning as the adolescent accommodates to his or her inner upheaval. This constant process of adjusting both tone of approach and content of intervention to suit the adolescent *now,* presents an enormous challenge for the health care professional.

Perspectives on Adolescent Health Care is a contribution to the current storehouse of knowledge about the healthy and ill adolescent. Its purpose is not only to help the health care provider to acquire a fuller understanding of the adolescent based on knowledge we already have but also to catalyze the reader to develop new insights and knowledge about the process of adolescence and the most effective methods for providing health care to its members.

BARBARA E. BISHOP, R.N., M.N.
Editor, *MCN, The American Journal of Maternal Child Nursing*

Preface

Although a wide range of skilled professionals are involved in providing care for adolescents, the variety in the points of initial interaction for the delivery of health care does not seem to alter the kind of basic information that is needed about adolescence. A broad base of knowledge is helpful in counseling the young man or young woman in his or her decision making for responsible action for optimal growth and health.

Adolescents present a special challenge to the health professional. They are not easy to work with. Is it because we project a stereotypic response and the adolescent in turn lives up to our expectations? Is it because our culture provides few guideposts and few models for expected behaviors in accomplishing unknown goals? Or is it the unpredictable behavior of this age group that unnerves us and makes us feel uncomfortable? Do we identify uncomfortably with the adolescent as we recall our difficulties at a similar time ourselves? Or is it because we represent the parent or authority figure to the young person and, thus, arouse stereotypic responses in him that he projects to us? Perhaps all of these factors, and more, contribute to some of the difficulties we experience in our work with adolescents.

The idea for this book originated while I was conducting a workshop for professionals who were working with pregnant adolescents and adolescent parents in a variety of community settings—schools, health clinics, and hospitals. Following the workshop several participants remarked, "One book that pulled all of this information together would be most helpful." These remarks provided the stimulus to begin outlining the content for this book. Dialogue with Karen Hoxeng, Associate Editor with the Nursing Department of J. B. Lippincott Company, prompted extending the content to include additional perspectives on health care, apart from childbearing. This meant that a search for contributors who had expertise in these additional perspectives was necessary. The positive response of the contributors who are actively involved in their own research projects and clinical work with adolescents provided additional stimulation for my own work. Their enthusiastic commitment to health care for adolescents is evidenced by their unique ideas, cogent questions, and helpful suggestions. There are no easy, pat answers, but through sharing knowledge and experiences, much can be gained. This book represents this kind of sharing.

The purpose of this book is to pull together some of the major ideas and issues about adolescent health. It is intended as a resource for those who work with adolescents in a variety of settings—the nurse in acute care or ambulatory settings, the teacher, the social worker, the chaplain, the physician, or others who counsel the young person. The student should find the book helpful as a supplement to professional texts, particularly the adolescent health, family, maternity, or pediatric nurse practitioner or the clinical specialist student whose clients are adolescents. Although the non-nursing professional will not be utilizing many of the detailed clinical descriptions, the information can be helpful in interpreting health care to the adolescent. This book does not purport to be all-inclusive; however, it offers perspectives about the adolescent in a variety of situations which call for special skill and helpful guidance from the health professional.

Several major themes continue throughout the book. These themes include the interdependence of the major tasks of adolescence and their concomitant emotional impact on the adolescent, an emotional impact that perhaps is reflected by two of the leading causes of death for this age group—accidents and suicide. The special psychosocial and counseling needs of the adolescent and the influence of the interrelationships of the family group and the larger cultural and societal context on the adolescent's evolving sexuality and adult identity recur in each chapter. These needs are discussed in relation to a specific perspective on adolescent health.

Selected perspectives that focus on some of the major health concerns for this age group are organized into four sections. Section 1, The Well Adolescent, focuses on the adolescent as a person and adolescence as a social entity. Selected adolescent tasks as they relate to the early, middle, and late adolescent are explored as an introduction to the book: acceptance and achievement of comfort with body image; determination and internalization of sexual role; development of a personal value system; preparation for productive citizenship; achievement of independence from parents; and development of an adult identity.

Lois Welches shares her views on adolescent sexuality and on alternatives and indicators in sexual behavior, based on her work and research with the adolescent. Dr. Welches is Nursing Coordinator of the Interdisciplinary Adolescent Health Training Program at the University of California, San Francisco. The impact of the ethnic group on the adolescent is explored: Carnie A. Hayes, Jr., maternity nurse practitioner, discusses the task of the black family in promoting self-esteem in young blacks; Teresa A. Bello, community health teacher and researcher, astutely outlines the strong family impact on Latino adolescent mores and values; Carolyn M. Fong, pediatric nurse practitioner and pediatric instructor, describes the experience of being Chinese and American as an adolescent.

Yolanda Gutierrez, a nutritionist with extensive experience in counseling young women in antepartal and postpartal clinics and in teaching health professionals, speaks to the special nutritional needs of the adolescent from the perspectives of the adolescent's rapid growth and development and dietary habits, and also considers the unique nutritional needs presented by pregnancy, sports and activity, oral contraceptives, and chronic illness.

Diana Taylor, maternity nurse clinical specialist, has worked several years as a nurse practitioner in adolescent contraceptive counseling and in organizing adolescent contraceptive clinics. She shares several special approaches in contraceptive counseling for the young person. Both her creativeness and her sensitivity to the adolescent client are reflected in the clinical examples and suggestions for care.

Section 2 focuses on the adolescent with a health problem. Health problems commonly encountered in the adolescent are succinctly presented by a team from the Interdisciplinary Training Program for Adolescent Health at the University of Alabama Medical Center, Birmingham: William A. Daniel, Jr., M.D., Director; Robert T. Brown, M.D., Assistant Director; and Carol L. Garrison, pediatric nurse practitioner, core faculty member from the School of Nursing. The nurse practitioner particularly will find the special approaches to the history taking and physical examination most helpful.

Marilyn Savedra, who teaches pediatric nursing and is researching coping patterns of ill school age children, discusses the adolescent who is hospitalized and how the adolescent's developmental concerns and cognitive operations interact with his response to hospitalization and to illness. Implications for nursing care and for the hospital setting are focused upon.

Eugenia H. Waechter, researcher, nurse educator, and child development specialist, has studied children and their families during grief and chronic illness extensively. She discusses some of the special problems of the adolescent who has a chronic illness and special concerns of the adolescent and his family when faced with a life-threatening illness.

Frederick Meyers, physician, pharmacology professor, and researcher, is the founder or cofounder of several treatment programs for substance abusers. His expertise in pharmacology and treatment programs is reflected in his consulting services to the Senate subcommittee (the "Kefauver Committee") whose investigations led to the revision of the Food and Drug Act in 1962, and to the technical Advisory Committee on Drug Abuse of the State Department of Health, California. In discussing drug use among adolescents Dr. Meyers presents reasons for taking drugs, patterns of use and abuse, the drug, individual, and group or sociological factors. His challenge for prevention of drug abuse among adolescents is both provocative and a stimulus for self-reflection.

Sister Penny Prophit for much of her career has studied the enigma of adolescent suicide in the United States. She approaches the problem from a theoretical and research base and offers suggestions for working with the troubled young person and for those counseling the family who is left behind following adolescent suicide. The over 300% increase in adolescent suicide during the last decade speaks to the need for all professionals to become increasingly sensitive to the masked depression and the emotional problems of the adolescent, who usually cries out for help long before attempting suicide.

Section 3 deals with the special health and social problems presented by the childbearing adolescent. As a maternity nurse clinical specialist, I have had extensive clinical experience with pregnant adolescents and adolescent parents. During the last decade I have studied these areas more formally. The pregnant adolescent is viewed from the perspectives of physiological, psychological, and sociological risks, in the context of some of the crucial decisions she faces—abortion, adoption, marriage. Needs of the youthful father are discussed. Prenatal care for the adolescent encompasses the special risks of the adolescent client who is pregnant and the special counseling needs which both she and her partner have. The adolescent experiencing labor, delivery, and early postpartum is viewed from the perspectives of the risks involved during these processes and the responses of the early, middle, and late adolescent. Special needs of the mother who relinquishes her infant for adoption and the importance of continuity of care for all adolescent parents are discussed. Vignettes from a study of the teenager's first year of motherhood dramatize some of the problems encountered by adolescent parents as well as some of their strengths in resolving these problems. The process of maternal role attainment and the promotion of role attainment of the teenage mother are discussed.

Section 4 examines the interrelationships of the adolescent, the health care professional, and the health care system. The health professional's role and response as well as special hazards for professionals who work with adolescents are viewed. Some of the weaknesses of the health care system are explored, along with some of its potential strengths and assets.

Rich clinical examples are offered throughout the book to illustrate theory about the adolescent and about health care for the adolescent. The creative and practical suggestions offered may be utilized in most settings with alterations adapted to each professional's style and unique situation.

RAMONA THIEME MERCER

Acknowledgments

Although one person organizes and writes much of a book, the contribution by others is always profound, and this book is no exception. Appreciation is expressed to the contributors who wrote chapters on the various perspectives on adolescent health care and to several persons who contributed in other ways. Many shared clinical illustrations which greatly enhance the section on the childbearing adolescent: Leslie Carey, Peggy Goebel, Susan E. Japar, Rose Lacki, Mary E. Müller, Jean Muncrief, Anne McCormick, Patricia O'Malley, Diana Taylor, Catherine R. Tobin, and Lois Welches.

Special thanks are extended to Connie Stockdale for her critique of the section on the childbearing adolescent and to Carol Howe, who proofread and reviewed the entire book. Mary Ann Whitemore, Associate Editor, Nursing Department, J. B. Lippincott Company, provided both editorial criticism and encouragment. Their suggestions added much to the content and its clarity. Appreciation is expressed to Lewis P. Mercer for his artwork in the illustrations. Margaret L. Oakley performed the miracle of typing the ''collages'' and rendering them readable; for this transformation, I am very appreciative.

To the adolescents who have shared their anxieties, joys, doubts, and fantasies, I am deeply grateful. Care has been taken to assure their anonymity by altering environmental situations. All names used in the text are fictitious; the one exception is Lorraine, my niece, who wrote all of the treasured letters shared in Chapter I.

To be productive, one must enjoy one's work and colleagues. Betty L. Highley has created an enjoyable, stimulating milieu for productivity through the exchange of ideas and mutual support of peers. Her leadership is gratefully acknowledged.

Special acknowledgment and appreciation are extended to the publishers of the following journals and books for permission to include selected copyrighted material: The American Journal of Nursing Company, The National Dairy Council, Birth and the Family Journal, The Alan Guttmacher Institute, Harper and Row Publishers, Inc., National Council on Family Relations, Hart Publishing Company, Inc., W. W. Norton and Company, Inc., Doubleday and Company, Inc., and the C. V. Mosby Company.

R.T.M.

The Well Adolescent

Perspectives on the Adolescent and Adolescence

Ramona T. Mercer, R.N., Ph.D.

The adolescent and adolescence are concepts that are difficult to describe. The paired antonyms commonly used in referring to this period of life reflect this difficulty, as well as some of the conflict experienced by adolescents. At times adolescence is called painful, at times pleasurable. It is a period filled with many doubts and fears as well as a time of certainties and joys. It is a period of heightened expectancy in which one experiences for the first time some of the adult privileges that were taboo in childhood. Longed-for, anticipated first experiences may include driving a car, going to restricted movies, dating, or drinking a first cocktail. A first ''true'' love or first sexual intercourse may be experienced. Much nervousness, fear, and anxiety accompany first experiences, along with appreciation, thrill, and excitement. First experiences are often nostalgically etched into our memories as prototypes that can never be recaptured with a similar intensity of feeling and excitement.

When addressing adolescents, or speaking about them, there is often hesitancy as one searches for the best or most acceptable word to use. Are they young women and young men? They are not ''kids.'' They are not children. The difficulty in choosing a term of address for the adolescent reflects the uncertainty and ambivalence that exist within the adult frame of reference about this age group. Adolescents are sometimes viewed as children; at other times their body size and sensitivity allow them to be viewed as adults. This ambiguity is also communicated to the adolescent who is experiencing the growth process. One young woman stated, ''I call and make my own appointments for a check-up; I drive myself to the appointment. I do not want to be treated like a child when I arrive.''

Adolescence is a process of evolving from childhood to adulthood. Process connotes progression, continuing development, constant change or unfolding. Within this progression from childhood to adulthood are phases, or stages. It is good to keep in mind, however, that with any development or progression there is a certain degree of fluidity. There are points at which a temporary plateau is reached, accompanied by a reaching backward or reverting to earlier, more comfortable styles of relating and behaving. This kind of fluidity may be seen in the ocean wave: as it crests and rushes forward onto the shoreline there exists beneath its surface a swift, retreating undertow pulling backward into the ocean. In a developmental process, there is an observable forward movement toward higher specificity and greater differentiation in all of the thinking and behavioral responses, but the undertow, or pull, to earlier modes of thinking and behaving is there. This forward-backward movement of trial and error continues as the individual moves forward to a new and higher plateau of development.

This chapter examines the adolescent as a person in the process of becoming an adult, an individual who is distinguished from others by his unique and characteristic way and style of interacting with others and with the environment. Knowledge about the process of evolving toward adulthood and the nature of its inherent tasks provides baseline data for assessing, planning, intervening, evaluating growth, and facilitating health care. Relevant, meaningful health care for adolescents has both a synergistic and a markedly catalytic function in the process of evolving to adulthood. The phases of adolescence and their developmental tasks provide a conceptual framework from which therapeutic intervention with adolescents may be approached. Reasons for concern about adolescents, varying concepts of adolescence as a cultural entity, and phases in the process of evolving are discussed. Selected tasks and related theory within physiological, psychological, and sociological contexts of development are discussed.

Why So Much Concern About Adolescents?

Why do we hear so much about the adolescent? *Why* do we bother with special conferences on adolescent health? What is the significance of the problem—if there is a problem?

In the United States one-fifth of the population is between the ages of 10 and 19.[1] The adolescent population doubled from 20 million to 40 million in the years from 1950 to 1970.[2] A precipitous growth rate such as this has created problems not only in the educational institutions in which this age group seeks preparation for a life's profession, but also in the health care system. The health needs of this large group of our citizens have far exceeded the available health care systems to the extent that the majority of this population are not receiving adequate health care.[1]

For some specifics about the kinds of health problems that have increased, one in every ten girls in the United States becomes pregnant while she is of high school age or younger.[3] Approximately 918,000 school days are missed each year by young women who have gonorrhea and related complications. This means that approximately 5,750 young women miss school daily because of gonorrhea.[4] Teenagers from 15 to 19 are the second highest risk group for gonorrhea; this age group is the fourth highest risk group for syphilis (based on age-specific case rates).[4] Approximately one third of the abortions performed in 1974 were for women under 20.[5] A study[6] of 255 "healthy" females, ages 11 to 17, found that almost two thirds of them had undiagnosed medical conditions requiring treatment and that over one half had psychosocial problems.

According to available research and statistical reports, one fifth of our current adolescent population has a wide range of undiagnosed diseases—including malnutrition and gynecological, urinary tract, and cardiovascular diseases. Adolescence has been stereotyped as a healthy period of life. Is the gap between myth or stereotype and reality too broad to close? Health care professionals who deal with young adults are raising these and other questions as they try to ameliorate these conditions. Nursing and other service-oriented professions and organizations are sponsoring workshops on adolescent sexuality, health, pregnancy, and parenting in attempts to close the gap.

Adolescence: A Combination of Cultural, Historical, Physiological, Psychological, and Sociological Factors

Adolescence as we know it—a period spanning the years between childhood and adulthood—is a phenomenon of industrialized, developed societies. Developing countries or primitive cultures rarely have a recognized period in which the child gradually assumes adult responsibilities. If a specific rite or preparation for adulthood does exist, it is usually much shorter than the lengthy period of 8 to 12 years with which we are familiar in the United States. An example of a cultural rite of passage may be seen in the popular book *Roots*[7] in the story of Kunta Kinte, a youth of the Mandinka tribe in Africa. For Kunta Kinte the process of transformation to adulthood began with the traditional gift of a cloak to hide his nakedness, after which he was expected to assume the responsibility of herding the goats. The final transition occurred when, upon reaching his twelfth rain (year), he was secreted away, circumcised, and trained rigorously for his new role as a man. For Kunta Kinte, however, there were no doubts about the responsibilities that he was to assume in his community or the method by which he was to assume them after the completion of the rites of passage. He was well prepared for his role as a man in his culture—although he had occasional fears and doubts about his capabilities.

Contemporary complex societies with extended time periods of adolescence do not offer such specific guideposts or end-points at which one becomes an adult. The young person knows he will achieve independence from his parents eventually, but the method or manner in which he will do so is vague and ill-defined, both to himself and to his parents.

In the United States, adolescence as a specific period of life evolved with the social changes that occurred during the latter half of the nineteenth and the beginning of the twentieth centuries.[8] Legislation has given recognition to the entity of adolescence as the newly emerging urban, industrial society required it. Laws for compulsory education, child labor legislation, and criminal procedures for juveniles all served the purpose of distinguishing and separating a portion of the population.[8]

Therefore, prior to the early twentieth century, there were no references to problems with adolescent parents or health problems of the adolescent. Children, as little adults, were expected to learn adult roles early. It was not unusual for a girl of

16 to marry; in some states the legal age for marriage without parental consent is still 16. Social conditions are drastically different now than they were then, however. Then, teenagers often grew up on the farm as productive, valuable contributors to their families' welfare. They worked hard, shoulder to shoulder with the rest of the family. The teenager today has difficulty finding a job either for the summer or when he graduates from high school. He is usually isolated from his father's occupation, and in general feels rather superfluous as far as his family's welfare and security are concerned. Conversely, he may be reminded that he is a financial drain on family resources, which in reality he is, and he may be chided for his laziness in performing chores around the house.

Conditions for child-rearing were also different some hundred years ago. Families lived in homes, often with three or four generations in one household, in smaller communities where everyone knew and cared about everyone else's children. Mothers had access to the wise and experienced amateur counsel of family or friends rather than the professional specialist. The harshness of disease and the lack of immunizations took their toll in children's lives, and the death of a family member was a common experience.

As social conditions have changed, parent, child, and adolescent roles have changed. The young person's needs for internal acceptance of an adult body with new functions and the resolution of conflicts experienced in moving from childhood to adulthood have not changed, however. Young people have always experienced the sexual urges that emerge with physiological maturation as well as restlessness and awkwardness with their growing physical bodies. How the young person behaves or copes with these changes depends, in large measure, upon what his society provides as acceptable avenues of expression at his particular historical moment.

Adolescence is socially defined according to the context within which the youth lives. The culture, or totally learned way of life transmitted from generation to generation, is learned both directly and indirectly by the youth as he works at the process of becoming an adult. Within the socially defined behavioral expression of the transition from childhood to adulthood, an interdependent self-development occurs which involves biological, psychological, and sociological maturation.

The terms "development" and "maturation" are often used interchangeably. *Development,* as used in this text, refers to a forward-moving process of growth or advancement to a higher level of functioning and adaptation. *Maturation,* in this text, refers broadly to the adult or mature state as opposed to childlike behavior or childhood. Development does not end with adolescence. Physical maturation occurs at adolescence, but psychological and sociological development continue throughout life as an individual evolves through varying phases of adult development.

Physiological development during adolescence begins with the acceleration of the individual's growth and the development of secondary sexual characteristics. It ends with the fusion of the epiphyseal plates of the bones and the completion of sexual maturation. The ranges are not discrete; physiological development may begin as early as 8 years or as late as 18 years and may reach completion as early as 15 or as late as 25 years. Many factors, such as gender, familial traits, and nutritional and health status, have an impact on the timing for physiological growth.

Psychologically, during adolescence a different cognitive style develops. The adolescent progresses from the concrete and egocentric thinking of childhood to abstract conceptualization and the development of an ability to view the world from another person's perspective.[9,10] The individual has to deal with feelings, attitudes, and values as they relate to his goals in life. The attainment of a sense of identity and of comfort with his perception of who he is and where he is going suggests that the young person has reached young adulthood. The individual's feelings about himself are firmed up as he resolves conflicts about his decisions for choices and values up to that point in life.

Sociologically, the individual moves from a dependent child role to an independent adult role. The individual reaches adulthood sociologically when he is accorded full adult prerogatives and status. The ability and willingness to play the role of an adult consistently occur when sufficient healthy maturation and experience have accrued.[11] Psychologically and socially, some persons never fully meet these criteria of adulthood—as is indicated by their frequent vacillation between the adolescent and adult states.

Many young people in this culture have a psychosocial moratorium or experimental period in which to find themselves.[12] There are some, however, who at very early ages must assume the responsibility of fending for themselves, and sometimes for an ill or handicapped parent as well. The social assets or liabilities of a family can drastically facilitate or hinder the youth in his work of evolving to adulthood.

In addition to the handicaps or assets imposed on the teenager by his social status, many conflicting messages are transmitted to him. For example, many of the rites of passage to adult prerogatives occur at different ages in different states—or even different localities within the same state. In most states, the young person can obtain a driver's license at 15 or 16 years; in all states, the privilege to vote comes at 18. The young man may be drafted in time of national emergency when he becomes 18. Yet, the adult prerogative of purchasing alcoholic beverages is not accorded until age 21. Since these adult privileges are awarded at different points in his development, the youth gets the message that he is wise enough to choose his leaders and mature enough to die for his country—yet not mature enough to know what he should drink until some three years later. If the adolescent's family moves from a state which permits driving a car at 15 to a state which does not grant licenses until 16, he may be disappointed and frustrated.

The changing social definitions of acceptable behaviors for various roles create dilemmas for parents and health care workers alike. Parents have to unlearn in order to relearn what is currently appropriate to existing roles. This sort of discontinuity* exists for the teenager also. For example, as he was growing up, the child asked permission or approval from his parents about matters related to where he went or what he did. As an adult he must assume responsibility for these choices and make such decisions for his own child. A current example is the young woman who chooses to remain a virgin until marriage, who has been restraining her sexual urges and saying, "no, no." When, on the night of her wedding, it is suddenly all right to say, "yes, yes," she has to immediately discontinue restraining or redirecting her

---

*The concept of discontinuity in which cultural learning of the child inevitably fails to meet the role requirements of later life is from Ruth Benedict's classic article "Continuities and Discontinuities in Cultural Conditioning," *Psychiatry* 2:161–170, 1938.

sexual urges, and is expected to consummate these urges in sexual intercourse. In this discontinuity she is equally frightened about appearing uncooperative and about her ability to perform well.

Phases in the Process of Evolving

Early, middle, and late adolescence seem to provide some general and practical, although indiscrete, dimensions of the process of becoming an adult. Early adolescence may be roughly designated as including the period from about 12 to 14 years of age. Middle adolescence spans the ages from 15 through 16 years, and late adolescence extends from 17 years until adulthood. The normal variation between individuals precludes the idea of distinct boundaries for a phase, and there are also fluctuations in characteristic behaviors between phases.

EARLY ADOLESCENCE

Blos[13] views the phase of early adolescence as the most crucial phase, since it sets the stage for progression within later phases. He points out that because biological maturation has been occurring four months earlier every ten years, an individual has evolved who has a child's mind and an adult's body. This early adolescent is often pushed ahead by well-meaning parents and teachers into relationships for which he or she is unready.

Blos[13] notes that adolescent development progresses by a process of detour and regression. The young male usually deals with this unsettling regression of his disorganized psyche through sloppiness in appearance and habit. He needs and seeks out close, idealized friendships with other boys. Parents often become frightened that this is homosexual behavior, and attempt to push him toward interacting with girls. Whereas the boy in early adolescence usually exhibits slovenly habits, girls may maintain a neater personal appearance. Blos[13] observes, however, that the young male's struggle with his strange bodily sensations and his control of these sensations arouse the unconscious struggles of bodily regulation that he experienced when he was an infant; he resists the mother of his infancy to such an extent that he becomes leery of all females. The formation of an ego ideal through his relationship with his father enables him to make later choices for career goals and helps him to overcome his fear of women so that he can enter the phase of middle adolescence.

The girl in early adolescence uses her girlfriends as mother substitutes in her early attempts at detaching from her mother.[14] This is difficult for her since she usually has a strong desire to remain in a dependency role with her mother.[14] Her newly emerging feminine body creates ambivalence about her preadolescent activity as a tomboy. She may have a great crush on her teacher or the popular star of the time as she leads a rich fantasy life.

The young adolescent's cognitive thinking is dominated by descriptive comments of current circumstances.[9] An excerpt from *The Diary of Anne Frank,*[15] written during the time when Anne was with her family in hiding from the Nazis during World War II, illustrates some of these points:

I think what is happening to me is so wonderful, and not only what can be seen on my body, but all that is taking place inside. I never discuss myself or any of these things with anybody; that is why I have to talk to myself about them.

Each time I have a period—and that has only been three times—I have the feeling that in spite of all the pain, unpleasantness, and nastiness, I have a sweet secret, and that is why, although it is nothing but a nuisance to me in a way, I always long for the time that I shall feel that secret within me again.

Sis Heyster also writes that girls of this age don't feel quite certain of themselves, and discover that they themselves are individuals with ideas, thoughts and habits. After I came here, when I was just fourteen, I began to think about myself sooner than most girls, and to know that I am a "person." Sometimes, when I lie in bed at night, I have a terrible desire to feel my breasts and to listen to the quiet rhythmic beat of my heart.

I already had these kinds of feelings subconsciously before I came here, because I remember that once when I slept with a girl friend I had a strong desire to kiss her, and that I did do so. I could not help being terribly inquisitive over her body, for she had always kept it hidden from me. I asked her whether, as proof of our friendship, we should feel one another's breasts, but she refused. I go into ecstasies every time I see the naked figure of a woman, such as Venus, for example. It strikes me as so wonderful and exquisite that I have difficulty in stopping the tears rolling down my cheeks.

If only I had a girl friend!

Yours, Anne*

MIDDLE ADOLESCENCE

During middle adolescence the young person manages to disengage from his or her parents and make a decisive turn toward heterosexual relationships.[16] The parent is renounced as a love object finally and completely. The revival and resolution of the oedipal conflict may lead to sexual experimentation with peers. Homosexual episodes may also occur during this phase.[16]

An increase in narcissism occurs, along with a deep appreciation for beauty and nature. Fantasies entertain the young person as he shares his attachments and infatuations. The middle adolescent may fall in love very deeply and the love object often resembles the parent.[16] Emotions vacillate both in range and from moment to moment with little predictability; drama and creativity are prevalent.[14]

Around the age of 15 years, the young person begins to reason deductively from hypotheses in problem solving and has the power to maintain an argument.[9] Gradually he realizes that others' thoughts are not all directed toward him.[17] Under pressure, however, his cognitive functioning returns to earlier levels of operation.

*Excerpt from *The Diary of a Young Girl* by Anne Frank. Copyright 1952 by Otto H. Frank. Reproduced by permission of Doubleday and Company, Inc., p. 117.

LATE ADOLESCENCE

During late adolescence, the young person achieves the ability to maintain stable relationships; chosen life tasks and goals are acquiring shape. The work of defining and articulating social roles has been accomplished although there is still some uncertainty about the new, more consistent emerging patterns.[18] Blos[16] refers to the achievement of relative maturity as a phase of consolidation. The closing phase of adolescence, according to Blos, is recognizable by the following psychological features: a unique and stable repertoire of ego functions and interests; an extension of independence with less conflict; an irreversible sexual identity with genital primacy; respect for self and an ability to form attachments to another; and a stabilization of mental functioning capable of safeguarding his integrity.

The person in the late adolescence phase no longer has to show that he is an individual through indiscriminate protest; behavior is less chaotic and much more predictable.[18] Cognitive functioning is fairly stable and is seen in the ability to view problems comprehensively and to reject remote possibilities.[9]

Tasks of Adolescence

Tasks during the developmental phases of adolescence vary somewhat from culture to culture and with each young person's goals for his life. Many tasks could be enumerated for this period of development; however, six tasks are eclectically chosen: (1) acceptance and achievement of comfort with body image; (2) determination and internalization of sexual identity and role; (3) development of personal value system; (4) preparation for productive citizenship; (5) achievement of independence from parents; and (6) development of an adult identity. The tasks were chosen for their universality and for their scope. The theoretical basis for the selection of each task is incorporated in the discussion of the task.

ACCEPTANCE AND ACHIEVEMENT OF COMFORT WITH BODY IMAGE

The body image is a mental picture of the way the body appears to the self.[19] The self begins as a bodily self: the infant first knows and experiences bodily sensations. All senses that receive external and internal stimuli become integrated into the body image.[20] The individual interprets and integrates the many sensations or impressions (percepts) and internalizes these as a general notion (concept) of self.[21] Perceptions of body image may not reflect actuality. Fisher and Cleveland[22,23,24] found that attitudes and expectations played a large part in an individual's perception of body boundaries.

The body image aids in defining the reality of the world through defining the relationship of the body to the environment. Individual peculiarities or differences in the body image contribute to unique perceptions of the world; this could in part explain an artist's ability to paint previously unknown and different perceptions of the environment.[25]

Bodily changes are usually met with strong emotional resistance. Alterations, losses, and changes within the body may be comprehended as danger.[26] Thus, the adolescent is keenly interested in the size and shape of his developing body. Although the body may be well within the normal range of development, the young person will frequently have great concern about some aspect of his appearance.

One study[27] found that early adolescents from 12 to 13 years of age had heightened self-consciousness, less stability of the self-image, lower self-esteem, and perception that others held less favorable views of them to a greater degree than any other age group from the third through the twelfth grade. The self-image disturbance appeared suddenly between the eleventh and twelfth years when the physical growth spurt usually begins. The self-image disturbance also seemed to be related to entry into junior high school, since 12- and 13-year-olds in the seventh grade were more disturbed than those in the sixth grade. Both physical and social variables seem to be interacting in ways that contribute to the difficulty of this early adolescent phase.

Heunenmann and associates[28] found that ninth to twelfth grade adolescents' self-images were unrealistic when compared with actual measurements. Large numbers of girls described themselves as fat; more than half of the girls wanted smaller hips, thighs, and/or waistlines, in that order. The boys were concerned about being underweight and expressed a desire for larger biceps, chest, wrists, shoulders, and/or forearms. Although black girls seemed more satisfied with their figures than white girls, the black youths seemed anxious for increases in all body dimensions.

A study[29] of late adolescents enrolled in an introductory psychology course in college found male-female differences in the self-concept. The young women's self-concepts were more strongly related to their physical attractiveness, whereas the young men's self-concepts were related more to their physical effectiveness, although attractiveness of body parts was correlated with both male and female self-concepts. Whether gender leads to a particular personality orientation, or whether social learning that rewards and punishes these differences is the deciding factor, continues to be questioned.

Getting acclimated to the new body size and its appearance and function takes much energy and concern on the youth's part. In Salinger's[30] novel *Catcher in the Rye,* Holden Caulfield at 16 blamed his shortness of breath on his heavy smoking and on his having grown six and a half inches the year before. There may be some resistance to the discomforts of the emerging physically mature body, along with awkwardness and hesitancy about accepting it.

If the reader has ever gained 30 pounds within six months, as during pregnancy, or, conversely, has had a sudden loss of weight following delivery or after dieting, she may recall that she looked for a size 14 or 16 dress for some time before she automatically went to the size 12 dress rack again. Somehow, the internalization of body changes takes much longer than the actual change. In adolescence, the randomness and the variability in the timing of changes bring disappointment and anxiety to many.

A study[31] of women aged 13 to 64 years found that the highest frequency of symptoms usually associated with menopause occurred at two developmental stages, adolescence and menopause. Psychological symptoms were higher in the 13 to 18-year-old group than in any other age group. Somatic symptoms were higher in the

45 to 54 year age group. These findings led the researchers to conclude that the menopausal woman, because of her maturity, probably copes more effectively with bodily change than the adolescent.

The adolescent's body image also reflects his sexual identity. In addition to the male's basic concern with his height, strength, and muscular development, he is concerned with the length of his penis, the prescence of testes, and hirsutism.[32] When a 16-year-old is able to grow a beard before his 18-year-old brother who has always been the pacesetter for him, this is a satisfying victory for the younger brother. The youth who has hypertrophy of mammary tissue, or is short, or who has undescended testes and delay in onset of adolescence is seriously hampered psychologically and socially.[33] In girls, the absence of breast development, amenorrhea, and facial and body hirsutism create equally distressing disturbances.[33]

If a person feels different from most of the others in his social group, he usually feels inferior. Twelve-year-old Yvonne was thrilled and excited when her menses began. Others in her class were already experiencing menstrual periods; she felt that she was at last admitted to an exclusive sorority.

Along with the cognitive internalization of bodily changes, however, come the very practical problems of having longer arms and longer legs. Balance is thrown off, a feeling of awkwardness is prevalent as the adolescent struggles with where to put the longer arms or legs—either standing or sitting.

The sporadic and highly individualized growth rate also presents problems for the adolescent within the peer group, where conformity is stressed.[34] The stresses evolving from appearance that is different or from being a social reject because he does not meet peer standards may hamper the young person's total activities. The late maturer may be penalized socially, while the early maturer with an adult body and behavior like a child's may be looked down upon accordingly.

The adolescent growth phase is unique because of its finality. The young person has to come to terms with the reality of permanent differences. As the final physical growth occurs, this signals not only adulthood, but also strength and independence. If, during this last chance to grow, the individual's height levels off at five feet two inches, he may feel inferior, weak, and saddened at the permanent loss of childhood. His hopes of becoming a tall man someday are demolished.

The state of flux of the adolescent's body image makes him especially vulnerable to other persons' judgments of him. His self-awareness and body image are based in large part on how his parents, peers, and society see him and how he interprets their evaluation of him. Advertising media also tell him what he is or should be, and how he should behave with the opposite sex. Parents can easily create feelings of inadequacy and anxiety in a youth through statements or by glances which in reality reflect their own inadequacies.[33]

The adolescent formulates an ideal body image from his real and fantasied experiences, perceptions, comparisons, and identifications with others.[33] The heightened narcissism that is associated with an ego ideal is nonetheless a normal state of the adolescent as he exhibits a certain degree of self-glorification in projecting a model of what he would like to be.[35] The newly formulated ideal includes social, cultural, and peer values with a view toward future roles; it is both more than and different from any earlier ideals or role models. Although the adolescent may formulate fantasies in which he solves all problems and eliminates weaknesses and imperfections, he is aware of the irrationality of any excessive self-glorification and of the quasi-reality of his goals.[36] This is why parental expectations, peer values, or social demands may be experienced as coercion by the adolescent; they remind him of demands he is already making on himself in his attempt to actualize his ideal image.[35]

DETERMINATION AND INTERNALIZATION OF SEXUAL IDENTITY AND ROLE

Sorting out the sexual identity and determining the role of that identity requires role-taking behavior, as for any other role. In taking roles, there are various levels of involvement;[37] however, in taking on the masculine or feminine identity and role in a heterosexual relationship, maximal involvement of self occurs. Role taking is not done in isolation; it occurs in interaction with another person. Behaviors are tried and cues from the significant other are read to determine the acceptability of the behaviors. The adolescent working at his sexual role first uses many persons of the opposite sex, as well as parents, friends, and other role models, such as popular stars or sports heroes. A lot of fantasy precedes role-taking behavior. This is especially true with young people who avidly listen to stories told by older friends about their love lives. A certain amount of role playing is then tried. The adolescent's parent of the opposite sex may be used, in part, for this. However, the reemergence of the oedipal conflict makes the adolescent uneasy, and older teachers may be used more safely for this purpose. Peers of the opposite sex are used in many situations of fantasy and role playing, and role models are used for internalizing behaviors that are desirable to the individual in that role. After much fantasy, role playing, introjection, and projection of self in the role, a role is finally internalized and becomes a part of the individual's identity.[38]

To illustrate this process in a young woman's life, some letters from Lorraine, written to her aunt during her thirteenth to eighteenth years, are shared and discussed. Lorraine is the oldest of three children; she has a sister five years younger and a brother seven years younger than she is. She grew up in a happy, child-centered, intact, middle-class home. Her letters poignantly illustrate a normal young girl's fantasy, pain, and anxiety in becoming a young woman. The spelling, vocabulary, and style are as Lorraine wrote them.

April 2, 1971
[Day after 13th birthday]

It was very nice of you to remember a little brother's daughter. Daddy must have been a wonderful little brother. "Little Brother" When you were younger you translated that word into everything imaginable (slave, brat, tag-along, cissy). I know because I have one. But everyone grows up and starts to cherish him.

. . . Twelve is a nice age but one must look ahead to the years called teens. Thirteen. That age seemed a long way off but it came; it finally came.

Daddy's a model airplane nut now. (But I follow him in this field) but he is always getting smarter and smarter.

. . . I have a boyfriend he is real nice. He gave me a bracelet like this. Pretty isn't it? [Lorraine draws a picture of it.] Another boy at school likes me too. Some boys are still cissys though, they hate girls.

[Lorraine then wrote a history of moves the family had made since she was four and a half years old.]

Love,
Lorraine

Lorraine was ambivalent about becoming a teenager, although she had anticipated it. Becoming a teenager meant entry into a special period of life, but the transition evoked a thoughtful, sobering affect leading to a review of her family history.

Lorraine's admiration for her father was evident, but she was uncomfortable elaborating on her feelings for him and moved directly to describe a boyfriend. This suggests her work on resolving the reemerged oedipal conflict. She could safely fantasize about her evolving sexual identity in relationship to boys at school. Her observation that some boys hated girls supports Blos's description of the young male who rejects all females.

May, 1971
[13 years, 1 month]

I am sorry I have not written you in so long. I am very upset and Mom doesn't understand. I suppose I am too old to be crying but I still cry. The main reason I am upset is my boyfriend. I'll start at the beginning so you can understand fully. A boy named Joe likes me I like him too. But it was pretty clear he liked another girl too. We were together almost always, he went to football games with me and bought drinks for me, and opened the door for me. We didn't hold hands or anything like that, but he liked me and that was all that mattered.

I began to like him more and more. Soon I was in love with him. I was very happy until the "other" girl acted like she liked him. She was everything I was not, I was not sophisticated or anything. He found out she liked him "soon". Without a word he began going around with her. He never said a thing to me. This cut my heart like fire, it hurt as much! I couldn't bear to see him and her. I almost cried every time I saw them. She got mad at him all the time, though with me we never fought at all. They broke up, it was the same until one day, the kids in my class started a fad. We married boys just for the fun of it. Some of the kids were the Justice of the Peace! He asked me to marry him. This is a month later. I did, soon he said he liked me. I was glad. I thought I liked him again. He never paid as much attention to me as before. He only said "hi" and opened doors for me. Then a good movie was playing. This is now. He asked me to go with him. I said yes. He even asked me to go to the prom with him. I got all dolled up. He never came for me. I was very upset, I cried so hard Mom told me to quit it. I just couldn't stop crying.

I cried because my heart was cut deeper. I knew I would never be able to be his girlfriend unless he treated me like a girlfriend. I think I will just call off the prom unless he changes his attitude otherwise we can just be friends. My heart cannot stand one more hurt from him. . . .

Please ''sympathize''.

Love,
Lorraine

At 13, Lorraine was not allowed to date, so much of that letter seemed to be fantasy. Nevertheless, she was working at boy-girl roles very hard. Lorraine expressed her painful feelings of inferiority to her boyfriend's new girlfriend. The happiness of her love for her boyfriend plunged to deep pain when she saw (or fantasized) a rival winning him. The role-play of marrying illustrates the early adolescent's role-play for later roles.

March 6, 1972
[3 weeks before 14 years]

. . . Guess what, I got a secret admirer note. It says, ''My dearest Lorraine'' (on the front of it) Then it says, ''Dearest Beauty of God. You are the most neatest person I have ever met. Not much to say now but I will write more later. Love, Your Secret Admirer'' That's the way he wrote it. If a girl wrote it for a joke its not very nice. (But I do hope its a boy!) Some girls do that but it really could be a boy., He wrote so neat and tidy. Next time I get a note I'll write you right away and tell you what it said.

I won a science fair, 2nd place! I dissected a fish and put it in solution of formaldehyde (I think thats how its spelled.) I also was in a spelling bee too but I lost. I was so scared and flustered in front of everyone. There has also been a school dance. I couldn't go but I'll probably get the gossip about it from the girls. They always talk about everything that goes on.

My boyfriend is pretty nice. He isn't a bad boy. He's always telling me that he loves me. And he goes to the show if he knows I'm going, or if he thinks I will be there. I hardly get to see him, but when I do he acts like I haven't seen him in years. He kisses really nice. You may think I'm pretty young for all that but that's the way girls are about their boyfriends now-adays.

I like to write poetry. Its my thing! I have millions of ideas for stories but I just can't write them the way I want to. Most of them would be good children's books if I could get them written down the right way.

Daddy still builds model airplanes. Lots of boys come to my house to see them. They really are interested. Daddy likes that a lot.

Love,
Lorraine

Almost a year later, at 14, Lorraine's feelings about her feminine identity were more positive. The note from a secret admirer pleased her, even though she recognized the possibility that a girl could have written it. Although Lorraine couldn't go to the school dance, she and her boyfriend arranged to meet at the movie theatre. Whether in reality or fantasy, in one year Lorraine progressed in her boy-girl interactions from not even holding hands to kissing. Although she felt she was young for kissing, she conformed to her peer group. Lorraine's creativity is illustrated in her interest in writing poems and children's books. Lorraine's feelings about her father and boys continued to be interrelated. She projected her feelings to her father in indicating that *he* liked having the boys come to her house.

March 14, 1973
[2 weeks before 15 years]

How are you? I'm fine, the weather here is so dreary. I feel so *trapped* in by winter. I want to feel all the sunshine and warm evenings. We've had a long winter and it doesn't look as if it will go away for quite awhile.

. . . School is fine. We had a Sadie Hawkins Dance at our school and I went and had lots of fun. This time girls asked boys and picked them up and paid for everything. I didn't ask anyone. (But I did have fun.)

Love,
Lorraine

As a middle adolescent at 15, Lorraine felt trapped by weather that restricted her activities. She had been allowed to go to a school dance, but had not invited a boy. Apparently her fantasy and role-play in boy-girl interactions had not bolstered her confidence to the point where she would invite a boy.

November 8, 1973
[15 years, 7 months]

. . . I used to read a lot but lately I haven't had enough time for anything! Between housework, homework, school, and church, I try to squeeze in time to goof-off. I'm not really as dedicated as it sounds, in fact maybe I goof-off too much.

. . . I went to the homecoming game and dance with my boyfriend and I really had a good time. His name is Carl. We got along all right, but now we're just friends after the fight we had. A fight seems the easiest way out to explain, but I think we really got tired of each other or maybe I'm just boring. Well anyway that's over.

Sometimes I wonder if school is worth the hassle. [She goes on to explain all of her teachers' idiosyncrasies.]

Well that's most of my teachers. My favorite is *coach*. He's the football coach and a great Spanish teacher. Everyone gets along with him. Everyone! . . .

Love,
Lorraine

As Lorraine neared 16, her activities were keeping her busy, yet she was critical of herself regarding use of time; perhaps she was too critical.

She looked at girl-boy relationships more realistically in her breaking up with her boyfriend. At 13, she dramatically described her breakup as very painful. At 15½, she speculated that they were tired of each other. Some feelings of inadequacy still remained, however.

Lorraine had a crush on the coach, a much safer masculine ideal than her father. The crush on the coach suggests that she was distancing herself from her father.

[Family has moved to another state.]

> August 8, 1974
> *[16 years, 4 months]*

. . . Guess what!! Daddy bought me a ten-speed bike! I'm really excited to see what it looks like and everything. He ordered it and also one for my mother.

. . . I babysit four days a week for a nine month baby boy. He's really cute. blond, and blue-eyed and a real good baby. So far from just babysitting I've gotten about $42.00. I plan on using it for school clothes. My Mom is buying my shoes.

. . . I'm also going to school away from home. The school here isn't as good as where I went before. I'm going to be living with my best friend.

. . . I guess I haven't told you about any of the boys I've met this summer. First I'll tell you about my boyfriend (Wow!) He's 6 foot 1 inch, brown hair, brown eyes, 16 years old, and his name is Ted. He lives in Salt Lake and was up here working for the forest service, but he writes me. Then there's Larry. He's 17 and really good-looking! He's like a brother to me. He wants to come to visit me next year. I hope we still live here. I've met more boys than this but I haven't got enough room to tell about all of them! I think I've gotten a little bit more mature this year but most of all I've had the greatest summer ever! I've come to love my home and family a lot more. I've especially come to appreciate all the beautiful wilderness here. My Mom and I get along really good now and rarely fight at all. There's really no generation gap here, unless I make one! I've really been trying to make a better person out of myself and to be a little less selfish.

You know, suddenly education seems so important to me. I just hope the feeling lasts till school starts. I plan on working hard this year.

. . . I feel sometimes I waste all my time doing nothing. I probably have wasted at least two years of my life already. Do you know anything about being a stewardess? I've been thinking about it as a career. I want to travel and grow up some before I go to college. . . . One thing that's certain for me. I don't want to get married right away. Or get into trouble and have to get married. There's so much that I want to do and experience. I'm trying not to think of my life as starting tomorrow or after high school. I'm starting everything today!

I've got lots of things to occupy me until I leave. I have a shirt to finish, two skirts to hem . . . Packing to do . . . I'm going to leave lots of prize possessions!

Life seems to be grabbing and swallowing me all at once! I'm sure that you're enjoying your "age" as much as I'm enjoying mine. I think I'll be sixteen another year! I must close now but wish you happiness in all that you do.

> Love,
> Lorraine

By babysitting Lorraine could role-play the mothering role, but making money to buy school clothes seemed to have been the priority. Lorraine viewed herself as more mature, and her mother, who "didn't understand" her heartbreak at 13, had now become her ego ideal. She enjoyed her many boyfriends at this age and had established that she did not want to have to get married.

Although she was so busy that life was "grabbing and swallowing her all at once" she was critical of herself for wasting time. She was also perhaps appreciating her home and family more because she was leaving to go away to school. This move helped to facilitate the usual middle-adolescent task of becoming more independent of both parents. Her appreciation of the wilderness is characteristic of the middle-adolescent's awe of nature.

[Family has moved back to former place and Lorraine is living with her family again. She has just returned from vacation.]

September 1, 1975

[17 years, 6 months]

. . . I had a happy reunion with my boyfriend when I got back. He sure missed me! I was with him every night until he left for college. He was home for Labor Day weekend so we've only been apart for a week. He just left today for school. He had his car finished and was planning to take it with him this weekend but it broke down.

You ought to see the necklaces he bought for me. One was a turquoise and heeshi shell choker, that's an expensive necklace. And a sterling silver pendant with his college emblem. He brought me a T shirt with the colleges name too. He can't really afford it but he does things like that a lot.

. . . I'm going to work for a year after school, get a car and go to college after that. My Mom isn't too excited about me becoming 18 and going away. But I guess that's normal for all parents. I'm not in a hurry to grow up, but it seems like it happened so fast.

Love,
Lorraine

At 17½, Lorraine had moved into the older adolescent phase. Her desirability in the feminine role was reinforced by both her boyfriend's attentiveness and gifts. The fact that the gifts were expensive added to her self-concept as a valued person. Lorraine was beginning the separation from her parents and sensed her mother's difficulty in seeing this happen. Growing up happened all too fast for Lorraine.

June 28, 1976

[18 years, 3 months]

If you missed your invitation to my graduation its because I forgot to order some. I was so busy with everything else I forgot. I'm sorry I haven't written. Everything has been happening all at once.

It seems like I don't keep up with anything. I was so excited about graduating then, and now I'm engaged to be married! Mike and I went down to Flagstaff and found a ring. My whole set has 3 diamonds, one large and two small ones. Its really pretty. We're planning on getting married in August. I'll send you an invitation as soon as we decide a definite date. I've been working for about a month and a half so far.

Love always,
Lorraine

P.S. Have any advice for a couple starting out?

July 21, 1976

[18 years, 4 months]

. . . I'm sure it (marriage) won't be easy, but we're happy going steady, engaged I mean. I haven't gotten used to that yet! We haven't fought with each other very much at all. We disagree and talk about whatever is bothering us. Mike and I have good communication between us. We don't always agree, but we talk about it.

I think he is a little nervous about getting married, but isn't everyone? We've gone for our blood test and I see that as a great achievement. He's funny when it comes to blood. He can't stand the sight of it especially his own. If they had to use a syringe I think he would have balked but he held up real well! I was scared to go to my premarital examination but we have a real good doctor. He's straight forward and honest and he made me feel at ease right away. I was so glad.

You should see my wedding dress! Its so pretty! Its got a real long train and lace all over . . .

Love,
Lorraine

At 18, Lorraine had a firm feminine sexual identity and made a stable commitment. Life continued to move quickly for her—graduation, engagement, and marriage. Her conceptualization of marriage suggested a sense of sureness with little conflict about her decision. Although the premarital examination was dreaded the doctor had put her at ease. A series of rites of passage seemed to have facilitated Lorraine's attainment of her confirmed feminine identity in marriage: gifts, the engagement ring, the blood tests, premarital examination, and the traditional wedding dress.

Lorraine did a great deal of role-playing in early adolescence and fantasized about what dating would be like for her. By middle adolescence, she felt more mature and noted that she appreciated her family more. Preparing to go to school in another state may have precipitated her serious thinking about the family that she was leaving for a short while. Lorraine noted that life was grabbing her, swallowing her up, but she liked 16 so well she wanted to be 16 another year. At 18, in late adolescence, she was engaged to be married immediately after graduating from high school, something which she had said she would not do two years earlier. Her letters suggest, however, that she began fantasizing and role-playing for marriage at 13. Within six years, Lorraine internalized her heterosexual identity and feminine role and moved into the young adult stage of life described by Erikson[12] as intimacy versus isolation. Although Lorraine still seemed childlike in some ways, she moved into her role of wife with no more observable outward difficulty than other young women.

Lorraine's internalization of her heterosexual identity went along smoothly. For other adolescents this transition is not so easily made.

For some teenagers, the movement from the bisexual orientation of early adolescence to a confirmed heterosexual role can be painful and may be accompanied by anxiety and fear. If the body image is not in keeping with the ideal sexual image currently in vogue, the youth may feel powerless and defeated. The boy whose penis has not grown may be reluctant to go to gym class because of the necessity of undressing and showering with other boys. The tight-fitting jeans that are worn by men today enable them to display their genital size as women have always done with breast size.

The feelings and emotions that a youth experiences as he attempts to overcome the reemerged oedipal conflict may be quite traumatic. Examples from literature illustrate some aspects of the conflict experienced by males in working on their heterosexual roles. It is not an accident that Alex in *Portnoy's Complaint*[39] talked at length with his psychiatrist about watching his mother seductively slip on her nylon hose and attach them to her garter belt. Alex recalled his preschool incestuous conflicts and described his current incestuous fantasy at age 25 rather vividly. He mused about what his father's response would be, if all of a sudden he and his mother tumbled to the floor in the act of sexual intercourse.

As it was in the fictional case of Alex, the arousal of unresolved oedipal feelings may account for some of the sexual acting-out of the teenager. Alex recalled that he spent half of the time he was awake in the bathroom masturbating.

Masturbation plays an important role in tension reduction; however, it often revives castration fears and evokes guilt conflicts.[40] Masturbation may intensify confusions and distortions in the adolescent's sense of identity or it may positively accentuate his feelings of self.[41] The adolescent fears that everyone knows his secret by his acne (or "pud bumps"), the uncontrollable bulge of his erections, or his long stays in the bathroom. Other common myths are that masturbation leads to blindness or insanity, or causes hair to grow in the palms of the hands. These myths were probably begun by well-meaning parents who wanted to discourage masturbation.

The threat of homosexual encounters also may "unglue" a youth. Holden Caulfield, the central figure of *Catcher in the Rye*[28] became very frightened by an approach made by one of his teachers and ran out of the teacher's apartment late at night. Holden reacted physically to this encounter by shaking and perspiring heavily, reflecting his intense fear and anxiety about the experience.

In the novel *Ode to Billy Joe,* Billy Joe McAllister's death plunge from the Tallahatchie Bridge was the result of a homosexual encounter when he was drunk at the Saturday night jamboree.[42] Accidents are the leading cause of death for the 15- to 24-year-old age group. The 1972 fatality rate for all accidents was 68.1 per 100,000 in the 15- to 24-year age group, or 53% of all deaths. The death rate for all causes was

127.7 per 100,000.[1] Suicide accounted for 11.4 per 100,000 deaths.[1] How many accidents might be suicide? Millar[1] noted that the fact that suicide is a leading cause of death for older adolescents reflects the increasing incidence of such mental health disorders as depression, impulse disorders, and acting-out behavior. Achieving sexual identity is not easy even for the young woman or young man who is not mentally ill. The pain of early romance is acute; rejection or separation causes temporary depression and emotional upset. A newspaper account of a 14-year-old boy and 15-year-old girl who attempted to run away on a sailing yacht stated that the boy had threatened suicide before deciding to run away after his parents had forbidden him to see his girlfriend.

DEVELOPMENT OF A PERSONAL VALUE SYSTEM

Before personal values can be determined, certain conditions must be met; among these are the development of a conscience, competence in abstract thought, the ability to make judgments, and the ability to view the world from another person's perspective. As the individual emerges into adulthood, he brings with him a value system by which he intends to live. Adolescents are idealistic in their thinking and work hard at determining a code of behavior.

Josselyn[43] described the individual's development of values as a merging of the ego ideal with the superego into a mature conscience, occurring with cognitive maturation. She described the ego ideal as a representation of self-image that can be loved and respected. Failure to live up to one's ego ideal results in a loss of self-respect and the development of a sense of shame, which is alleviated either by changing personal goals or by exerting greater effort to achieve the goals. The superego represents the internalized values of parents or other important persons, but is also influenced by culture. Feelings of guilt represent internalized fear of or actual punishment by parents during childhood.

Blos[44] described four developmental tasks which ''collaboratively and synergistically'' lead to the closure of adolescence and stable character formation. The first task is the second individuation process (the first occurring at the end of the third year when the toddler individuates from his mother) in which the individual achieves independence from family and takes responsibility for his actions. According to Blos, the superego becomes less rigid and less powerful as the ego ideal becomes better established and more influential. The adolescent's peer group allows him to try out roles without permanent commitment, and enables him to share and alleviate the guilt feelings that he is having from wanting to be rid of childhood dependencies and prohibitions. A temporary self-aggrandizement and overestimation of power occurs, with the result that reality testing may be affected adversely. This phenomenon could be one explanation for the increased rate of accidents among teenagers.

A second task for closure of the adolescent process and a stable character formation is the resolution of earlier trauma (trauma being any conditions which were unfavorable or injurious to the previous development). Internalizing or dealing with earlier trauma helps to render it ego syntonic (harmonious with self), in that anxiety is lessened and there is no longer a feeling of helplessness at the memory of the trauma. Anxiety does not disappear, but it can be managed by integration and adaptation.

A third task for establishing stable character formation is a sense of ego continuity. Blos observed in his study of adolescents in analysis that the ego moves forward only if a historical continuity is established; this historical continuity seems to have an integrative and growth-stimulating effect. Perhaps this precondition of character formation explains why so many adoptees seek their biological parents during adolescence. At developmental milestones, the young person seems to need to recapitulate his entire life from birth. Many parents report that their adolescents ask to have the story of their birth and childhood repeated rather often.

The emergence of the sexual identity is the fourth task in Blos's schema that brings to a close the period of adolescence and adult character formation. As long as ambiguity or ambivalence of sexual identification lasts, the ego cannot escape being affected by the ambiguity of the drives. The extent to which the four tasks or challenges have been fulfilled will determine the defensive nature of the character that evolves. Defenses are unconscious responses developed by the ego to protect the self.

Asceticism is a major defense developed at puberty. In the ego desire and attempt to maintain the character developed during latency, self-denial of many instincts occurs.[45] Asceticism was observed in young people during the sixties when so many of them rejected the luxuries of their parents' middle-class standards and moved to various forms of communal living, where they often lived off the land and dressed simply. The adolescent's move from asceticism is indicated by a swing to excess. A 14-year-old may become an avowed vegetarian for a few days, then suddenly eat all meats that are available. Currently, various cult groups seem to be appealing to youth's asceticism. Many cult groups, however, exert powerful influence on the adolescent, controlling every facet of his life.[46] Johnson[46] notes that most cult groups meet all of the needs usually met by a family, except that in cult groups there is no autonomy; therefore, adolescence does not end. Shapiro[47] observes that the cults are harmful to the adolescent's physical and mental health, as is evidenced by a syndrome of personality change, loss of personal identity, change in mannerisms, and intense psychological fear. Deterioration, rather than intellectual development, seems to occur in those cases.

Intellectualization evolves as a defense in adolescence along with cognitive development. Intellectualization is seen in verbalization or thought that represents fantasy more than reality; it is a way of avoiding emotionally disturbing feelings.[45] The intellectual content of daydreams may offer gratification as a process of thinking, but behavior is not necessarily changed.[45]

Kohlberg and Gilligan[48] define six stages in the development of moral thought; two stages occur in each of three levels—preconventional, conventional, and postconventional or autonomous. At the preconventional level in stage one, orientation is to unquestioned dominant power, and the physical consequences of an action to the self determine whether an action is good or bad. In stage two, selected action satisfies needs of the self and the needs of others when the self benefits. At the conventional level in stage three, good behavior means conformity to the majority. One is good in order to be accepted by the group. Stage four orientation is directed toward concern for social order; respect is earned by keeping rules and maintaining order. At the postconventional level in stage five, the entire society determines rights and standards. Laws are changed for the good of the majority. In stage six the orientation is toward universal principles concerning justice and human rights for all mankind. These stages in moral reasoning are seen by Kohlberg and Gilligan as always developing in this sequential order; steps may not be omitted in the developmental sequence. The preconventional level is usually reached between the ages of four and ten, the conventional level in preadolescence, and the postconventional level in adolescence.

The individual's personal value system develops concurrently with his thought processes, character, and moral judgment. The initial orientation toward self expands to include concern for others and orientation toward universal ethical principals. The idealistic adolescent is vulnerable to proselytizing groups.[46]

PREPARATION FOR PRODUCTIVE CITIZENSHIP

This task combines the selection of and preparation for one's life work and the cognitive preparation for skills needed in negotiating with the social system in general. The adult, through his vocational role and participation in the social and political aspects of the community in which he lives, is a vital, contributing member of society.

Choosing an occupational role for his or her lifetime is a frightening task for a young person. Furthermore, rapid social change makes the choice even more difficult. Technology has created more job opportunities and at the same time has made other jobs obsolete. A person with a new baccalaureate degree in education may have difficulty finding a teaching position and may return to school to prepare for another occupation. The changeable nature of the contemporary job market may be the impetus for some change in career direction; for others, changing majors after completing a college degree may mean that, with greater maturity, life's goals have changed. Parents often nag adolescents during the freshman year of college to choose a major. One young woman responded to her parents' prodding by stating, "I'm too young to know what I want to do the rest of my life."

Major motivations for selecting and preparing for an occupation include self-fulfillment, challenge, and the achievement of independence. But with choices more numerous than ever before, educational preparation for occupations more expensive, and the promise of a future in a particular field of employment less sure, the young person has to select and plan carefully.

The parent, on the other hand, often cannot understand the difficulty which the young person faces. When the parent was choosing his or her life's work, there were fewer choices; consequently the task was perhaps easier.

Given the state of the world's energy supply, environmental pollution, and the necessity to maintain defenses against nuclear war, the young person may wonder what he can realistically do *in* and *with* the world that he is inheriting. He questions which political decisions need to be made, and which problems should be solved first. The problems of today are quite different from those of yesterday; every era has its challenges. The rapid changes in world and social conditions may be dramatized if the reader who is over 30 will momentarily recall her life at 16 or so. What was happening in the world at that time? What were the major crises confronting youth? The newly evolving adults of the late 1970s have a life's work and challenge cut out for them.

ACHIEVEMENT OF INDEPENDENCE FROM PARENTS

This task includes the achievement of both psychological and financial independence from parents. Gould[49] in his study of sequential change over adulthood observed a loud, repetitive theme — "We have to get away from our parents" — among 16- to 18-year-olds and 18- to 22-year-olds. At the earlier age, little is done to carry out the desire expressed in the theme, and even attempted close relationships with peers are short-lived as the adolescents make temporary rebounds to their parents. The 18- to 22-year-old is actively implementing the theme but fears being pulled back into the family circle. He resents an intimate peer who cannot meet his needs as his family did earlier.

As was stated earlier, one of the greatest motivators for choosing a vocation and preparing for it is the desire to become financially independent from the family. College provides an opportunity for practice in making decisions on one's own, setting priorities for and managing one's time, and managing one's own money. Our society, however, does not define or describe the specific steps involved in the process of moving from the dependent child status to the status of independent adult. For the middle-class or upper-class youth, there are better-defined and more gradual steps, such as coming-out parties or college. For the lower-class youth, the transition may occur abruptly. He may be told that he has to drop out of school and find work in order to help buy food for the family or to help with other expenses. Thus, he gets the message that he is no longer going to be cared for even minimally, and that he must move to a contributing or adult status. A daughter in a family from a lower socioeconomic group may choose a premature marriage or quitting school and going to work as the only way out of deprivation.

A child is a legal and a financial liability; there are indeed few parents who do not look forward to their child's financial independence. Parents more often fail to look forward to, or to acknowledge, social and psychological or emotional independence, however.

As the adolescent breaks the ties to his parents, he may do so harshly or impulsively. The majority of adolescents, however, are able to achieve independence without the total devaluation and negation of their parents.[50] The first argumentative disagreements between parent and adolescent are often trials in asserting independence. The adolescent refuses to carry out the garbage because his mother wants him to. The adolescent often decides what he will do in response to what his parents do not want him to do; his negative assertion of independence or rebellious attempt at emancipation reflects the conflict that he is experiencing.[50]

The adolescent becomes increasingly involved with peers who can share his emotional experiences. Deutsch[51] points out that what the adolescent cannot do individually he can permit himself to do in a group. The group provides a true peer society whose major goal is a search for identity. In groups, adolescents avoid isolation and conquer anxieties.

It is hard for some parents to understand the adolescent's rebellion as a painful assertion of independence and the trial of new wings—and to understand and accept the fact that the adolescent needs these trials. Many parents see their usefulness in life diminishing as their adolescent leaves home. Other parents, however, have reached a point in life at which they can enjoy togetherness and the fruits of lifelong labors in renewed relationships. When parents experience letting go as difficult, this makes the youth's task of achieving independence all the harder. Many teenage mothers have described a new kind of relationship developing with their own mothers. In this new relationship, their mothers treat them as equals, really understand them, and talk to them differently. Perhaps much of the energy we expend in promoting the independence of the young could be directed toward supportive understanding of their parents—toward helping them to take a new look at life, which promises new richness as they enter into adult relationships with their children. An adult-to-adult relationship with one's child can be very rewarding.

DEVELOPMENT OF AN ADULT IDENTITY

The task which encompasses the development of an adult identity is derived from Eriksons's[52] "sense of ego identity," described as the major developmental task of adolescence, and from Levinson's[53] stage of early adult transition. The development of an adult identity is an interdependent aspect of all of the tasks of adolescence. Identity evolves from earlier experiences and identifications and is integrated with basic biological drives, native endowment, and social and vocational roles.[54]

Erikson[52] noted that adolescent love is largely an attempt to arrive at a definition of one's identity by projecting one's diffused self-image on another and by seeing it thus reflected and gradually clarified. This is why so much of young love is conversational. Lorraine's letters contain a lot of work towards her achievement of a sense of identity.

The sense of ego identity is gained by the accumulation of confidence in one's ability to maintain inner sameness and continuity; this ability is verified by interactions with significant others.[52] The emerging ego identity gradually turns from the early childhood meaning of self and of others and is tempered by a variety of social and cultural definitions which become increasingly coercive with age.[54]

Levinson[53] observed "twin developmental tasks" in the early adult transition period from 17 until 22 years. They include beginning to move out of the preadulthood era and making preliminary steps into the adult world. To accomplish this transition a reappraisal and modification of self and of existing relationships are required. To enter this new phase of life, adulthood, it is necessary to consolidate an initial adult identity and to make choices about adult living. The initial adult identity is a culmination of development in all of the tasks chosen for discussion.

Summary

In the process of becoming an adult, the young person works arduously at accepting a new adult body, identifying and internalizing a sexual role, determining a value system by which he can live, preparing for productive citizenship, and, finally, at achieving both his adult identity and his independence. These tasks are helped or hindered by such available societal supports as role models, rites of passage, stability, and respect within the social system for individuality.

It is helpful to view the transition from childhood to adulthood as occurring in three phases—early adolescence, middle adolescence, and late adolescence. The dramatic physical and psychic growth that precedes and continues throughout early adolescence seems to reach a level of some stability at middle adolescence so that the young person consolidates these new maturational processes into a comfortable self that is uniquely his during late adolescence.

The rich years of adolescent turmoil that bridge the world from childhood to adulthood have lasting meaning for all of us. Helene Deutsch[55] in her ninth decade of life wrote:

> The biological destiny of old age varies from one individual to another. Like all developmental periods of life, it depends greatly on the events of adolescence. To our stereotyped way of thinking, the process of growing up is identical with the conquest of the stormy forces of adolescence. Yet I feel that my *Sturm und Drang* [storm and distress] period, which continued long into my years of maturity, is still alive within me and refuses to come to an end. This feeling is supported by the continuation of relationships that span three generations. I find that there are still ecstasies and loves in me, and that these feelings are rooted in my adolescence. They may be reaction formations against the threat of death, but at the same time they represent the generous impulses of the most energetic period of my life.
>
> . . . All the best human impulses can be traced back to adolescence. I believe that these persistent adolescent forces are the best aspect of my own old age.*

Perhaps some of the difficulties encountered by those working with adolescents—nurse, social worker, physician, or teacher—stem from the reexperiencing of some of the old pains and conflicts of their own adolescence. However, if, along with the reexperiencing of some of the struggles, we also relive some of the love and the ecstasy of this period, we have a dimension of richness added to our ongoing development.

REFERENCES

1. Millar, H. E. C. *Approaches to Adolescent Health Care in the 1970s*. Rockville, Md.: U.S. Dept. Health, Education and Welfare. DHEW Pub. No. (HSA) 75–5014, 1975.
2. McCoy, K. "Adolescent Sexuality: A National Concern." *Report of a Wingspread Conference*. Racine, Wis.: The Johnson Foundation, 1974.

*Reprinted with permission of W. W. Norton & Company, Inc., 500 Fifth Avenue, New York NY 10036.

3. Williams, T. M. "Childrearing Practices of Young Mothers: What We Know, How it Matters, Why It's So Little." *Am. J. Orthopsychiat.* 44:70–75, 1974.
4. *VD Fact Sheet 1976.* Atlanta, Ga. 30333: U.S. Dept. Health, Education, and Welfare, Center for Disease Control. DHEW Pub. No. (CDC) 77–8195.
5. Baldwin, W. H. "Adolescent Pregnancy and Childbearing—Growing Concerns for Americans." *Population Bull.* 31(2):12, 1977.
6. Fiedler, D. E., et al. "Pathology in the 'Healthy' Female Teenager." *Am. J. Pub. Health* 63(11):962–965, 1973.
7. Haley, A. *Roots.* New York: Doubleday & Co., Inc., 1976.
8. Bakan, D. "Adolescence in America: From Ideal to Social Fact." In Kagan, J., and Coles, R., eds. *Twelve to Sixteen: Early Adolescence.* New York: W. W. Norton & Co., Inc., 1972, pp. 73–89.
9. Peel, E. A. *The Nature of Adolescent Judgment.* New York: Wiley-Interscience, 1971.
10. Piaget, J. "The Intellectual Development of the Adolescent." In G. Caplan and S. Lebovici, eds. *Adolescence: Psychosocial Perspectives.* New York: Basic Books, Inc., 1969, pp. 22–26.
11. Horrocks, J. E. *The Psychology of Adolescence Behavior and Development.* 3rd ed. Boston: Houghton Mifflin Co., 1969.
12. Erikson, E. H. *Childhood and Society.* 2nd ed. New York: W. W. Norton & Co., Inc., 1963.
13. Blos, P. "The Child Analyst Looks at the Young Adolescent." In Kagan, J., and Coles, R., eds. *Twelve to Sixteen: Early Adolescence.* New York: W. W. Norton & Co., Inc., 1972, pp. 55–72.
14. Hatcher, S. L. "Understanding Adolescent Pregnancy and Abortion." *Primary Care* 3(3):407–425, 1976.
15. Frank, A. *Anne Frank: The Diary of a Young Girl.* New York: Doubleday & Co., Inc., 1967, p. 117.
16. Blos, P. *On Adolescence.* New York: Free Press, 1962.
17. Elkind, D. "Egocentrism in Adolescence." *Child Dev.* 38:1025–1034, 1967.
18. Josselyn, I. M. *Adolescence.* New York: Harper & Row, Pubs., Inc., 1971.
19. Schilder, P. *The Image and Appearance of the Human Body.* New York: International Universities Press, Inc., 1950.
20. Gorman, W. *Body Image and the Image of the Brain.* St. Louis: Warren Green, II, 1969.
21. Kolb, L. C. "Disturbances of the Body-Image." In Arieti, S., ed. *American Handbook of Psychiatry,* Vol. 1. New York: Basic Books, Inc., 1959, pp. 749–769.
22. Fisher, S. "A Further Appraisal of the Body Boundary Concept." *J. Consult. Psychol.* 27(1):62–74, 1963.
23. Fisher, S. "Body Boundary and Perceptual Vividness." *J. Abnorm. Psychol.* 73(4):392–396, 1968.
24. Fisher, S., and Cleveland, S. E. *Body Image and Personality.* New York: Dover Pubns., Inc., 1968.
25. Peto, A. "Body Image and Archaic Thinking." *Inter. J. Psychoanal.* 40:223–231, 1959.
26. Rochlin, G. *Griefs and Discontents.* Boston: Little, Brown & Co., 1965.
27. Simmons, R. G., et al. "Disturbances in the Self-Image at Adolescence." *Am. Soc. Rev.* 38:553–568, 1973.
28. Huenemann, R. L., et al. "A Longitudinal Study of Gross Body Composition and Body Conformation and Their Association with Food and Activity in a Teen-Age Population." *Am. J. Nutrition* 18:325–338, 1966.
29. Lerner, R. M., et al. "Physical Attractiveness, Physical Effectiveness, and Self-Concept in Late Adolescents." *Adolescence* 11(43):313–326, 1976.
30. Salinger, J. D. *The Catcher in the Rye.* New York: Signet Books, 1951.
31. Neugarten, B. L., and Kraines, R. J. " 'Menopausal Symptoms' in Women of Various Ages." *Psychosomatic Med.* 27(3):266–275, 1965.
32. Schonfeld, W. A. "Body-Image in Adolescents: A Psychiatric Concept for the Pediatrician." *Pediatrics* 31:845–855, 1963.
33. Schonfeld, W. A. "Adolescence: Inappropriate Sexual Development and Body Image." *J. Am. Med. Women's Assoc.* 22(11):847–855, 1967.
34. Dwyer, J., and Mayer, J. "Psychological Effects of Variations in Physical Appearance During Adolescence." *Adolescence* 3:353–380, 1968.
35. Rubins, J. L. "The Self-Idealizing and Self-Alienating Process During Late Adolescence," *Am. J. Psychoanal.* 25:27–37, 1965.
36. Rubins, J. L. "The Problem of the Acute Identity Crisis in Adolescence." *Am. J. Psychoanal.* 28:37–45, 1968.

37. Sarbin, T. R., and Allen, V. L. "Role Theory." In Lindzey, G., and Aronson, E., eds. *The Handbook of Social Psychology,* Vol. 1, 2nd ed. Reading, Mass.: Addison-Wesley Pub. Co., Inc., 1968, pp. 488–567.
38. Rubin, R. "Attainment of the Maternal Role." *Nurs. Research* 16(3):237–245, 1967.
39. Roth, P. *Portnoy's Complaint.* New York: Bantam Books, Inc., 1969, pp. 50–51.
40. Laufer, M. "The Body Image, The Functions of Masturbation and Adolescence—Problems of Ownership of the Body." *Psychoanal. Study of the Child* 22:114–137, 1968.
41. Francis, J. J. "Masturbation." *J. Am. Psychoanal. Assoc.* 16:95–112, 1968.
42. Raucher, H. *Ode to Billy Joe.* New York: Dell Pub. Co., Inc., 1976.
43. Josselyn, I. M. "Value Problems in the Treatment of Adolescents." *Smith Coll. Studies in Social Work* 42(1):1–14, 1971.
44. Blos, P. "When and How Does Adolescence End: Structural Criteria for Adolescent Closure." *Adolesc. Psychiat.* 5:5–17, 1977.
45. Freud, A. *The Ego and the Mechanisms of Defense.* New York: International Universities Press, Inc., 1966.
46. Johnson, A. B. "Drifting on the God Circuit." In Esman, A. H., ed. *The Psychology of Adolescence.* New York: International Universities Press, Inc., 1975, pp. 524–534.
47. Shapiro, E. "Destructive Cultism." *Am. Fam. Phys.* 15(2):80–83, 1977.
48. Kohlberg, L., and Gilligan, C. "The Adolescent as a Philosopher: The Discovery of the Self in a Postconventional World." In Kagan, J., and Coles, R., eds. *Twelve to Sixteen: Early Adolescence.* New York: W. W. Norton & Co., Inc., 1972, pp. 144–179.
49. Gould, R. L. "The Phases of Adult Life: A Study in Developmental Psychology," *Am. J. Psychiat.* 129(5):521–531, 1972.
50. Offer, D., and Offer, J. "Four Issues in the Developmental Psychology of Adolescents." In Howells, J. G., ed. *Modern Perspectives in Adolescent Psychiatry.* New York: Brunner/Mazel, Inc., 1971, 28–44.
51. Deutsch, H. *Selected Problems of Adolescence.* New York: International Universities Press, Inc., 1967.
52. Erikson, E. H. *Identity: Youth and Crisis.* New York: W. W. Norton & Co., Inc., 1968.
53. Levinson, D. J. "The Mid-Life Transition: A Period in Adult Psychosocial Development." *Psychiatry* 40:99–112, 1977.
54. Erikson, E. H. Identity and the Life Cycle, *Psychological Issues* 1(1), Monograph 1, 1959.
55. Deutsch, H. *Confrontation with Myself: An Epilogue.* New York: W. W. Norton & Co., Inc., 1973, pp. 215–216.

2

Adolescent Sexuality

Lois J. Welches, R.N., D.N.S.

The so-called Sexual Revolution that has been sweeping the country in the past two decades is considered by many to be little more than a liberalization of attitudes. Few would dispute the existence of greater tolerance with respect to the sexual behavior of others, or greater openness in discussion. However, the extent to which these more liberalized attitudes have influenced the sexual behavior of adolescents is not fully known, and the definition of normal sexual expression during adolescence in this society is a source of controversy and confusion for adolescents, the parents of adolescents, and health professionals providing services to them.

In this chapter some of the conflicting views, theories, study findings, and interpretations of adolescent sexual behavior will be examined. Initially, the importance of the developmental tasks of adolescence as they relate to a young person's decision regarding his or her sexual behavior will be emphasized. A discussion of some of the major concerns of adolescents and their parents will follow, and will include masturbation, homosexuality, peer pressure, dating and going steady, and sexual intercourse. An examination of parental influence as it relates to sexual behavior will be presented and will encompass findings from my own study related to the young person's perception of the relationship both with and between the parents and the decision to have or not to have sexual intercourse. A discussion of implications for the improvement of services and clinical treatment of adolescents and their families will conclude the chapter.

Factors Influencing Decisions about Sexual Behavior

In Chapter 1 both the internal factors—physiological and psychological changes—and the external factors—social and cultural influences—with which the young, emerging individual must cope in his struggle for autonomy and adulthood have been outlined. Adolescent sexual behavior must always be viewed within the context of all of these demands. Let us consider briefly the effects of some of the internal factors on an individual's ability to make decisions regarding sexual behavior during the teenage years.

The reader will recall from Chapter 1 that the onset of puberty is accompanied by relatively drastic changes in both physical growth and hormonal functioning. These changes force the young adolescent to cope with new feelings of a sexual nature with which he has had little previous experience. The manner in which the adolescent perceives his or her body, and the responses to the changes which are perceived by others, may indirectly influence decisions regarding the manner in which sexual feelings are expressed. For example, the early-developing female may feel ''different'' and hence isolated from her own age peers. She will often seek older friends, both male and female, who are socially and perhaps sexually more mature. Similarly, the older male who finds himself nearing physiological maturity and continues to be five feet five inches tall, may respond to his shortness, if he perceives shortness to be ''unmanly,'' by acting out his feelings of inadequacy in attempts to prove himself sexually.

Cognitive development during adolescence may also have bearing on the teenager's sexual behavior. Piaget defines intellectual development during adolescence in terms of the transition from concrete operations—a logic relating to objects or ideas within the individual's past or present experience—to formal operations, which involve the person's ability to understand ideal or abstract theories and concepts that allow him to consider alternatives to problems not yet experienced at the concrete level.[1]

Although it has been generally assumed by Piaget that adolescents have reached the stage of formal operations by age 15 or 16 years, Hamburg[2] has observed that even young people who have reached the stage of formal operations tend to revert to concrete operations when confronted with an unfamiliar or unusually difficult problem. For the teenager who is operating primarily at the stage of concrete operations, decisions regarding such sexual behaviors as masturbation or sexual intercourse will be made on the basis of past experience. This experience will be primarily determined by parental or societal values. Thus the young persons may not be intellectually mature enough to consider alternatives or even the possible outcomes of their decisions, beyond this limited experience, without assistance.

The young person's own personality traits may also influence decisions about sexual behavior. In my study of teenage girls,[3] a personality inventory, the *Personal Values Abstract,*[4] was administered to determine whether it was possible to differentiate, by personality traits, sexually active from sexually inexperienced young women. The possibility that two different themes might be related to earlier sexual experience emerged in the findings. One sexually active group could be described as energetic, impulsive, emotional, and variety-seeking. The other sexually active group appears to include conventionally feminine young women who lack verve, self-confidence, and spontaneity.

Concerns of Adolescents and Parents

The far-reaching influences of society and culture will also be discussed as additional factors that may influence an adolescent's decisions regarding sexual behavior. Behaviors such as masturbation, homosexuality, and the like, are often deemed problematic by the adolescent, his parents, teachers, health professionals, and the society at large.

MASTURBATION

In a recent study of sexual attitudes and behavior patterns in a middle-class adolescent population, Chess and associates[5] reported that masturbation was not mentioned by either adolescents or their parents during interviews. Neither did they find masturbation to be a problem in their psychiatric practice with adolescents and their families. The authors interpret these findings as follows:

> This lack of mention, . . . of masturbation does not reflect any anxiety and consequent avoidance of the issue. . . . It appears to reflect such a matter-of-fact acceptance . . . that it is not necessary to report it in their repertoire of behavioral activities . . . (p. 697)[5]

Although it may be acceptable, in fact in many instances an ''in'' thing, to be able to talk about sex, adolescents do not voluntarily talk about masturbation. In my experience, only after a group discussion of the harmless effects of masturbation, when individuals who were worried about their masturbatory behavior were encouraged to discuss their concerns, were teenagers able to openly express these concerns, often with some difficulty and embarrassment. Restrictive puritanical attitudes still exist in this country, even among the middle class. Rumors are still prevalent regarding the harmful consequences of masturbation and are often given credibility by disapproving and prohibitive parental attitudes. Gallagher[6] has found college students today who are guilt-ridden and deficient in overall effectiveness because of their struggle to stop masturbating.

Blos[7] defines adolescent masturbation as a phase-specific developmental task that must be mastered to achieve adult genitality, and believes that the total absence of masturbation during adolescence indicates an incapacity to deal with pubertal drives that must be experienced. In such instances, according to Blos, parental attitudes of prohibition regarding sexual activity in infancy and early childhood have so influenced the child's attitudes and behavior that his normal sexual development is impaired.

Masturbation during adolescence is often accompanied by fantasies that may be tinged with violence and aggressiveness. Feelings aroused by such fantasies are frequently frightening to the inexperienced and naive young person, especially if he feels his parents disapprove.[8]

Most uninformed adolescents will be relieved to hear that masturbation is an essentially normal activity. It is a normal response to their sexual development and can facilitate control and integration of new desires. Masturbation may provide a means of experimenting with emerging biological capacities and relieving tension, and may ultimately lead to the working out of new relationships through trial acting in fantasy.[8]

HOMOSEXUALITY

During adolescence, when the establishment of sexual identity becomes a major task, fears surrounding the issue of homosexuality may be present in both the adolescent and his parents. The incidence of frank homosexuality among adolescents is not great; there are, however, large numbers of young people, especially early in adolescence, who do not yet feel comfortable relating to members of the opposite sex. It is not unusual for young teenagers to experiment with newly discovered sexual feelings in relationships with members of their own sex. Boys and girls in pairs or boys sometimes in groups, may practice mutual masturbation and body caressing. These transitory homosexual episodes may evoke anxiety about homosexuality, but nearly always, as young people acquire more experience relating to the opposite sex, they become more assured about their gender identity and ultimately choose mates of the opposite sex.[8]

Psychoanalytic literature defines the onset of frank homosexuality as an arrest of emotional development during the early years of life (4–5 years of age).[7] According to Bieber,[9] frank homosexuality results from adverse life experiences where, in most cases, an unhealthy relationship existed with and between the parents.

In the case of the male, Bieber describes the mother as having been overprotective, overcontrolling, and often inappropriately intimate with her son. The father usually spent little time with his son, preferred other children in the family, and was seen by the son as rejecting and a competitor for the mother's love and attention.[9]

In the case of the female, a rejecting and critical mother, often jealous of her daughter's relationship with her father and brothers, resulted in the girl's identity confusion. In other instances the mother was seen as highly possessive, dominating, and controlling of her daughter. Fathers of lesbian daughters were described as detached and rejecting or overprotecting and seductive. In the case of the latter, the father frequently formed an alliance with the daughter which excluded the mother.[9]

When parents are uncertain of their own identities, when dissension exists between them, and when the affection normally expressed within the marriage bond is displaced to the child, the process of identification with the same-sex parent may become distorted. This distortion often leads to narcissism, indecision regarding the parent with whom to identify, and lack of wholesome inner controls. This young person may then love others like himself or herself and may only be able to establish same-sex love relationships.[9]

Though the basis for the developing gender identity is formed during childhood, generally it is not believed to be irreversibly set by the adolescent period. The flexibility and transitional nature of development during this period provides opportunity for the treatment of individuals expressing concern and requesting assistance. Early identification of such individuals leads to a more hopeful outcome.[9]

Increasing support is being given to the concept of homosexuality as a normal variant of sexual behavior. Proponents of this belief consider homosexuality to be a choice of life style rather than a pathological state, and hold that it is society's prohibitive attitude which creates conflict within the homosexual regarding his sexual identity.

Among adolescents there are some who do express preference for their own sex. These young people, by the age of 18 or 19 years, have elected to express their sexual needs exclusively with members of the same sex and often are identified with the homosexual subculture. Acceptance and understanding of these young people by heterosexual peers, parents, and health professionals will enhance their opportunities for a less conflict-ridden and a richer life experience.

PEERS

The adolescent peer group is seen as constituting a subculture with its own language, customs, mode of dress, economic power, musical tastes, and social institutions. The peer group provides for the adolescent a source of empathy and a sense of belonging during the period in which he or she is neither child nor adult. This close, more intense relationship with peers compensates for the "loss" of parents, as the adolescent moves to a position of more autonomy and less dependence upon parents.[8] To be accepted by the peer group the adolescent will go to great lengths in conforming to the group's modes. Therefore, group pressure from peers may be a strong force in either discouraging or encouraging sexual experimentation.

Sixty percent of a sample group of post-abortion adolescents reported having few, if any, girlfriends.[10] Having few female friends is considered to be an important variable contributing to a high risk for pregnancy during adolescence.[11] In my own study of adolescent girls, the number of close girlfriends did not differentiate girls who reported having sexual intercourse from those who reported they had not.[3] However, studies have shown that sexually active teenagers choose friends who are sexually active, and those who were not sexually active tended to choose friends who were also inactive.[12,3]

During my interviews of adolescent girls, sexually inexperienced young women reported feeling "pressure" from their sexually active peers to have sexual intercourse. Interestingly, the opposite was not true. No sexually active young woman reported feeling "pressure" to stop having sexual intercourse.[3] Kanin[13] found that college males who tried to force their female dating partners into sexual intercourse were most influenced by pressures from their male peers. It appears from these findings that peer pressure today supports sexual "doing" rather than "not doing." For these reasons, the questions of whether dating and going steady will lead to sexual intercourse is often problematic for parents.

Recent studies of the relationship of dating and going steady to the incidence of sexual intercourse are virtually absent in the literature. In my study of 75 adolescent girls who attended high school in a conservative community of central California, sexually experienced young women reportedly went out more often and had gone steady with more boyfriends than the sexually inexperienced. However, from responses of young women who were interviewed it appeared that going steady had different meanings for the sexually active and sexually inexperienced young women. Statements of sexually experienced subjects included such comments as: "It can be a hassle to go steady. You get too close and get your feelings hurt." "No one has ever treated me the way he does. He has really helped me a lot." In contrast, girls who reported never having had sexual intercourse stated: "It's OK to go steady, everyone does." "I can't date yet, but going steady is great. It gives you someone to talk to."[3]

Sexually experienced young women tended to go steady for longer periods of time, whereas the sexually inexperienced teenager often broke up with a steady after a week or two. For the sexually active, going steady seemed to be a serious and very intimate affair, and the sexually inexperienced appeared to be experimenting with a variety of relationships on a less intense level.

These findings can be misleading unless seen within the context of the adolescent's total life experience. As Wickes has pointed out,'' . . . parents ought to be far more worried over absence of the opposite sex than their appearance even with some problems attached'' (pp. 107–108).[14]

Opposite sex attraction among peers is born in adolescence and provides for the socially developing individual an opportunity to practice and experiment with male-female relationships. Young people, especially in their late teens, who have been unable to establish any relationships with the opposite sex are often beset with doubts and anxiety concerning their sex-role identity and inability to socialize. These individuals should be identified early by the health care professional and offered counseling assistance with their socialization.

Nearly three quarters of the sexually inexperienced young women in the study mentioned above reported having gone steady with at least one male. The important question is not whether dating or going steady leads to sexual intercourse. It seems reasonable to assume that an intimate sexual relationship between two adolescents would lead to more dating and a more intense steady relationship. The more important question is why some adolescents choose an intimate sexual relationship while others do not. Perhaps the answer to this question can be better understood within the context of intrafamilial relationships and interaction.

Sexual Behavior and Relationship with Parents

Sexual acting out among adolescent young women is believed to reflect the breakdown of parental control, a rebellion against authority, and an acute disturbance in the parent-adolescent relationship.[15] In his work with families of sexually active teenage girls, Friedman found mothers to have excessive emotional investment in their daughters; nearly half of the mothers in his group encouraged their daughters to take over significant aspects of their own mothering role.[15]

Domination of the adolescent by her mother is frequently mentioned as a forerunner of teenage pregnancy in studies. Most of the adolescent girls in Babakian's study[15] were reported to have a strong identification with their mothers, and three girls reported that they were responding to their mother's wish for a baby by becoming pregnant. Lipper[17] found 63% of post-abortion teenage girls to be mother-dominated, and Hetherington[18] described mothers of daughters from broken homes as being overprotective and solicitous.

In contrast, when comparing 30 antepartum adolescents with 20 never-pregnant subjects, Curtis found that fewer than half of the antepartum teenagers had a close relationship with anyone in their immediate families, whereas 19 of the 20 young women who had never been pregnant named their mother as the person to whom they felt closest.[19]

Fathers have been described as seductive to their daughters, caught up in the daughter's oedipal feelings, and seeking excessive attention from the daughters.[16] In some instances daughters were found to be alienated from their mothers while in an intimate relationship with the father.[11,16]

In a four-year longitudinal study of the transition from virginity to nonvirginity among high-school-aged young people, nonvirgins were found to have less parental support, fewer parental controls, and less disapproval of problem behavior. Parents of virgins were more apt to approve of the friends of their teenagers than were parents of nonvirgins.[12]

In my study of adolescent girls, items were included which related to the young woman's perception of her relationship with each of her parents and her perception of the relationship between her parents. On the average, the subjects who reported never having had sexual intercourse felt close to both parents, but closer to their mothers than to their fathers. They also perceived their parents as being close to one another. Those subjects who reported having had sexual intercourse, on the average, felt close to their mothers, but not as close as their inexperienced peers. They felt more distant from their fathers, and were not certain that their parents loved each other.

When the relationships were viewed within the context of all other variables in the study and related to sexual activity, four groups of young women emerged. Table 2–1 presents the young women's perceived relationships with their mothers and fathers and the percentage of sexually active women in each group.

TABLE 2–1. *Perceived Relationships with Parents and Percent Sexually Active*

RELATIONSHIP	% SEXUALLY ACTIVE
Mother + Father +	6.4
Mother − Father −	37.5
Mother + Father −	44.0
Mother − Father +	66.7

KEY: + above-average relationship
− below-average relationship

Before discussing each of these groups it may be useful to reexamine the development of the adolescent within the context of the family and the influence of parents upon the emerging teenager. Throughout childhood, independence has been developing; during adolescence it begins to unfold into individuality. The young person must now be given progressively more freedom to find new friends, to make his own decisions, and to develop his life goals. A new form of comradeship develops between parents and offspring. If the parents have depended primarily upon their children for life satisfactions and have neglected their own individual life interests and their relationship with one another, they cannot be sufficiently separate from the child during adolescence to face this new relationship, which is necessary for the child's growth.[14]

The mother provides, in many ways, the psychic pattern for her daughter. If the mother has a healthy and well-adjusted love relationship, the daughter will take over the inner attitude that her mother expresses. However, if the mother is unsatisfied and unhappy in her marriage, the girl will find her own love path beset with doubts. The mother provides not only the pattern for the daughter's relationship with men but also for her friendship with women, and her understanding and acceptance of the woman's role in life.[14]

The young woman must also have a satisfactory relationship with her father. An important aspect of this relationship is the mother's attitude toward the father and her influence on the child. The father's own attitude provides a pattern of what the daughter accepts or rejects in a man. If the father lavishes upon his daughter the love that should normally go into his marriage relationship, the daughter may either find herself unable to break the bond or she may reject him — and thus lose a foundation of trust and love which is necessary for her own love life. If her father neglects her, she may feel resentment and hate and may rebel by becoming involved in love relationships that can only end in disaster.[14]

Within this framework, each of the four groups is now considered: (1) above-average relationship with both parents; (2) below-average relationship with both parents; (3) above-average relationship with mother, below-average relationship with father; and (4) below-average relationship with mother, above-average relationship with father.[3] The relationship between the parents varied within the groups and will be discussed in following sections.

Above-average relationship —both parents: Thirty-eight percent of the subjects in the study reported an above-average relationship with both parents, and all subjects in this group perceived the relationship between their parents to be above average. Only 6.4% of the young women in this group reported having had sexual intercourse. They included subjects of all ages (14 through 18 years).

Two subgroups emerged from this group. One group had few friends of either sex, few hobbies, seldom participated in extracurricular activities at school, and reported that most of their social life was enjoyed with the family. It would appear that, for this subgroup, the family ties were very strong and the daughter seemed to have greater difficulty moving beyond the family to establish relationships outside the family framework.

The other subgroup in which subjects felt close to both parents reported having many friends of both sexes, were doing well in school, had many hobbies, and were active in extracurricular activities. For these young women the closeness of the family seemed to provide a secure base from which to move out of the family and form friendships with members of both sexes.

Below-average relationship —both parents: Twenty-three percent of the sample reported a below-average relationship with both parents, and 37.5% of the group reported having had sexual intercourse. They were members of large families, seldom reported having many friends, and had few interests outside of school. Some reported pouring much of their energy into their studies to meet the high expectations of their parents. However, those who were the youngest in very large families reported having the poorest relationships with their parents, and in addition to having limited interests they were doing poorly in school.

When subjects who were sexually active also perceived the relationship between their parents as being below average, they reported having a series of partners and seldom, if ever, using reliable contraceptives. When, however, the relationship between their parents was perceived to be above average, they reported having sexual intercourse with only one partner and always using reliable contraceptives. The importance of the relationship between the parents was particularly striking in this group.

Above-average relationship—mother; below-average—father: Twenty-four percent of the sample of young women reported an above-average relationship with their mothers and a below-average relationship with their fathers. Forty-four percent of this group reported having had sexual intercourse. All subjects in this group perceived the relationship between their parents as being below average. They reported that their mothers frequently discussed with them the problems they were having with their fathers. It was pointed out earlier that the young woman's attitude toward her father is most influenced by the mother's attitude toward him, and frequently the daughter's behavior with men becomes the working out of her mother's marital problems.

The sexually experienced young women in this group tended to be careless in their sexual relationships, seldom using a contraceptive. Many of both the experienced and inexperienced young women appeared to be struggling with a poor feminine identity, dependency, and rebelliousness.

This group of subjects seemed to have great difficulty establishing healthy relationships with either sex outside the home. They were often in a coalition with the mother against the father, and might be considered at high risk, not only for early pregnancy, but in terms of their future development and happiness.

Below-average relationship—mother; above-average—father: Only 13% of the study subjects reported an above-average relationship with their fathers and a below-average relationship with their mothers. Two thirds of this group reported having had sexual intercourse. The group was, on the average, older; they were having sexual intercourse on a more regular basis, and over half were using a reliable contraceptive. Because the number of subjects in this group was so small and the percentage of sexually active subjects was so high, a more extensive examination of all subjects who reported feeling closer to their fathers was done. Some subjects who reported above- or below-average relationships with both parents also reported feeling closer to their fathers than to their mothers. In fact, 33 sexually inexperienced and only 8 sexually experienced young women in the sample reported feeling closer to their fathers than to their mothers. Six of the eight sexually experienced subjects fell into this last group. From these findings it can be generally concluded that a closer relationship with the father is not an indicator of sexual acting out, except in those instances in which the relationship with the mother is seen as below average.

Because of the small number of subjects in the groups, generalization to a larger population is not possible. However, the study has, I believe, demonstrated that both the child's perception of her relationship with her parents and her perception of the relationship between her parents influence her decision to have or not to have sexual intercourse.

Unfortunately, no similar study of male adolescents is available. In general, adolescent males in our culture have been found to experience more intense conflict with parents in their efforts to become independent.[20] However, study of the influence of the adolescent-parental relationship on the sexual behavior of males has been sadly neglected. It may be that the long-standing double standard for teenage males and females, especially in regard to sexual behavior, has led to less concern about this topic in males. However, when viewed from the developmental stance—considering the important influence of sexual behavior in relation to identity formation during adolescence—the need for such studies of males, as well as females, takes on increasing importance.

Today, two prevalent attitudes exist in relation to the sexual behavior of adolescents. On the one hand, sexual mores are regarded as outdated. Teenagers are not only believed to be biologically, psychologically, and socially ready for sexual intercourse, but are believed to need this experience to establish their sexual identity and to learn to develop healthy relationships with the opposite sex. Others feel that adolescents, particularly of high school age, may be biologically ready for sexual intercourse, but are psychologically and socially too immature to deal with the complexity of sexual intimacy in a relationship.

Erikson[21] identifies adolescence as a period during which the integration of the biological and psychosocial aspects of past experience lead to greater stability in an individual's sense of self, and he believes that sexual intimacy prior to identity formation leads to a crisis of premature commitment. Identity formation provides for the individual sufficient ego strength and sex-role identity to experience sexual intimacy without risk of identity diffusion—which is the outcome when complexities which the young person is ill-prepared to handle are introduced into a relationship.

Maddock[22] argues that the "uniqueness of adolescent sexual expression lies in combining mature genitality with an incomplete self structure." He believes that adolescent sexual expression provides the possibility of experiencing intimacy prior to the achievement of identity, and might be expected to be utilized by adolescents who are engaged in a mutual search for identity.

Though Maddock acknowledges that forms of sexual expression which precede identity formation without precipitating a crisis of premature commitment have not been identified,[22] even if such knowledge were available, there is no assurance that adolescents could be convinced that they should behave accordingly.

At the present time identity formation as described by Erikson takes place, for the most part, within the circle of the family. A review of the studies presented throughout this chapter will reveal as a common theme the interaction of the adolescent with the parents. Masturbation emerges as a problem when related to prohibitive attitudes of parents regarding early sexual behavior. Homosexuality is attributed to sexual identity confusion in early childhood. Peer pressure to have sexual intercourse is prevalent, but seems most influential, at least among girls, in those instances in which a disturbed adolescent-parent relationship exists. Sexual intercourse early in adolescence is more prevalent among young women when dissension between the parents and with one or both parents is identified.

Implications for Health Professionals

What implications, then, does this knowledge have for those who work with adolescents and their families? For many years emphasis has been placed on the early identification of problems within the family. Health care professionals who work with pregnant couples and young children and their parents should continue their efforts at early identification. However, increased effort should be devoted to the development of more sensitive instruments for the assessment of family interaction and functioning. At present, many problems, though they may have been insidiously developing over the years, are not identified until the onset of adolescence, when they are more overtly expressed.

Parenting is a complex developmental task in and of itself, and the attainment of the ''parent-self'' is frequently an all-consuming experience. Many parents, in their effort to be ''good'' parents, neglect the need to maintain their relationship with one another and the need for their own continued personal growth. The parents' success then becomes dependent on their offspring's behavior. In those instances in which the parent cannot be sufficiently separate from the adolescent, development is stifled and the adolescent's sexual behavior becomes an acting out of the parents' problems or an effort to pull away from a too close and all-absorbing relationship at home. If adolescents feel rejected or neglected by their parents, they may seek in sexual partners the love which they feel has been denied them at home.

The entire family should be considered in the treatment of an adolescent's problems. Family therapy may be ideal for those families in which all members are willing to participate. Some adolescents, in their struggle for autonomy, cannot see the value of working within the family and may refuse to cooperate. In these instances, it is possible that the health professional's time will be spent most productively in working with parents. It is by helping parents—helping them to see their teenager's need for more space and freedom in which to grow and to see their own needs for growth and separateness from their adolescent—that the health care practitioner may ultimately pave the way for constructive changes within the family and an improvement in the adolescent's behavior.

This focus on parents of adolescents does not, of course, exclude the need for working with the troubled adolescent. Adolescents will, in fact, frequently seek out adults other than their parents with whom they will, if given the opportunity, discuss their most intimate feelings.

Often the young adolescent's concerns regarding his or her sexuality will be masked by a series of all too frequently occurring symptoms such as headaches, stomachaches, menstrual cramps, etc. School nurses frequently hear such complaints voiced by students who wish to be excused from physical education classes. The practitioner who is knowledgeable about the needs and concerns of adolescents may find that an understanding and nonjudgmental, but direct, confrontation of these observations will ultimately be welcomed (with great relief) by the adolescent. This is especially true when the practitioner provides an opening for the adolescent with a statement appropriate to the situation such as, ''It is not unusual for boys who are just starting high school to feel a little embarrassed in gym class, especially in the showers.'' Such openings may lead to discussions of concerns regarding body image in physically immature or obese young people.

In other instances, especially when the professional has been identified as trustworthy, teenagers will seek information regarding contraceptives, pregnancy, or abortion. These requests may appear to be casual and impersonal, and may take the form of comments such as ''My friend Mary says the Pill can really hurt you. What do you think?'' The skillful practitioner may take this opportunity to assist the young person by providing information about contraception; she can, more importantly, encourage the teenager to discuss her own feelings and worries regarding her sexual behavior. During such discussions various possible outcomes related to sexual behavior may be considered which could motivate the adolescent to take greater responsibility for the decisions she makes regarding her sexual life.

Many health professionals have great difficulty discussing ''sex'' with any age group. Adolescents in particular are extremely sensitive to the slightest indication of discomfort or of judgmental attitudes on the part of an adult. Professionals who deal with adolescents and sexuality are most effective when they are secure in their own sexual identity, are aware of their biases related to sexual behaviors, and are able to relate to young people in a warm and sympathetic but objective and matter-of-fact manner.

Summary

To summarize, many questions remain unanswered concerning the sexual behavior of adolescents in today's society; however, studies of the sexual behavior of adolescents have as a common theme the adolescent-parent relationship. Early identification of family problems and greater efforts to develop more sensitive instruments for assessing the family seem of utmost importance. Assistance to parents, in addition to the treatment of adolescents, may be the most productive use of the health professional's energy and time.

REFERENCES

1. Piaget, J. ''The Intellectual Development of the Adolescent.'' In A. H. Esman, ed. *The Psychology of Adolescence*. New York: International Universities Press, 1975.
2. Hamburg, B. A. ''Early Adolescence: A Specific and Stressful State of the Life Cycle.'' In Coehlo, G., Hamburg, D., and Adams, J., eds. *Coping and Adaptation*. New York: Basic Books, 1974.
3. Welches, L. ''Factors Influencing Decisions Regarding Sexual Behavior of Adolescent Girls.'' Unpublished doctoral dissertation. San Francisco: University of California, 1976.
4. Gough, H. G. *Manual for the Personal Values Abstract*. Palo Alto, California: Consulting Psychologist Press, 1972.
5. Chess, S., Thomas, A., and Cameron, M. ''Sexual Attitudes and Behavior Patterns in a Middle-Class Adolescent Population.'' *Am. J. Orthopsychiat.* 46:689–701, 1976.
6. Gallagher, J. R., and Harris, H. I. *Emotional Problems of Adolescents*. New York: Oxford University Press, 1976.
7. Blos, P. *On Adolescence*. New York: Free Press, 1962.
8. Group for the Advancement of Psychiatry: Committee on Adolescence. *Normal Adolescence*. New York: Charles Scribner & Sons, 1968.
9. Bieber, I. ''Homosexuality.'' *Am. J. Nurs.* 69(12):2637–2641, 1969.
10. Martin, C. D. ''Psychological Problems of Abortion for the Unwed Teenage Girl'' *Genetic Psychol. Monograph* 33:23–110, 1973.
11. Abernathy, V. ''Illegitimate Conception Among Teenagers.'' *Am. J. Pub. Health* 67:662–665, 1974.
12. Jessor, S. L., and Jessor, R. ''Transition from Virginity to Non-Virginity Among Youth: A Social-Psychological Study Over Time.'' *Developmental Psychol.* 11:473–488, 1975.

13. Kanin, E. A. "Reference Groups and Sex Conduct Norm Violations." *Sociolog. Quarterly* 8:495–504, 1967.
14. Wickes, F. G. *The Inner World of Childhood.* Rev. ed. New York: Appleton Century, 1966, pp. 100–123.
15. Friedman, A. *Therapy with Families of Sexually Acting Out Girls.* New York: Springer Publishing Co., 1971.
16. Babakian, H. M., and Goldman, A. "A Study of Teenage Pregnancy." *Am. J. Psychiat.* 126(6):111–115, 1971.
17. Lipper, I., Cvejic, H., Benjamin, P., and Kinch, R. A. "Abortion and the Pregnant Teenager." *Calif. Nurses Assoc. J.* 109:852–856, 1973.
18. Hetherington, M. "Girls Without Fathers." *Psychol. Today* 6(9):47–52, 1973.
19. Curtis, F. "Observations of Unwed Pregnant Adolescents." *Am. J. Nurs.* 74(1):100–102, 1974.
20. Kelly, D. H., and Pink, W. T. "Status Origins, Youth Rebellion, and Delinquency: A Reexamination of the Class Issue." *J. Youth & Adol.* 4:339–347, 1975.
21. Erikson, E. "Identity and the Life Cycle." *Psychological Issues* 1(1), 1959.
22. Maddock, J. W. "Sex in Adolescence: Its Meaning and Its Future." *Adolescence* 8:325–342, 1973.

3

The Adolescent from a Different Ethnic Group

Ramona T. Mercer, R.N., Ph. D.
Carnie A. Hayes, Jr., R.N., M.S.
Teresa A. Bello, R.N., M.S.
Carolyn M. Fong, R.N., M.S.

Culture, the way of life learned from birth and transmitted from generation to generation, is a complex phenomenon. The habits, skills, and learning of a particular cultural group are unique characteristics by which the group is identified and often stereotyped. The cultural shaping of the young is multifaceted; there are many variables, all interacting with one another. The adolescent may live in a home in which his parents speak a native language and hold to "old traditions and values," and may attend a school where he learns "WASP" (White Anglo-Saxon Protestant) values and traditions. The youth is shaped by both the microculture and the macroculture, and he in turn shapes both cultures as he adapts to the social world in which he participates. The macroculture refers here to the larger social system (the United States) in which many microcultures are subsystems (the family network, church, and ethnic groups).

The impact of cultural shaping on individual response is profound. The individual has been reinforced from birth regarding desired behaviors and attitudes within his family. He has learned the values, rules, regulations, and priorities of his family and ethnic group; he has also learned survival tactics. These all relate to how health is perceived or valued and the means by which health is maintained.

This chapter focuses on the adolescent in the macrocultural context of the United States. The impact of the macroculture, the historical time, poverty, and the ethnic group are discussed. The black, Latino, and Chinese groups are examples selected as representative of larger populations in the United States. Each contributor presents sensitive insights into some of the formal and informal cultural shaping that takes place within each of the groups discussed. These sections of the chapter demonstrate the many kinds of learning and values that adolescents in the United States may have which may be quite different from those of the professional who seeks to help them. The goal is to increase the professional's sensitivity to differences and to highlight the importance of respecting the richness of those differences.

Impact of the Macroculture

The political and economic climates of the macroculture have an influence on the adolescent through his ethnic, family, and religious affiliations and the educational system. The multiplicity of microcultures within the larger macroculture reflect some of the complexities a young person faces in defining his identity, establishing his own values, and preparing for a life's work within the setting. That he will experience conflict seems inevitable. In resolving conflict, the young person helps to shape the social environment at both the micro- and macrocultural levels.

An example of the young person's impact on the macroculture is seen in the more casual style in dress adopted in the middle to late 1970s. Fifteen years earlier a well-dressed man always wore a tie; over the years turtleneck sweaters or open shirt collars and lavish necklaces became acceptable. Youth "hippie" cultures rejected many of the ways of their parents; one form of rejection was choosing longer hair styles and beards. Within ten years the father who had earlier complained of his son's long hair and beard frequently had longer hair and a beard himself. Some youth groups concerned with food and environmental pollution have adopted styles of living comparable to life as it was at the turn of the century. They are growing their own foods to avoid food additives that are used in many commercially prepared foods. Because of the dwindling supply of the world's energy and other grave ecological concerns, the macroculture may follow the pattern set by young people, if alternate supplies of energy and ways of controlling pollution are not found.

Macrocultural factors have the potential for both a healthy and an unhealthy impact on an individual through parental attitudes, child-rearing practices, reinforcement or inhibition of desirable attributes that contribute to self-concept and identity, and language.[1] Rubins[1] pointed out that psychopathology varies from country to country and according to historical periods. Examples cited by Rubins include the hysteria and neurasthenia of the 1900s, which are rarely seen today; cardiac and muscle neuroses observed during World War I, which disappeared during World War II, when intestinal and phobic forms of psychopathology were more frequently observed; and the evidence that depressions seem to occur more frequently in higher socioeconomic classes and in Westernized societies than in poor or primitive societies.

Leff[2] observed a strong link between the existence of appropriate words within a culture for different emotions and the ease with which persons within the culture can distinguish these emotions. Persons in developed countries in which the language includes a greater range of emotions show a greater differentiation of emotions than persons in less developed countries. Persons learning a second language usually do not learn the cultural modes of thought for the language, which makes it difficult to communicate as accurately in the second language. For example, Laplanders have an extensive vocabulary for types of snow—different kinds and conditions which are of very practical importance to them—that the Englishman with very limited words for snow would have difficulty learning and communicating.[2]

A study of Soviet and American youth suggests that the influence of both the sociopolitical system and the cultural system leads to different personality types among adolescents.[3] Rollins[3] noted that Soviet young people tend to conform to adult values in their society—obedience, dependence, industriousness, and warm personal relationships. The highly variable American youth reflects his country's historic revolutionary values, which are characterized by a striving to remold society or to find a better life. In promoting individual achievement adults have been more permissive and have stressed competitiveness and independence.

However, the American adolescent conforms more to his peer group, which results in a protean, or fluid and diffuse, personality style. This fluidity is reflected in carelessness about personal appearance, anxiety, guilt, anger, and suspiciousness, which, were it not for the macrocultural context, could be considered pathological.[3] It is more difficult to diagnose psychopathological behaviors in such a fluid personality type group than in a conformist personality type group.

The macrocultural context also seems to have an impact on the youth's emerging value system. White and associates[4] have challenged the universality of Kohlberg's six states in the development of moral reasoning that represent the individual's perception of rights and obligations for the social welfare of self and others (see pp. 22–23 for description of stages). They observed in a study of 426 Bahamian male and female school children, ages 8 through 17, that no individual reasoned beyond Stage 3 and the great majority reasoned at Stages 1 and 2. The Bahamian school system requires obedience to rules. These findings suggest that the development of moral reasoning is a consequence of the cultural-social development, and not all cultures value or reinforce autonomous reasoning.

The great variability of adolescents worldwide led Opler[5] to conclude that the cultural context is responsible for the adolescents' characteristics and their assets or liabilities.

Society's use of age as a criterion in allocating roles, privileges, and priorities has an impact on adolescence as an entity. In general, the simpler the organization of a society, the greater the likelihood that the age specifies the role. Mead's[6] field research in Samoa illustrates a society that has clear distinctions concerning age-specified roles; older persons always command the younger persons. Boys and girls are ignored until they are 15 or 16, at which time they are given adult roles with corresponding obligations and privileges. Children grow up observing specific role behaviors that they will be expected to assume as adults.

The adolescent from a minority ethnic group in the United States faces greater difficulty in his identity formation than does the adolescent in the majority group. The adolescent from a minority ethnic group sees less role modeling by members of his group via television commercials, newspapers, magazines, and other communications media. Further, the individual experiences conflict on those occasions when he chooses to emulate certain behaviors or responses of the majority group which are different from or in opposition to those of his family. Research substantiates that exposure to rejection and deprivation leads the individual to perceive that his successes and failures are due to forces beyond his control.[7]

The place of residence, urban or rural, has an impact on the minority adolescent through his choice of role models.[8] Oberle and associates[8] observed that 2% of the rural black males preferred close friends as role models and 49% preferred glamour figures, whereas 12.9% of the urban males chose a close friend and 39.6% chose a glamour figure. Twenty-six percent of the rural black females chose a glamour role model and 14.9% of the urban females did so. This research suggests that rural adolescents have difficulty finding role models among friends with whom they can identify; their friends are more likely to be in circumstances similar to their own.

When the adolescent is a member of a depreciated ethnic group, his self-image may be depreciated and become the center of his system of defenses.[9] In studying identity disorders among young men with dual cultural membership who were World War II veterans, Sommers[9] found that the young men had denied their native cultural group when they observed that it was being treated as inferior. In their attempts to take on the macroculture's way of life many changed their names, refused to speak their parents' language, and rejected their parents' religion; however, the price was great, as is evidenced by the inner conflict and psychoses that resulted.

A study of black students from a population enrolled in a predominantly white university who had sought mental health counseling, revealed four modes of adapting to the dominant culture in response to identity conflicts resulting from ethnic or sociocultural marginality.[10] Just over a half of the sample used withdrawal, a movement away from the dominant culture, which was characterized by feelings of depression, helplessness, and alienation. Most of this group were from a lower socioeconomic class, had attended a predominantly black high school, had difficulty with academic tasks, and felt less than adequate. Separation, or movement against the dominant culture, was the second most likely coping measure chosen by non-middle-class blacks; one eighth of the sample were in this group. Separation behaviors included hostility toward, contempt for, and rejection of the dominant group. One fourth of the sample responded by affirmation, or movement with the culture, and attempted to merge cultural patterns from both groups that did not conflict with their personalities and goals. They had a positive ethnic identity, high motivation, and self-actualization behaviors. None of the lower-class sample coped by affirmation. Students who concealed their black identity and avoided other blacks coped by assimilation or movement toward the dominant culture; one eighth of the sample used this mode. Earlier childhood experiences related either to school or to socioeconomic class seemed to influence their modes of adaptation.

Brim[11] stressed the need for examination of macrostructural influences on child development so that public policy changes and legal steps can be initiated to improve the health of American children. The national support of maternal and child health programs must receive greater priority for monies for programs and research. Policy change can be accomplished by various means; Zigler[12] pleaded for greater political involvement of child advocates in efforts to have Congress legitimize the Office of Child Development and to expand it to the "Office for Child and Family Development." Careful study of our macroculture's programs for parental and child health indeed seems warranted.

Historical Time

Our society has passed from a time in which little was known about—and little attention was paid to—adolescence to a time in which adolescence is a popular topic and is often depicted as the favored age.[13] Adolescence was not a serious field of study before the twentieth century. G. Stanley Hall's two-volume book on adolescence, published in 1904, was the first major publication in this country to focus on this age group.

Depending upon the time in which one was born and grew up, little or no attention may have been afforded the individual as an adolescent. As the culture changes, the position of the adolescent in the culture changes.[5] The more rapid the change in society, the greater the generation gap between the parent and teenager.

In societal change, any one change leads to additional change; change in turn forces individuals to adapt.[14] For example, if schools close two weeks earlier than usual, parents must plan for child supervision in the home or plan earlier vacations, and students also seek activities to fill the two-week period. In times of rapid change, increased stress and reduced tolerance to stress occur.[14] The adolescent faces different stressors at different points in history. As standards of conduct or values change, the adolescent has to evolve his own values, often only with naive peer support. Levine and Salter[15] found in a study of 106 youthful members of nine nontraditional religious groups that the young person perceived the group as offering security, a sense of belonging, and a reason for existence. When traditional social structures did not seem appropriate, the young person found his own.

In *Culture and Commitment, a Study of the Generation Gap,* Margaret Mead[16] described three kinds of culture—postfigurative, cofigurative, and prefigurative. Mead described the postfigurative culture as one in which children learn largely from their ancestors. In these cultures, change occurs so slowly that the parents cannot dream of any future for their children other than one similar to their own. The children follow their ancestors' way of life. In the United States some of the Indian tribes, particularly in New Mexico and Arizona, have postfigurative cultures.

In cofigurative cultures the adults set guidelines and are the authority figures, but they expect that the child will have a different style of life than they had. Both children and adults learn from their peers in a cofigurative culture. A cofigurative culture may be illustrated both by immigrants to this country and by our WASP culture. Children are expected to improve on their parents' style of life and parents learn about the new style of life from their children. Peers are better role models for the new style of life than are the parents who are leaving old ways behind. Mead points out that grandparents are absent in cofigurative cultures. Old and young move frequently, and the old may be placed in special homes. The frequent transfer of families by businesses and companies and a concomitant rapid growth in the number of homes for the aged reflect this phenomenon in the United States.

Mead described the emerging cultural form as prefiguration. In the prefiguration culture parents and adults learn from the young. Mead described a break between generations that is universal, involving the entire world, and suggests that we are moving toward one worldwide culture. The rapid movement from horse-and-buggy days to the satellite and exploration of the universe has occurred within a lifetime. No other generation has ever faced such rapid change. All previous certainties about the world and its future were swept away as rockets propelled man into space and weapons were designed to destroy cities at the push of a button. Consequently, the generation that has witnessed this change and the generation born after World War II were born into such different worlds that neither generation can ever know just how the other experienced growing up in its particular historical moment. To bridge the gap between these generations calls for listening and communication between the two, and for the willingness of the older to learn from the younger.

Experiencing and growing up with a set of values derived from one's family of origin, that were shaped by the social conditions of that family's time, clouds one's view and one's ability to perceive or understand the response of another individual who represents a different set of values and a different historical moment. The stock market crash in October, 1929 was a national event that deeply affected every household in this country. Children in the 1930s grew up hearing about and seeing the necessity for hard work, careful planning, thriftiness, and conservativenesss. Perhaps this atmosphere provided motivation for the children growing up during the thirties and forties to strive for better education and for better and more secure jobs. The pervasiveness of this climate of "hard times" and the struggle for survival so shaped the individual's early childhood during the thirties that later on these persons often had a total lack of understanding of their adolescent children of the sixties and seventies. Intellectually, parents during the middle seventies knew that their child who was born in the sixties had grown up in a very different atmosphere from that of the 1930s. With a rapidly growing economy and items of luxury more accessible, a different style of life existed. Yet these parents often found it difficult to avoid judging the child who chose not to compete or struggle for what the parents grew up defining as "security" in life. This example dramatizes the importance for health professionals who work with individuals from different ethnic, social, and age groups (because of the historical shaping) of becoming cognizant of the unconscious tunnel vision and the unconscious ethnocentrism that each brings to a client situation.

In a longitudinal study of 1,800 adolescents aged 13 to 18 from 1970 to 1972, developmental change was influenced more by the historical moment than by age.[17] Regardless of age level, adolescents decreased in superego strength, social-emotional anxiety, and achievement from 1970 to 1972. Conspicuous during that period were the Vietnam war and the ethical, moral, and political issues it raised. Females showed higher stability than males, leading the researchers to suggest further examination of underlying genetic and enviromental interactions. Girls were not as directly affected by the Vietnam war, however. They faced no draft or disruption of education, so that the threats they perceived were quite different. Also, the girl's feminine role model was not as likely to be drafted and sent to battle as was the boy's masculine role model.

The Impact of Poverty

Young people from homes in which the language spoken is not English are twice as likely to be living in poverty.[18] The 14- to 18-year-old non-English-speaking group is much less likely to be enrolled in or to complete high school. In grades 9 through 12, 86% of students from English dominant households are enrolled, as opposed to 65% of students from non-English dominant households. Almost half of the children of Spanish heritage live in households in which Spanish is spoken as the usual language, and about a third of Asian children live in households in which an Asian language is spoken predominantly.[18] Thus, the dual-culture adolescent may be penalized by a culture of poverty and may have less opportunity for an education, the most common vehicle for upward social mobility in this culture.

Regardless of his or her ethnic origin, a subculture of poverty may exist for the individual. The impact of the culture of poverty is pervasive. Economic deprivation contributes to poor health, disorganization, and the absence of most of the comforts of life—particularly the recreational and creative pursuits that are more readily available to the middle-class population. Pearlin and Schooler[19] found that the poor and the poorly educated have fewer effective coping mechanisms for warding off stresses resulting from hardship than those who are more affluent. They pointed out that some human concerns, such as occupational problems, may require collective efforts and resources for coping, since many stem from powerful social and economic factors that cannot be influenced by personal efforts for change. Considering the harsh negatives of poverty—insecurity, lack of privacy, starvation, illness, high death rates—the fact that strong humans manage to cope suggests that man's potential is indeed profound where opportunity exists. Approximately one in five Americans live at the poverty level. What impact do these imposed hardships have on adolescent development?

Six focal concerns of lower-class cultures were identified by Miller,[20] who collected data from 21 corner groups—black, white, male, and female in early, middle, and late adolescence—in a slum area of a large city. These concerns take up much time, energy, and emotion; they include trouble, toughness, smartness, excitement, fate, and autonomy. Miller concluded that the dominant concern of lower-class cultures is trouble, whether one is law-abiding or non-law-abiding. Membership in certain adolescent gangs that break laws may be considered prestigious. Getting into trouble leads to additional attention from others and provides excitement. Toughness seems particularly important for the male's masculine identity; he must appear hard and undemonstrative and denounce stereotypical feminine traits or values. Outwitting another, or smartness, is likewise valued and respected. The search for excitement follows extended periods of inactivity and boredom about once a week. Excitement seeking often involves danger or the possibility of trouble through fights, drinking, or gambling.

The concept of destiny, or fate, is related to the belief held by most persons in the lower classes that their lives are subject to forces over which they have no control.[20] Gambling is popular and often involves other concerns of toughness, smartness, and excitement, in addition to "Lady Luck" or fate. Although they express a desire for autonomy, actually lower-class young persons often actively seek controlled care: they tend to seek out highly restrictive social environments with stringent rules and regulations, such as the army or the disciplinary school. Belonging to a street-corner gang may mean status and acceptance.

The six focal concerns described by Miller offer the deprived adolescent something positive. The adolescent's self-esteem may be promoted considerably by his peers' recognition of his toughness, his smartness, and his contribution to excitement in the life of abysmal deprivation that they share.

The health care worker who works with the disadvantaged adolescent cannot compete for his attention unless he also fosters the adolescent's self-esteem. Unless a sincere effort is made to understand, know, and communicate with the poor person, he is not likely to be affected by health care attempts. The lower-class language is different; words are direct and not concerned with subtleties. The health care worker cannot react judgmentally to directness and must use terms that are readily recognized—without "talking down"—in order to communicate effectively. Health professionals tend to use a lot of jargon in everyday usage that is misunderstood by most lay persons, regardless of socioeconomic level.

The poor person's priorities are different from the affluent adolescent's. He cannot think of his future security or the trip to the clinic next week if his belly is empty and cramping and his children are crying from hunger. If he has no decent clothes to wear, he may feel more comfortable staying home.

Family patterns in the poverty culture have been observed to be different from middle-class family and child-rearing patterns.[21] Some family characteristics that have been observed among all of the urban poor, regardless of ethnic group, include mother-centered families, high incidence of abandonment of mothers and children, male superiority, frequent use of violence in settling quarrels, physical punishment in training children, wife beating, early initiation into sex, and free unions.[21]

From the moment of birth, a poverty child is bombarded by stimuli from which the middle-class child is protected. A stark light bulb from the ceiling and the loud quarrels or joyful conversations of his relatives may be commonplace. The poverty child learns early to block out sensory overload. If the health care worker is not sensitive to and understanding of the deprived youth, or does not attempt to communicate meaningfully, the adolescent who has grown up in poverty has little difficulty in blocking out the health care worker's advice.

The Black Adolescent: Attitudes and Reflections

CARNIE A. HAYES, JR., R.N., M.S.

The migration patterns of blacks that developed around the beginning of World War II were or should have been expected. Blacks from South Carolina, Georgia, eastern Alabama, and Florida sought routes north, and many ended up in Washington, D.C., Philadelphia, or New York. Those from Mississippi, Arkansas, and Tennessee tended to migrate to St. Louis, Chicago, or Detroit. Blacks from Louisiana and Texas often went West. This migration pattern shows that a southern background and heritage are shared by many blacks living in urban ghettos.

The black family, in its move from the rural setting to the city in search of employment and the fulfillment of hope for an improved life style, has experienced many obstacles in its struggle to achieve these goals. This section focuses on some of the unique problems that the black family faces; some of these are misconceptions that have evolved from research reports and others are problems that minority groups face in instilling confidence and promoting self-esteem in their adolescents.

Misconceptions about Black Families

Research reports about blacks have led to many misconceptions that are widely held. The different ideological perspectives (and biases) of researchers studying the black family have contributed to diverse and conflicting conclusions.[22] Allen[22] identified three ideological perspectives—the "cultural equivalent," the "cultural deviant," and the "cultural variant"—which characterize black family research. Allen pointed out that the *cultural equivalent* perspective of deemphasizing the distinct cultural qualities of black families and highlighting the common, shared qualities of black and white families, overlooks the validity of distinct cultural characteristics. The cultural equivalent perspective recognizes black family structures only in relationship to the organization and function of white middle-class families. Although the researchers from the *cultural deviant* perspective recognize distinct cultural patterns, these patterns have been labeled "pathological" when they were at variance with white dominant cultural patterns. The cultural deviant perspective is probably responsible for many of the misconceptions about the black family—i.e., that black males are dominated by matriarchs and that the family pattern is unstable and chaotic.[22] The Moynihan report,* "The Negro Family: The Case for National Action," published by the United States Department of Labor in 1965, is probably the most controversial report of this nature, and has contributed greatly to widespread misconceptions.

The *cultural variant* perspective views the different social and cultural environments as contributing to differences in the structure and functioning of black and white families; situational variables have impact on universal family functions.[22] In addition to social and economic inequalities, the black family has had to cope with stereotypes emanating from research that reflects these diverse perspectives. These stereotypes based on research from small populations have been generalized to all blacks. An example is the common belief that all black families are matriarchal.

The reported number of black families headed by females may be inaccurate because some females may report (as a survival tactic) that they are the sole providers for their families. If the husband has seasonal work or another low-paying job, the husbandless classification serves as insurance for periods when the husband is out of work, since it allows the wife to collect welfare. Kriesberg[23] observed that the absence of a husband did not always mean that the family was without income and had to depend on either the mother's work or public assistance. Staples[24] noted that shifts among black women to roles as family providers were responses to economic conditions, and as such deserve praise and compassion.

* A very good critique of this report by Alex L. Swain, "A Methodological Critique of the Moynihan Report," is published in *The Black Scholar*, June, 1974, pp. 18–24. The reader working with middle-class or poor blacks is encouraged to read it.

The belief that black females dominate households has not been upheld by research. Hammond[25] reported that 60% of the husbands and 57% of the wives studied rated their marriage as egalitarian. Scanzoni[26] suggested that the more secure the male's position, the more willing he is to participate in a partnership marriage. It may be that the egalitarian relationship is more prevalent in black working-class families than in those of whites; the man is considered the head of the household in the white working and middle-class family—contrasting with the view of marriage as a joint venture.[25]

Because of the increasing mobility of black families—both geographic (Jackson, Mississippi, to Los Angeles, California) and vertical (socioeconomic)—the accepted belief that an extended family is always available for support is no longer true. The isolation of the nuclear family from the extended family adds to nuclear family stress in that the casual visiting, joint holiday events, ritual celebrations, support of aging parents, and help from the larger family are missed.[27] The upward-mobile black often must build a life around a family of orientation and deny contact with his family of procreation.[27] The black individual who aspires to achieve despite the social cost may be labeled "uppity." Those individuals who assign a higher priority to their careers than to having a family may be ostracized by the extended family.

Young nuclear black families who have moved away from the extended family often bring friends and neighbors into their family circle, however, to combat this loneliness and to make up for the loss of the warmth and loving support of their extended family.[28] It is not unusual for the young couple's children to call the friends and neighbors who are brought into the family circle in this way, "aunt" or "uncle." [28]

Confidence and Self-Esteem

Knowing where one's ancestors came from is important. This knowledge is especially important to the adolescent working on his identity. Many people argue that the past is not important. Uncertainty and confusion about one's past leads to ambivalence and less assertiveness about the future. Black awareness can come from many sources; it is evidenced by the brother handshake or a raised Black Power fist. Knowing one's ancestors' achievements and familial history can help bolster one's confidence.

I cannot trace my "roots" back to Africa but I do have enough knowledge of my heritage so that I feel secure in my identity. My great-grandfather was born in slavery, but he was an achiever. He homesteaded 160 acres of land and reared a large family. Back in the early 1900s he had a shed large enough to make syrup in all types of weather. Having knowledge about my own family history and other aspects of my heritage helped build my confidence.

Confidence is an "ego trip" that manifests itself in many ways, but it is also built in subtle ways. In my own farm upbringing, I had to work. I fed the hogs and helped with the milking. I knew these jobs were important to the farm, and knowing the importance of these jobs boosted my self-confidence. Today, with more people living in cities than in rural areas, there is a challenge to urban parents that is unparalleled in history. The adolescent in an urban setting has few, if any, chores he can do to prove his value to the family economic unit. The individual's knowledge that he can achieve is a great "shot in the arm" for confidence and self-esteem. Yet, confidence and adolescence are often at different ends of a continuum. An adolescent has lived only a short time, 13 to 18 years, and the confidence gained by much trial and error is denied him. Considering the fact that confidence and maturity allow one to make better and sounder decisions it is not hard to see why urban adolescents often lack confidence in making decisions and in being assertive.

Brown[29] compared poverty-stricken black high school students with black college students, using Holland's Vocational Preference Inventory and Gough's Adjective Checklist. The poor black adolescent perceived himself as incompetent and ineffective in contrast to the black college student, who saw himself as more competent and successful. The poor adolescent was willing to attempt to achieve characteristics that were rewarded by society. The overall low self-concept of poor black adolescents, when coupled with fewer learning opportunities, promotes a vicious cycle of feelings of low self-esteem.

Research comparing black and white senior high school students found that black students had lower self-confidence, were defensive in their descriptions of themselves, and were confused about their identities.[30] These findings reflect the impact of prejudice on minority youth.

The challenge to rear black young people so that they have positive identities and are free of prejudice must be met if progress is to be made. Prejudice is a two-edged sword that hurts both dominant and minority groups by depriving them of their potential in contributing to society. Since black youths know that their odds for summer jobs are seven to one, bitterness is understandable. The unemployment rate for black teenagers is consistently twice that for white teenagers.[31] In the face of considerable odds the black youth needs additional encouragement in order to succeed and to gain the confidence to achieve. Brown's[29] study of teenage blacks in a summer work program for poverty-level youth found general self-deprecation among the group. Their commitment to the summer program indicated their desire to become more competent and effective.

The job of black parents is not an easy one. Rearing a well-balanced, normal child is a challenge for the black family. Dr. Alvin F. Poussaint has identified this problem precisely:

> Black parents . . . must rear their children free of prejudice as they help them develop a positive Black identity in the face of prejudice and social handicaps.[32]

How can black parents instill in a child the desire to succeed? There are no easy answers. A child may begin to learn confidence by being given the responsibility for some chore around the house. Handling his own allowance with some supervision and guidance until around age 12 may also contribute to self-confidence. Individual projects with parental guidance may be utilized. Age-grouped activity such as the Brownies or Cub Scouts may also help. Although adolescents may denounce parental attempts to help, black parents must look beyond the rhetoric of their adolescents and help them to achieve. Instilling self-confidence and self-esteem begins early, long before adolescence.

Seeing black role models in the community and larger culture can foster self-esteem for a black child. The increasing numbers of black performers and blacks in television commercials during the last decade has perhaps had a positive effect on the self-esteem of black young people. Teplin[33] found in a study of black, Anglo, and Latino third- and fourth-grade children that the black child chose pictures of black children and the Latino and Anglo children chose pictures of Anglo children. This finding is in contrast to earlier studies in which both black and white children chose white dolls and puppets, or photographs of white children.

When dealing with any adolescent, it is of paramount importance to respect his or her self-confidence. The need to show respect for the individual's self-confidence is often taken more lightly with regard to adolescents than it is in the case of adults. Society as a whole tends to consign adolescents to an almost nonexistent state. Pediatricians often stop seeing children around 14 to 18 years of age, depending upon the individual's psychological and physical development. Gynecologists often do not see young female patients until well after menarche, if at all, so that many adolescents remain for a long time in limbo with regard to health care and information. Awareness of these and other societal factors leads many teenagers to feel abandoned by the health care system. Any activity the teenager engages in is viewed with suspicion by his parents, his friends are not understood, and he remains distant. As they are batted to and fro in their not-child/not-adult state, it is no wonder that teenagers have serious doubts and react negatively. This negative reaction may also carry over in attempts to function sexually, since all the components to do so are present. Ambivalence emerges and indecision is paramount. The possibility of parents' finding out about sexual activity often overrides the fear of becoming pregnant; consequently, contraception seems less important.

Adolescent Pregnancy

The peer pressure felt by an adolescent often leads to his fumbling into the depths of human sexuality, and pregnancy or other complications are often the end result. The inability to say no and the knowledge that his peers expect him to "go all the way" are two factors behind many pregnancies. Sexual experimentation and sexual intercourse have been beginning at earlier ages.[34]

The notion that adolescents become pregnant because their peers are pregnant has perhaps been given too much credit as a reason for high black teenage birth rates. Furstenberg[35] found in interviewing 306 black disadvantaged mothers of teenagers who were illegitimately pregnant that only 4% approved of their daughter's pregnancy and 69% were decidedly negative. The majority of the teenagers, 65%, were also unhappy. The pregnant teenagers desired the approval of their close friends, however, and those who described themselves as very happy were more likely to have friends who had had illegitimate children themselves.

Gispert and Falk[34] studied 214 13- to 16-year-old black adolescents and their parents. The adolescents included three groups: a group choosing abortion, a group carrying pregnancy to term, and a control group of never-pregnant adolescents matched by age and socioeconomic status. The pregnant adolescents felt deeper despair and a greater sense of worthlessness than the nonpregnant controls. The group choosing abortion reflected a higher level of family disturbance. The adolescents who were having their babies were more socially isolated, both from peer and family interactions. The nonpregnant adolescents had fewer problems in school and had higher grades and higher educational goals than the pregnant adolescents.

Marrying after having a baby has many social connotations, and some stigma is attached to it by most ethnic groups. This has been somewhat less true of the black community—not because illegitimacy is desired, but because of the family's way of managing the problem. When the average black family discovers that an untimely pregnancy has occurred, the family neither moves away out of shame, disinherits the adolescent, nor sends her to Timbuktu. The family may send the adolescent to Kansas to live with an aunt for the duration of the pregnancy; the aunt may then adopt the infant. Black families seldom release infants for adoption, because of strong feelings of "self preservation and preservation of the family." [36]

Furstenberg[37] found in his study of pregnant adolescents (predominantly black) that only 6% were able to identify any method of birth control. Why do black adolescents from disadvantaged homes have poor or inadequate knowledge of contraceptive methods? Furstenberg notes that it is often a case of the blind leading the blind; the mother, aunts, and grandmother often have little knowledge about methods of contraception and how they work.

Why do black adolescents avoid family planning clinics? Fear of the setting, the effect of the setting on individual and family attitudes, are all reasons why black adolescents avoid family planning clinics. If the adolescent female is healthy, she probably has not had a physical examination since entering school some eight years earlier. Adolescents also fear that if friends or relatives know about their going to the clinic, or see them entering a family planning clinic, they will be labeled as "red letter" persons and everyone will know they are sexually active.

The absence of black role models or counselors in family planning clinics adds to the reluctance of blacks to attend these clinics. Although seeing a black practitioner would not eliminate the stress involved in going to the clinic, the presence of a black practitioner there would increase the adolescent's trust that her feelings would be understood, and could foster the aspiration that she too might hold such a position sometime in the future.

Adolescent Parenting

When black adolescents become parents, they often already have skills in child care. Blacks often provide child care at very young ages. Many teenagers know mothers who have babysitting problems—notably those in single-parent situations. Since their employment possibilities in the job market are very low, black teenagers are usually quick to capitalize on the opportunity to babysit. This helps the working mother and it provides the girl, who is often a very young adolescent, with experience in caring for a young baby. Once the mother is comfortable about leaving the baby with the babysitter, the teenager feels more comfortable in the role. This part of the cultural heritage began generations ago during slavery. When young girls could not get work in the fields, they could keep the babies quiet, under the eye of a grand, elderly black female who was too old to work in the fields.

After World War II, many black females found themselves taking care of families while all of the other family members were rallying to help the war effort. Often a baby sister was available to help an older working sister with her baby. Leaving an agrarian society for an urban one meant making many changes; one of those changes was in infant care for the single working mother. The black community used black teenagers as babysitters. The tradition of strong interdependence and reliance on family members for help is more characteristic of black families than it is of whites, who more readily utilize community resources.[27]

Babies are helpless and need care, love, and attention, and many teenagers are capable of giving them adequate care. Once a teenager is comfortable holding a young baby and changing its diapers under the mother's watchful eye, then other aspects of infant care can be learned. If a teenager has learned to expect certain infant behavior, she is more able to provide patient, understanding care for the baby. This kind of experience enables teenagers to adapt to the mothering role more easily if pregnancy occurs during their teens. Feeling comfortable in handling the baby is a factor in later feelings and attitudes of teenagers or any new parents in their new role.

Since many families today are small and the population is now so mobile, some teenagers may not have been around small infants in their growing-up years. The teenager may need to be taught how to care for a neighbor's baby by the mother or by a nurse in order to become proficient in her child care tasks. In most cases the mother of an infant is a good instructor for the teenager because she wants her child to be well cared for.

Young men are often very effective babysitters. This is often discovered when the oldest child is a boy and the family needs a babysitter; or a neighbor may like the way he handles his younger siblings. This exposure certainly helps the young man in his future fathering role.

Health Care Priorities and Implications

Health care is a low priority item for any adolescent, but for blacks it is even lower. The following schematic diagram illustrates this point:

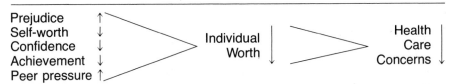

Variables affecting the black's feelings of individual worth and health care concerns.

Prejudice can be found in many public institutions in all parts of this country. Careless remarks made by the counselor can be devastating to an already frightened adolescent. For example, if a 16-year-old black girl comes in to a family planning clinic and innuendoes about promiscuity are made, she will be so embarrassed and upset that she will be unable to learn from any attempted counseling and most likely will not return to the clinic. Such innuendoes—which are based on some of the commonly held misconceptions about black families—reflect bias and prejudice. This is why "increased prejudice" is the first item in the diagram.

It is easily seen how a decrease in self-worth, confidence, and achievement feeds into the next level of decreased individual worth. What may be a bit more nebulous is the increase in peer pressure and how this fits into the pattern of decreased health concerns. Adolescents are very peer-oriented, and if a black teenager had an experience like the one described above, few if any of her peers would go to that clinic once the information was spread about the way she had been treated there.

Most family planning units give physical examinations to all who use the clinic's services. This is an opportunity for the health professional to communicate with the adolescent and to learn what he wishes to know. This can be a bit frustrating if straightforward questions are expected. Adolescents, both male and female, often ask questions obliquely or in the third person.

Example: "I have a friend who has been going steady with the same boy for over a year and she has never taken anything. She says she only has sex relations when her period is on. She says she can't get pregnant during that time. Can she get pregnant or not?" More often than not, a short, snappy answer is the initial response in a situation like this. A detailed, carefully worded answer would be more helpful; some graphs showing the menstrual cycle and hypothalamic activity would illustrate fertile and nonfertile periods and would increase the young woman's understanding of her body.

Teenagers may ask questions more comfortably anonymously. In a clinic situation this opportunity can be provided by having the young people write questions out in detail and place them in a box to be read by the nurse. This avoids embarrassment and allows for a full listening-learning experience. Health care personnel should make it clear that there is no such thing as a stupid or "dumb" question if a person needs to know that information.

Summary

Promoting the confidence and self-esteem of black adolescents is a challenge which must be dealt with if their health needs are to be met by the health care system. Achieving trust is a must if one is to succeed with the adolescent population, no matter what the ethnic background. A careful assessment of the black adolescent's family support system and recognition of the cultural diversity within the black population are important in meeting individual needs.

Experience is gained through exposure to life and its realities. Immaturity is a condition to be expected in the teenager. Today's society does not facilitate the adolescent's growing up as it should. The black adolescent's strengths must be given recognition; his weaknesses can be tactfully presented so that he can improve in those areas.

As sexual experience at earlier ages becomes more widespread in the adolescent population, more positive steps need to be taken to provide sound sexual information. Knowledge about family planning, contraceptive usage, and how pregnancy occurs must reach every adolescent. As adolescents receive more information and the health care system improves its efficiency, the adolescent birth rates should drop. Sound sexual information and contraceptive counseling are vital in meeting the adolescent's health needs.

Vigorous efforts must be made to increase the enrollment of blacks in programs preparing for health care careers. Though it is not advocated or necessary that all black clinics have an all-black staff, it is important that someone be available who can relate to the frustrated adolescent who may also be angry and distrustful. Health care professionals must "try harder" to meet the health needs of black and all other adolescents.

The Latino Adolescent

TERESA A. BELLO, R.N., M.S.

In this chapter, the reader is introduced to the ethnic/cultural variations among adolescents who are part of the diverse client population in the United States. Latino is used here as a broad category that includes Chicanos, Latin Americans, Mexican Americans, and Hispanics.

It is true that when one attempts to explain certain behavioral traits of particular ethnic or cultural groups for the purpose of increasing the knowledge and understanding of health professionals, there is a tendency to overgeneralize. For the purposes of this section, the author does generalize; however, the reader is reminded that within any particular cultural/ethnic group, there are behavioral similarities as well as variations. The generalizations are intentionally brief and are concerned only with the more common beliefs and demonstrated values of the culture that have been documented.

Socioeconomic differences, the length of time lived in this country, and geographic location are factors to be considered when working with a Latino family. Generally speaking, high socioeconomic group status and greater length of time in this country correlate with a greater degree of acculturation and decreased adherence to the traditional cultural beliefs and practices. Depending upon the geographic location, the nurse may also find variations in methods of food selection and preparation, health beliefs and practices, and the like. This is similar to the diversity one finds between Americans from the West Coast and Americans from the South.

This section will describe some of the characteristics of Latino adolescents and the nurse-client process that may be helpful when working with a Latino adolescent and his family and community.

With all of the above in mind, the author hopes that this section will serve as a base for appropriate and creative individual interventions and that it will also increase the reader's desire to seek more information about her individual Latino adolescent client.

Diverse Cultural Patterns

Varying degrees of acculturation between generations are not unique to the Japanese Issei (first generation, immigrant), Nisei (second generation, born and educated in the United States), and Sansei (third generation). Because of the continuous influx of citizens from Mexico and Latin America, one finds within the Latino population wide variations in behavior and in adherence to the traditional cultural beliefs and practices. Dorsey and Jackson[38] write that acculturated Latino/Chicano people accept the dominant culture's beliefs and practices and usually deny the existence of the practices of the ''mother'' country (Mexico or Latin American country). Some people may blend the culture of the ''old country'' with the ''new'' culture of the new country.

Whatever cultural pattern is followed, most Latinos are reared as Roman Catholics. Therefore, many attitudes about sex, marriage, and divorce are influenced by that religion. Attitudes about birth control and abortion are particularly affected by the teachings of Roman Catholicism. Healey and DeBlassie[39] found that Spanish-American adolescents scored higher than blacks or Anglos on measures of the moral-ethical self when they compared the self-concepts of these three groups. They postulated that this finding reflected the important role of religion in the Spanish-American culture; religion seems to be the domain least affected in the transition to a new culture.

The Family

Perhaps the most generalizable concept that may be applied to Latinos in general is their strong family orientation. The family, which includes not only father, mother, and siblings, but also grandparents, uncles, aunts, cousins, and godparents, provides the social, psychological/emotional, and often ''necessities-of-life'' support network. While sociologists ponder the ostensible demise of ''The Family'' in the white middle class, for the Latino, ''The Family'' is flourishing.

Children are regarded as treasures by Latinos. Although parents feel shock, shame, and anger when one of their unmarried daughters becomes pregnant, many parents do not consider abortion a viable solution. Usually, when the infant is born, there is no stigma attached to it and the infant is an accepted member of the family. The infant is reared by both the mother and grandmother.

According to Murillo,[40] the parents are permissive and indulgent with the younger children; however, children are taught to work for the welfare of the family.

Goodman and Beman[41] studied Mexican-American children in a Texas barrio to learn how school-aged children viewed their lives. They found that the children viewed the home and people at home as central to their lives and that they had a healthy respect for their elders. Their expressed affection and respect for people was confined to the immediate family and relatives.

Most authors who describe the Latino family write that the father is the disciplinarian and that the mother provides most of the warmth and affection. Rubel[42] observes that when the children begin to reach puberty, the affective relationship with the father decreases. The father usually becomes more authoritarian while demanding and expecting more respect.[40] It may be hypothesized that the father is attempting to prepare himself for the probably difficult adolescent period of the children. Most likely, the father is emulating the behavior of his father.

The relationship between the mother and the adolescent children continues to be warm and affectionate even into adulthood, although the female children are usually closer to their mothers as adults.

As with any family of any culture, sex roles are taught and learned in the home. Although it seems from observation that the women's liberation movement is having an effect on the college-bound middle-class Latino woman, at least as far as her attempt to reject the traditional sex roles is concerned, its effect on the Latinos at the lower end of the socioeconomic scale should be studied. Socioeconomically deprived Latino women may marry before the completion of high school or immediately after high school; therefore, their exposure to the philosophy of the women's liberation movement may be limited to the usually distorted comments they hear from other neighborhood women, their husbands, or television. Thus, the women may not realize the potential impact of the women's movement on their lives.

The female is expected to be respectful to her parents and elders; to avoid bringing shame to the family; to be a good wife and mother; and to be mindful of her duty to treat her father, brothers, uncles, and future husband with respect and devotion. Behavior considered shameful by the family is the loss of virginity before marriage.

The male is expected to be respectful to his parents and elders; to avoid bringing shame to the family (although his behavior would be regarded as less shameful than the female's behavior); to protect his sisters; to be a responsible father, husband, and breadwinner; and to expect that the female members of his family and his future wife will treat him with respect and devotion. In the literature, this type of behavior is usually labeled "macho." Some examples of male conduct bringing shame to the family are trouble with the criminal justice system and heavy drug usage.

The adolescent male usually spends most of his free time away from the home. He may work part-time or become involved in extracurricular activities. Conversely, the female is encouraged to stay close to the home and to avoid situations that might lead to intimate contact with males. Depending on the female's age and the situation at home, holding a part-time job is encouraged. However, if the female is responsible for babysitting and cooking dinner because both parents work, she will be discouraged from seeking a job. The same would hold true for extracurricular activities. The guiding principle involved is the benefit that will result for the whole family from the individual act. If the benefit to the family is minor, then the proposed act or behavior outside the home will be disallowed. This does not imply that the adolescent accepts the decision without the usual family disruption whenever a goal is frustrated. As the reader knows, any adolescent selectively chooses situations in which he wishes to be compliant.

Sex and Sexuality

Generally speaking, the open discussion of sex is forbidden in the Latino home. Boys and girls are separated early, and after the age of five or so, seeing the genitalia of brothers and sisters is expressly forbidden. Children's innocent sexual play is considered a grave offense and this behavior brings severe punishment. Children are not allowed to hear dirty jokes or ''adult talk'' about sex or to see anything that depicts nudity. The adolescent female is intensely modest about showing her body and may refuse to participate in school physical activities if she must expose her body to the other females while undressing or taking a shower. The adolescent female usually experiences terror at the thought of a male doctor or nurse looking at or touching her body. Although she is taught that being a wife and mother is important, the idea is ingrained in her that she must not let anyone touch her genitalia until marriage. Often, the Latino female is unaware of menarche until it occurs; thus, she may be frightened when it happens and may be afraid to tell her mother. The adolescent knows little about her body and how it functions.

The female is taught to handle relationships through submissive behavior because it is unfeminine and disruptive to the family to ''act like a man.'' She is also taught that the greatest shame to a Latino family is a pregnant unwed daughter.

The male, although not explicitly taught about sex or sexuality in the home setting, is taught that he as a male will be expected to carry on the name of the family. He cannot show weakness. Throughout his childhood, he is encouraged to play the male role and trained to handle relationships through dominant and assertive behavior.

Therefore, adolescents learn about sex from their peers, pornographic books, magazines, and other ''enlightened'' sources. Their information is piecemeal and contains many fallacies. Because the Latino adolescent, especially the female, has learned that the topic of sex is so obviously forbidden, the adolescent girl will shy away from discussing sex with adults, especially if the discussion is about the opposite sex and particularly if she thinks that the adult will tell her parents about her interest.

Given the movement toward dealing openly with sex in school and in the communications media and the abundance of pornographic literature, the Latino adolescent is now exposed to the topic of sex at an earlier age and is probably learning more about it, although the information may still be scanty and factually inaccurate. In either case, the Latino adolescent finds himself in a bind. At home he must contend with the strict code of silence about sex while being naturally curious about it. Even if he has learned about sex from a legitimate source, such as the school, the probable reaction of his parents to any discussion of the information will be negative.

On the other hand, peer pressure is forcing the Latino adolescent to ''make it.'' Both males and females are subject to this pressure, although a Latino female who is known to have intercourse with many ''guys'' develops a poor reputation. Males and females join in disparaging promiscuous sexual behavior in females. However, active sexual behavior on the part of Latino males is regarded as normal. The Latino adolescent females who do not engage in sexual activity usually fear that they will never have boyfriends. This gives rise to many dilemmas: should a girl engage in intercourse and bring feelings of shame and guilt to herself and her family or remain a virgin and worry about peer acceptance? On the other hand, she has also been taught that a woman who is not a virgin at marriage will be rejected by the male.

Implications for Nurses

Before a nurse interacts with Latino clients whose ethnic/cultural backgrounds may be dissimilar to her own, she should be aware of any of her beliefs and values that may conflict with the Latino clients' beliefs and values. Nurses would never begin delivering quality nursing care without knowing basic nursing skills and procedures; it is just as important for nurses to have relevant basic knowledge about the cultural foundations and beliefs of their clients—in this instance, Latino clients. A careless intervention may be just as harmful and ineffective as the administration of an injection using poor technique.

The following example related to the author by a client during a home visit for prenatal teaching illustrates the harmful impact of careless nursing intervention. Linda was 15 years old when she first went to an outpatient clinic with her father. Her mother was unable to accompany her. When Linda told the nurse that she came to see the doctor because of painful periods, the nurse asked the date of her last period. Linda replied that she could not remember it. The nurse flippantly remarked, "Everyone remembers the date of her last period." Beginning to feel intimidated, Linda began to wish that she had never come to the doctor's office. The nurse then asked Linda when she had last had sex. Shocked, Linda began to cry. Angrily, the nurse scolded Linda for crying and insisted that she tell her the last time she had been "with a boy." The nurse observed that Linda "couldn't be different from the rest of 'you people.'" When the doctor came into the room, the nurse went over to him and whispered into his ear. All of this time Linda felt a deep sense of shame. She had been accused of sex before marriage by a nurse and, although innocent, she worried that the nurse would tell her father that she was "bad."

The doctor pursued the same line of questioning. Fearing such an authority figure, Linda meekly replied "no" to his questions about premarital sex. Linda remembers that the doctor told her to "have babies" to stop her menstrual cramps, but he did not do a pelvic examination or ask her anything else about her cramping.

Aside from both the nurse's and physician's obvious lack of interpersonal skills, had they known about the Latino sex taboo for females and about the strong Latino family orientation they could have approached the adolescent differently. For example, the nurse could have begun her interview by validating with the adolescent that painful menstrual cramps must be distressful to her and must cause her family to worry about her. The nurse would have set the tone of the interview by accepting the adolescent's complaint as valid and by recognizing that her complaints might affect the family. The nurse could then have continued by telling the adolescent that she knew how embarassing it is to discuss a problem that affected such a personal and private part of her body. Once again, the nurse would be accepting the probability that the Latino adolescent could be feeling apprehension about discussing her periods and could convey the idea that to feel apprehension was acceptable. The nurse could have asked the adolescent how her mother handled her painful periods. Most likely the mother's painful periods would have been considered an illness; the Latino adolescent with menstrual cramps would be allowed to stay home from school, in bed, and would be relieved of home duties. Knowing this, the nurse would have realized how the family roles are shifted in order to help a family member and would have gained more insight into the health and illness practices of the adolescent and her family. The nurse could have used all of the information gathered to help develop a realistic and relevant care plan. However, Linda was now 18, married, and in her third trimester of pregnancy. She was referred to the Health Department by the local emergency hospital because she appeared in the emergency room with signs and symptoms of toxemia. Linda related that because of the treatment she had received three years before, she could never face a nurse or a doctor for fear that they would think she was promiscuous. She was also feeling embarrassed because when she delivered "so many people" would see her "private parts." The nursing error not only had a lingering impact for Linda, but also spread to others. Linda continued to relate her negative experience with the clinic to other adolescents.

APPROACH TO SEXUALITY

Many nurses working with Latino adolescent females make the mistake of limiting teaching to birth control and/or insisting on the use of a birth control device rather than dealing with the adolescent's feelings and knowledge about sex and intercourse, particularly if the adolescent still lives at home. If the Latino adolescent decides to have intercourse and use contraception, the guilt feelings may at times be overwhelming; figuring out a way to hide the pills or other device when one lives in close quarters imposes an extra emotional burden.

Recognizing the strong influence of the family upon the individual and the strong influence of religion upon the family, it would seem logical and appropriate for the nurse to take this information, together with a thorough assessment of the adolescent, and develop realistic interventions that would benefit the adolescent and the family. When the adolescent still lives at home, the implications are that the nurse will work with that adolescent, recognizing that the family, the community, and the church will exercise considerable influence on her beliefs and values. The nurse who wants to be beneficial cannot isolate the Latino adolescent from the family and expect total cooperation and change.

Female nurses working with Latino males may have a difficult time communicating effectively. For one thing an adult female, even a nurse, could probably not discuss sexuality without causing discomfort—because of the feeling that males should not need women to teach them anything about sexuality. To admit that they know almost nothing or that what they know may be incorrect would be to admit failure in that area. In this case, the nurse should seek out an enlightened male nurse, male physician, male community worker, or interested father to help her set up a group. A male lends credibility to the group for the male who grows up expecting females to look up to and be submissive to males. The approach should be "down-to-earth'' and nonthreatening to the male ego. When Latino adolescent males feel that the female nurse is not trying to dominate and impose her values as a female upon them, trust may begin to develop.

WORKING WITH PARENTS

Because of the strong family orientation, the nurse should include the parents in discussions about their adolescent children. Like other parents, Latino parents find that the tactics they utilized during the adolescent's earlier childhood now fail miserably. Also, our society has become more complex and makes more demands on adolescents than did the society that the parents knew. They often honestly do not know how to handle their adolescent children but recognize that they can exercise some parental control through the use of bribery—privileges connected to the automobile, spending money, dating, or going out with friends. However, conflict often arises when the Latino parent becomes overzealous in the exercise of parental control. The nurse may become involved after the adolescent has acted out by running away, getting pregnant, impregnating someone, leaving school without permission, or taking drugs. As a preventive intervention the nurse could easily begin discussion groups for these parents. Because of the usual problem of accessibility to agencies, the parents' discussion group meetings should take place in someone's home. The private and homey atmosphere often decreases the parents' anxiety about discussing the feelings of frustration or failure that they experience when trying to cope with their adolescent children. These meetings should also take place in the evening so that fathers and working mothers can attend. If nurses are truly committed to the future good adjustment of the adolescents and their families—and to the highest standards of nursing—such meetings could be arranged one evening a week.

Should the nurse feel insecure about setting up such a group alone, she should utilize the principles of community organization: seek out the informal and formal community leaders and present ideas to them; listen to their comments and suggestions and work *together* in establishing the groups. Not only will the nurse accomplish her objective, she will also have increased the broader community's awareness of the normally difficult adolescent period and the normal parental despair in handling this period, and she will have helped the community to recognize the helpful role of the nurse. Probably from all of this the parents will begin to realize that they are not alone in dealing with their adolescents and it will be possible to prevent irreparable emotional damage to parents and their adolescents.

The nurse may also include concerned people such as the social worker, the pharmacist, the parish priest, and the community worker during the planning stages and/or as co-discussion leaders.

Before the reader rejects such a suggestion because she has perhaps observed that "Latino families" and their adolescent children may not have attended similar meetings, the author asks the reader to consider that usually:

1. When parents' groups are started, there is no input from the community leaders, least of all the parents.

2. These groups are held at a time that is convenient for the nurse—usually from 8:00 A.M. to 5:00 P.M., Monday through Friday.
3. These group meetings exclude the fathers (even though it is common knowledge that Latino families are strongly family-oriented and that the father is the undisputed leader of the family).
4. These group meetings are held at some distance from the parents' homes and usually in an agency, which decreases privacy and increases the likelihood that friends, neighbors, or others will learn of the parents' difficulty with their adolescent children.
5. The group meetings are presented as "group meetings for ineffectual or bad parents."
6. The nurse has no group-organizing or group-leading skills.
7. The nurse who has little knowledge of and/or respect for the Latino family may often come across as judgmental and arrogant.

All of the above factors need to be considered when planning group meetings. One institution overcame the low attendance problem for a group of Hispanic prenatal clients by planning flexibility in group eligibility, publicizing meetings with colorful posters in Spanish, planning individual interviews prior to group participation—and by the leader's exploration of her feelings of ambivalence about her capabilities in leading the group.[43]

Summary

Understanding the strong family orientation will be helpful and is indeed essential to the nurse as she plans total, comprehensive care for a Latino adolescent. The nurse must decide if she wants to facilitate permanent positive changes within the total family or to continue to focus on the individual adolescent in the hope of effecting temporary changes, i.e., at least until the nurse leaves or is no longer involved with the individual. Does the nurse want to have a positive impact upon future adolescents and their families or wait until she sees them as "problem" adolescents?

The majority of nurses in this country are from the white middle class, and their values usually reflect those of the dominant society. Unless the nurse is conscious of potential value conflicts—because of her lack of knowledge about the Latino culture—she will be ineffectual and frustrated in her attempts to create change with the Latino adolescent.

The Chinese Adolescent

CAROLYN M. FONG, R.N., M.S.

By and large, the Chinese in America are still influenced by some vestiges of the traditional Chinese culture. Generalizations do injustice to the differences among people, but cultural groups do have certain common values. Knowledge of these common beliefs helps the health care worker to serve the Chinese adolescent more effectively. Ideally, the health worker is always aware of the diversity among adolescents and of the individuality of each.

Diverse Cultural Patterns

Chinese adolescents in America are not a homogeneous group. There is a wide variation in the degree of adherence to the traditional Chinese cultural beliefs and practices. Various factors influence the degree of acculturation and assimilation. These influencing factors include socioeconomic status, place of birth, age, length of time in America, citizenship, place of residence, political background, education, parental expectations, and personal experiences.

One must distinguish between Chinese adolescents that are:

1. American born and who have escaped overcrowded Chinatown
2. American born and who still live in Chinatown or among the Chinese by choice
3. Foreign born of middle- or upper-class parents
4. Foreign born and who are imprisoned in the ghetto due to language barrier or unmarketable skills

The degree of acculturation is highest among American-born Chinese youths, because the old world ways have been lost, weakened, or modified. Most are emerging and participating more fully in American life because of parental opportunities for economic advancement and social recognition. However, only when the problem of racial prejudice is entirely solved can total acculturation be effected.

Chinese adolescents who immigrate to the United States during their teens or who live among or near other Chinese people tend to retain or to be more influenced by traditional Chinese attitudes and norms. They may stay together in social and school groups for emotional security and social life.

The Adolescent

Chinese adolescents are taught to sacrifice self-expression for the welfare of the larger group. Development as an individual is not emphasized. Self-fulfillment, self-actualization, and artistic expression are secondary to family unity, conformity, and the maintenance of tight social control.

The Chinese adolescent sees himself as a descendant of a racial and cultural group, seldom as an American per se. Yet he cannot be totally Chinese because of questions regarding his place in American society. Therefore the adolescent must vacillate between two ways of life, two cultural heritages, and two racial groups, each of which is diametrically opposed to the other.

Cultural shock may occur when the individual is exposed to the social values and family life of American friends in later childhood or early adolescence. Often, Chinatown children grow up without knowing what American families consider to be necessities—e.g., allowances, separate sleeping rooms, stereos, vacations, trips, and cars. This sharpens the conflict of cultural loyalties. The degree of stress depends on parental support, the adolescent's coping ability, and the group by which he wants to be socially accepted.

An adolescent besieged with the problems of cultural transition, language limitations, or social rejection may become involved in antisocial behavior and juvenile delinquency. In some families, both parents work, so that there is less of the traditional parental guidance and limit setting. The adolescent may lack the home stimulation and close family relations that would lead him to adopt or maintain the traditional Chinese values.

The Family

In general, the traditional Chinese family is very strong and close-knit, with ties extending to several generations within the same community. The patriarchal (male-dominated) and patrilineal (vertically structured) Chinese family exerts great social control over its members. This control is usually enforced by shame or guilt-inducing techniques. Adolescents commonly hear, "What will the neighbors say? Don't lose face!" Youths are taught to "save face," to avoid bringing dishonor or shame to the family. Families tend to try to solve their own problems; outside help, which would cause embarrassment, is not wanted.

Filial piety, or loyal devotion to parents, obedience, respect for authority, family solidarity, responsibility, school and career achievement, and personal discipline are some traditional values deeply ingrained in the Chinese family. Upward mobility in social and economic status is very important to parents. America is the "Land of the Gold Mountain," the land of opportunity.

Parental sex roles in the Chinese family are rapidly changing in the direction of true equality. In the traditional family the father is the head; he earns the money, manages finances, makes decisions, and has absolute authority. The mother is the household manager and has inferior status. Because of urbanization, financial pressures, and the freedom and higher status of women in America, Chinese wives are now working outside the home. They now have educational, career, and personal ambitions contrary to the traditional roles. These more liberated wives may rebel against expectations that they be submissive.

Parent-Adolescent Relationship

To maintain dignity with, and respect from, adolescents, traditional Chinese parents tend to stand aloof in an authoritarian position. The parents command and decide what is best and expect unquestioning obedience. The parents do not invite confidences, discussion, or informal camaraderie, nor do they display emotional feelings with the adolescent. The American-born parents do tend to seek a warm rapport and open discussions with their adolescents, in which instances respect becomes secondary.

Cultural conflict over values is emotional and intense. Like other adolescents, Chinese adolescents may rebel against parental control. According to Fong,[44] Chinese adolescents complain that there is no communication between them and their elders—everything is a game, a ritual which they cannot escape and which serves no positive purpose.

Many Chinese adolescents are kept busy with family chores and Chinese language school, encouraged to work and study diligently, spurred on to higher academic achievement, and discouraged from adopting society's romantic tendencies. When parents see their adolescents deemphasizing academic work in favor of socializing with peers and extracurricular activities they may feel personally threatened. They view these as signs of disrespect to them as parents and to their traditional values.

The Chinese-American adolescent may be expected to chafe under any strict discipline that is imposed upon him, not so much because he is restricted, but because he compares himself with his American friends. "If Johnny can do it, why can't I?" The adolescent in disagreement with his parents will at first try reasoning with them, but the parents, shocked that their decisions are being questioned, refuse to listen. This prevents full communication and lucid explanation.[45]

Language may be another source of interpersonal conflict between parents and adolescent. Children grow up hearing and speaking Chinese. When they enter the American school, they become aware of deficiencies in communicating with peers and teachers. In self-defense they may refuse to converse with parents in Chinese, refuse to go to Chinese school, and resort to English at every opportunity. The developing children then cannot express themselves in Chinese and their parents cannot express themselves in English. Much is left unsaid and neither can understand fully the personality and values of the other.

Other conflicts may be dating, household chores, discipline, studies and allowances. These are common in most families of every race and culture in the United States, but must also be considered in their separate cultural contexts as well.

SOCIALIZATION

Parents feel that the primary goal in adolescence is to get a good education in preparation for college. Socialization and dating are secondary and not priorities. Conflict may arise when adolescents become involved in social activities away from home instead of studying, helping with the family business, or participating in family activities. To maintain family solidarity there is increased pressure from parents to attend family gatherings and celebrate Chinese holidays together.

In early adolescence, Chinese youths tend to date in groups. Common meeting places are school dances, the 'Y'', bowling alleys, churches, or simply the streets. Most Chinese parents discourage single dating until late adolescence. Dating and marrying a Chinese are highly desirable.

Among first generation Chinese parents, there may be very little discussion between parent and adolescent about school, dating, and social activities because of either the language barrier, the generation gap or a cultural gap. This may cause increased parental anxiety and apprehension. Parents are afraid that their adolescent may: (1) join a juvenile gang, (2) get pregnant or get someone else pregnant, (3) do poorly in school or (4) allow peer influence to erode their authority. As a consequence, Chinese parents may then become stricter about allowing extracurricular activity.

EDUCATION

Most Chinese parents are success and achievement oriented. Children are imbued with a love of learning and a respect for scholarship and higher academic achievement. An adolescent who does not complete high school brings shame and dishonor to the family.

Chinese parents value the educational opportunities of the American school system. But this system also undermines the traditional value of parental authority when it encourages assertiveness, independence, individual decision making, and extracurricular activities for self-actualization and fulfillment.

SEX AND SEXUALITY

Generally, sex and interpersonal relationships with the opposite sex are not discussed in the Chinese home. In the first generation family, adolescents see very little demonstration of affection or emotion between their parents. Physical intimacies are confined to the bedroom. This upbringing may affect the adolescent's own ability to share personal emotions and love with another.

Physical modesty is highly prized by Chinese parents. Children are taught to undress alone and are shamed when dressed "indecently." Innocent childhood sex play or even masturbation by infants is quickly curtailed.

Chinese adolescents are curious about their bodies, their bodily functions, and reproduction. Technical sex information is usually learned from peers, pornographic books, health films, family life class, 'R'' rated movies, or, occasionally, from older siblings. The accuracy of sex information from these sources may in some instances be questionable. Premarital relations for males and females are frowned upon by parents because of the chances for pregnancy. A baby born out of wedlock would bring shame upon the family. Alternatives considered acceptable by the family in response to such a pregnancy are early marriage or adoption. The family usually makes the final decision by coercion or demand. Unfortunately, the Chinese male adolescent may not be consulted in the decision. If the family is not aware of the pregnancy, viable alternatives for the couple are abortion, marriage, or adoption.

In general, physical sex is a very significant and intimate act to the Chinese male and female adolescent. They do not approve of casual sex encounters. If a couple engages in sexual activity they usually feel they must "go steady." Rarely do adolescents discuss sexual intimacies with friends.

The change in the status of women has had quite an impact on the Chinese female adolescent. With respect to education, it was formerly thought that it would endanger feminine virtue; a girl was expected to be a devoted helper to her future mother-in-law and a bearer of many grandchildren, preferably males. Ambitions for education have broadened for contemporary Chinese females, but the young women may still find that their emerging role is not fully accepted by all segments of Chinese society.[44]

In some Chinese families, the male is considered to be, and is treated as, superior to the female. There may not be an equal division of labor between brothers and sisters in the home. The brother may have more freedom to go out for work or play. The female generally has more home responsibilities, such as child care or household chores.

In the traditional Chinese family the male is highly treasured because he will carry on the family name and line. The son will also assure honor, respect, and support for the parents in old age. Generally, the males are free to work in the family business, or as paper boys, gas station attendants, waiters, etc. The relationship between the parents and son is especially emphasized. Even after a son is married, he must continue to obey his parents. Conversely, a married daughter must obey her in-laws.

Implications for Nurses

It is essential that the nurse or health care provider be aware of and recognize any of her own beliefs and values that may conflict with the Chinese culture. In working with Chinese families one must understand, respect, and accept the values and beliefs of both the parents' culture and the adolescent's culture to give quality nursing care. Any attempt by the nurse to force her values on the family may create a gap in her relationship, communication, and effectiveness in helping the family.

WORKING WITH FAMILIES

Conflict over parental authority heightens during adolescence. The following example illustrates the nurse's role in dealing with the frustrations of a Chinese adolescent and his parent. Mr. Lee was referred to the public health nurse for active tuberculosis follow-up. On her third visit, the nurse discovered that Harry, Mr. Lee's 16-year-old son, was in trouble for setting off a bomb at school. According to Mr. Lee, "Harry has shamed the family. I cannot control him anymore. He talks on the phone too much, watches TV too much, and stays out after school. He is going steady with one girl. I don't like that." Harry related, "There's a generation and cultural gap. I can't stay for after-school sports. I can't go out with girls now, but he expects me to marry when I'm 21. He keeps me in my room studying all the time. I feel like a prisoner. I made and blew up the bomb because I feel so frustrated. He never listens to what I have to say. He's from the 'old world'!"

The father was very discouraged because of his lack of authority and control over Harry. The nurse offered the father guidelines, positive reinforcement, and support for his belief that he was doing what he felt was right and best. She spent a great deal of time giving him insight into what it was like for Harry growing up in America and into Harry's concerns. She arranged for Mr. Lee to visit the school to learn more about the goals of the American educational system. She acted as a sounding board, listening and allowing Mr. Lee to find solutions at his own pace.

The nurse felt that Harry could benefit from personal psychiatric counseling. Harry wanted counseling but was afraid his father would object. The nurse offered to discuss this with Harry's father. It is important to maintain confidentiality with the adolescent. The nurse should get approval from the adolescent before approaching parents regarding any nurse-adolescent discussions. Because the nurse had established trust and rapport with the father she easily obtained parental consent. Most Chinese families generally do not approve of psychiatric counseling; they prefer to keep their problems to themselves.

Harry felt uncomfortable about seeking free community psychiatric help. He wanted an Asian psychiatrist but did not know the correct procedure to follow. Harry was also reluctant to take the initial step. The nurse made the appointment for the first meeting, but Harry followed through on his own for future appointments. The nurse continued to be a resource person to the family and a consultant to the psychiatrist.

Family therapy with a bilingual, bicultural nurse is ideal for a Chinese adolescent experiencing cultural shock. The Chinese-American nurse familiar with the Chinese family structure, language, and beliefs can help by acting as the intermediary between parent and adolescent. If a bilingual, bicultural nurse is not available, a nurse who shows empathy, concern, and a desire to learn about the culture and problems of the Chinese community can provide tremendous moral support.

Adolescents want to acculturate to the American way but their parents enforce the old Chinese way. Parents and adolescents need to join together, communicate directly, and explain their viewpoints and feelings. Parents must say, "I worry about your joining a street gang and getting killed in a gang war." Adolescents must say, "It hurts me when Peter goes on a camping trip and I have to stay home." This is a very difficult step for Chinese adolescents and parents because of the language barrier and the traditional "I say it, you do it" communication pattern. The nurse familiar with Chinese family structure, language, and beliefs can help by acting as the intermediary between parent and adolescent.

Chinese families generally do not air their "dirty linen" to people outside the family. For this reason, the nurse may find it difficult to initiate large parents' "rap groups." But Chinese parents do need to know that they are not alone in their problems. They need support in their efforts to maintain restrictions that are necessary and reasonable. It may be valuable for the nurse to introduce to each other the parents of two adolescents from whom she had gained trust, so that they may share their concerns and fears. It is also important to reiterate to both families the necessity for strict confidentiality.

WORKING WITH ADOLESCENTS

Chinese adolescents relate best to a nurse who is warm, sympathetic, and willing to listen to their fears, concerns, and aspirations. Because Chinese parents may not invite confidences or discussions with their adolescent children, the nurse may play an important role in helping the adolescent through a stressful period in life. Adolescents respond to people who are interested in them as individuals, as special persons.

The following example shows how a nurse established rapport and trust with Mary, a 16-year-old Chinese female. The nurse was very effective in meeting Mary's needs. Approximately one year ago, Mary obtained a release from the school nurse to go home because of menstrual cramps. Thereafter, the nurse greeted Mary by name in the school hallways, an important step toward increasing an adolescent's self-esteem and feeling of importance. Mary then began to visit the nurse several times a month with questions about vague physical problems. The nurse assessed Mary's problem as being more emotional than physical; she recognized that it might be difficult for Mary to share personal emotional problems because of her upbringing mandate to ''save face.'' The nurse asked, ''What's really happening, Mary?'' This released a flood of tears from Mary and a confession of suicidal thoughts. Mary was depressed because she had no friends.

The nurse scheduled regular sessions with Mary to offer support and guidance. Mary, being shy, refused suggestions to join clubs or sport activities. Also, any extracurricular activity was impossible because she had to return home after school to care for her two younger brothers. The nurse encouraged Mary to work in the school nurse's office during a free hours. Mary then met many more students and began to make new friends.

In working with Chinese adolescents, it is important to realize that many of them may not come to you for help when they need it. These adolescents have been taught to take responsibility for themselves and to avoid sharing problems with outsiders. Therefore, it is important that the nurse make every opportunity to meet and to maintain contact with adolescents. Suggestions for an outreach program may include (1) classes on personal hygiene and grooming, (2) classes on child care for potential babysitters, (3) classes in sex education and interpersonal relationships, (4) teen ''rap groups'' during school lunch hours, (5) a ''crash pad'' in the school nurse's offices where students can meditate on problems, and (6) setting up a program for Chinese adolescents to visit elderly Chinese shut-ins. The elderly are ideal for helping Chinese adolescents reidentify with the Chinese culture. The older generation can share many folk stories explaining Chinese values and beliefs.

As in working with any adolescent, the nurse must be sure to maintain full confidentiality regarding anything the Chinese adolescent may share. If the adolescent does not want the nurse involved with the parents, the nurse must abide by this wish. The nurse may find that sending a short note or making a telephone call during summer vacation will help maintain an established rapport with the adolescent. It increases the adolescent's self-esteem to know that someone from school with power remembers and thinks about her. The nurse really cares!

Summary

In this section, the author has shared some Chinese values and beliefs based on personal experience and observation. It is hoped that this information will stimulate more questions and concerns about the Chinese adolescent. An understanding and appreciation of the Chinese culture will contribute to the acceptance of health care by the Chinese family. The nurse must acknowledge the family's or adolescent's practices, then activate creative individualized nursing interventions which will not conflict with the personal values and beliefs of the clients. Only then will the nurse be giving the comprehensive, individualized, client-centered quality care which the Chinese adolescent deserves.

REFERENCES

1. Rubins, J. L. "The Relationship Between the Individual, the Culture and Psychopathology." *Am. J. Psychoanal.* 35:231–249, 1975.
2. Leff, J. P. "Culture and the Differentiation of Emotional States." *Brit. J. Psychiat.* 123:299–306, 1973.
3. Rollins, N. "Soviet and American Youth in a Changing World." *Austral. & New Zeal. J. Psychiat.* 8:149–153, 1974.
4. White, C. B., et al. "Moral Development in Bahamian School Children: A 3-Year Examination of Kohlberg's Stages of Moral Development." *Developmental Psychol.* 14(1):58-65, 1978.
5. Opler, M. K. "Adolescence in Cross-Cultural Perspective." In Howells, J. G., ed. *Modern Perspectives in Adolescent Psychiatry.* New York: Brunner/Mazel, 1971, pp. 152–179.
6. Mead, M. *Coming of Age in Samoa.* New York: William Morrow & Co., Inc., 1973.
7. Epstein, R., and Komorita, S. S. "Self-Esteem, Success-Failure, and Locus of Control in Negro Children." *Developmental Psychol.* 4(1):2–8, 1971.
8. Oberle, W. H. "Place of Residence and the Role Preferences of Black Boys and Girls." *Adolescence* 13(49):13–19, 1978.
9. Sommers, V. S. "The Impact of Dual-Cultural Membership on Identity." *Psychiatry* 27:332–344, 1964.
10. Gibbs, J. T. "Patterns of Adaptation Among Black Students at a Predominantly White University: Selected Case Studies." *Am. J. Orthopsychiat.* 44(5):738–740, 1974.
11. Brim, O. G., Jr. "Macro-Structural Influences on Child Development and the Need for Childhood Social Indicators." *Am. J. Orthopsychiat.* 45(4):516–524, 1975.
12. Zigler, E. "Who Will Speak for Children and Families? A Case for Strengthening OCD." *Am. J. Orthopsychiat.* 47(4):564–567, 1977.
13. Aries, P. "A Social History of Adolescence." In Esman, A. H., *The Psychology of Adolescence Essential Readings.* New York: International Universities Press, Inc., 1975, pp. 3–5.
14. Mathis, J. L. "Adolescent Sexuality and Societal Change." *Am. J. Psychotherapy* 30(3):433–440, 1976.
15. Levine, S. V., and Salter, N. E. "Youth and Contemporary Religious Movements: Psychosocial Findings." *Can. Psychiat. Assoc. J.* 21:411–420, 1976.
16. Mead, M. *Culture and Commitment A Study of the Generation Gap.* New York: Natural History Press/Doubleday & Co., Inc., 1970.
17. Nesselroade, J. R., and Baltes, P. B. "Adolescent Personality Development and Historical Change: 1970–1972." *Monographs of the Society for Research in Child Development* 39(1), 1974.
18. Hill, S. T., and Waggoner, D. "Children from Non-English Language Backgrounds." *Children Today* 6(3):24–25, 1977.
19. Pearlin, L. I., and Schooler, C. "The Structure of Coping." *J. Health & Soc. Behav.* 19(1):2–21, 1978.
20. Miller, W. B. "Lower Class Culture as a Generating Milieu of Gang Delinquency." In Winder, A. E., and Angus, D. L., eds. *Adolescence Contemporary Studies.* New York: Van Nostrand Reinhold Co., 1968, 189–204.
21. Lewis, O., quoted in Herzog, E. *About the Poor Some Facts and Some Fictions.* Washington, D.C.: U.S. Dept. Health, Education, and Welfare Social and Rehabilitation Service, Children's Bureau Pub. No. 451, 1967, p. 47.

22. Allen, W. R. "The Search for Applicable Theories of Black Family Life." *J. Marriage & Fam.* 40(1):117–129, 1978.
23. Kriesberg, L. *Mothers in Poverty*. Chicago: Aldine Publishing Co., 1972.
24. Staples, R. *The Black Woman in America*. Chicago: Nelson Hall Publishers, 1973.
25. Hammond, J., and Enoch, J. R. "Conjugal Power Relations Among Black Working Class Families." *J. Black Studies* 7(1): Sept., 1976.
26. Scanzoni, G. *The Black Family in Modern Society*. Boston: Allyn & Bacon, 1971.
27. McAdoo, H. "Family Therapy in the Black Community." *Am. J. Orthopsychiat.* 47(1):75–79, 1977.
28. Carrington, B. W. "The Afro-American." In Clark, A. L., ed. *Culture Childbearing Health Professionals*. Philadelphia: F. A. Davis Co., 1978, p. 37.
29. Brown, N. W. "Personality Characteristics of Black Adolescents." *Adolescence* 12(45):81–87, 1977.
30. Williams, R. L., and Byars, H. "Negro Self-Esteem in a Transitional Society." In Evans, E. D., ed. *Adolescents: Readings in Behavior and Development*. Hindsale, Ill.: Dryden Press, Inc., 1970, pp. 406–414.
31. Perrella, V. C. "Working Teenagers." *Children Today* 1(3):15, 1972.
32. Poussaint, A. F. "Black Child, White Child." *Parents' Mag.,* Oct. 1976, p. 40.
33. Teplin, L. A. "A Comparison of Racial/Ethnic Preferences Among Anglo, Black and Latino Children." *Am. J. Orthopsychiat.* 46(4):702–709, 1976.
34. Gispert, M., and Falk, R. "Sexual Experimentation and Pregnancy in Young Black Adolescents." *Am. J. Obstet. & Gyn.* 126(4):459–466, 1976.
35. Furstenberg, F. F., Jr. "Premarital Pregnancy Among Black Teenagers." *Trans-Action* 7(7):52–55, 1970.
36. Reiner, B. S. "The Real World of the Teenage Negro Mother." *Child Welfare* 47(7):391–396, 1968.
37. Furstenberg, F. F., Jr. "The Social Consequences of Teenage Parenthood." *Fam. Plann. Perspectives* 8(4):151, 1976.
38. Dorsey, P., and Jackson, H. "Cultural Health Traditions: The Latino/Chicano Perspective." In Branch, M., and Paxton, P., eds. *Providing Safe Nursing Care for Ethnic People of Color*. New York: Appleton-Century-Crofts, 1976, pp. 41–80.
39. Healey, G. W., and DeBlassie, R. R. "A Comparison of Negro, Anglo, and Spanish-American Adolescents' Self Concepts." *Adolescence* 9(33):15–24, 1974.
40. Murillo, N. "The Mexican-American Family." In Wagner, N. N., and Haug, M. J., eds. *Chicanos: Social and Psychological Perspectives*. St. Louis: C. V. Mosby Co., 1971, pp. 97–108.
41. Goodman, M. E., and Beman, A. "Child's Eye-View of Life in an Urban Ghetto." In Wagner, N. N., and Haug, M. J., eds. *Chicanos: Social and Psychological Perspectives*. St. Louis: C. V. Mosby Co., 1971, pp. 109–122.
42. Rubel, A. J. *Across the Tracks*. Austin: University of Texas Press, 1966.
43. Cooper, E. J., and Cento, M. H. "Group and the Hispanic Prenatal Patient." *Am. J. Orthopsychiat.* 47(4):689–700, 1977.
44. Fong, S. L. M. "Role of Chinese Americans." *J. Sci. Issues* 29(2):115–127, 1973.
45. Sung, B. L. *The Story of the Chinese in America*. New York: Collier, 1971.

4

Nutrition and the Adolescent

Yolanda Gutierrez, M.S.

The nutritional care of adolescents presents a special challenge. The adolescent's marked social, psychological, and physical changes, along with his social and psychological adjustments, all have repercussions on his nutritional status, nutritional needs, and food habits. In addition, the rapidly expanding scientific knowledge in nutrition requires special attention in order to keep abreast of advances in the areas of research, food industry, and food technology.

The health status of today's adolescent will have both nutritional repercussions on and genetic consequences for future generations. The expertise of all health care professionals is needed to meet the nutritional and counseling requirements of the active adolescent whose growing body has particular needs at particular times in this phase of development.

This chapter will present an overview of the adolescent's unique nutritional needs and special nutritional problems. Emphasis is placed on nutritional counseling with special approaches to improve the adolescent's diet.

Nutrient Requirements of Adolescents

Becoming informed about nutritional requirements is a first step in helping the adolescent meet his nutritional needs so that his continued healthy growth and development will be ensured. The Food and Nutrition Board of the National Academy of Sciences, National Research Council, has collected the best available data on the quantities of various nutrients required by normal persons, considering variations of body size, sex, age, and physiologic state. The latest recommendations derived from such data were published in 1974, and are commonly known as the Recommended Dietary Allowances, hereafter referred to as RDA. Because few studies of adolescent nutritional requirements have been done, the relationship between adolescent growth, development, and nutrition have been extrapolated from findings on the needs of children and adults.

74

   The RDA present safety margins for the amounts of 17 essential nutrients needed in the daily diet. There are 45 known essential nutrients which must be supplied in the diet because the body cannot synthesize them. The known essential nutrients consist of water, nine essential amino acids for adults (ten for children), linoleic acid (a polyunsaturated fatty acid), 14 vitamins, 21 essential minerals, and energy. However, the RDA should not be confused with an individual's *nutrient requirements*. Differences in the nutrient requirements of individuals, because of differences in individual genetic makeup, are ordinarily unknown. Therefore, there is no way of predicting whose needs are high and whose needs are low. The RDA (except for energy) are estimates that exceed the requirements of most individuals and thus ensure that the needs of most individuals are met. It is also important to note that the RDA do not take into account special needs arising from infections, metabolic disorders, chronic diseases, or other abnormalities that require special dietary treatment. These are problems that require individual attention.

   In adolescence, individual variations in the age at which physical maturation is completed are tremendous. Consequently, variations also occur in terms of nutrient requirements; requirements of a 12-year-old male who is beginning a growth spurt are different from those of a 12-year-old male who is not experiencing this rapid change. Because the adolescent growth spurt is markedly different for males than it is for females, separate recommended allowances of nutrients are provided for males and females beginning at 11 years of age. The highest nutrient and energy demands occur at the time of peak velocity of growth and decrease as the velocity of growth gradually decreases.

CALORIES

   There are many variables which determine the total energy requirements of adolescents. These requirements will vary with sex, age, body size and build, activity, and physiological state. Since weight and height reflect growth rate and body build more than age, they may be used as reliable predictors of total energy requirements. Females generally reach and pass through puberty at an earlier age than males, which means that they have a need for increased calories earlier and for a briefer period of time than males.

   The RDA tables recommend fewer calories for children over age ten (based on chronological age) than for infants and younger children. The recommended allowance for adolescent males is 45 kcal/kg; the maximum of 3,000 calories is suggested for 15- to 18-year-old males. For females, the recommendation is 38 kcal/kg; the maximum allowance is 2,400 calories for 11- to 14-year-old females.[1] The recommended energy allowance for obese adolescents is based on height for age, since the requirements for nutrients, including energy, for this group are related more to lean body mass than to total body weight. Adequate calories must be supplied if growth is to proceed normally. If calorie intake is below the requirement, protein foods will be used for energy needs rather than for their primary function of tissue building and maintenance.

PROTEIN

The protein requirement is considerably increased by the demands of growth; the highest need correlates with the growth spurt and later declines to the maintenance-level needs of adults. Food proteins provide amino acids for the synthesis of body proteins and nitrogen for the synthesis of many other tissue constituents. It is during the adolescent growth spurt that nitrogen retention and protein deposition are the greatest. Williams and associates[2] suggest 50 to 60 grams of protein per day to sustain daily needs and maintain nitrogen reserves, provided there is an adequate supply of energy for maximum protein utilization.

Reports indicate that protein in the adolescent diet ranges from 12% to 16% of total calories per day.[3] In the United States and Canada, reported intakes of protein usually exceed the RDA. However, adolescents on reducing diets that eliminate all animal products are at risk for suboptimal intakes of protein. In evaluating the adequacy of a diet in terms of protein, one must consider not only the quantity of protein, but also the quality. The quality of the protein is determined by the content of essential amino acids; therefore, the proteins of eggs, dairy products, and meats have high biological value because they contain all of the essential amino acids.

Proteins from plant sources are considered incomplete because one or more of the essential amino acids are in short supply. In grains such as rice, corn, wheat, oats, and barley, the limited amino acids are isoleucine and lysine. Legumes such as soybeans, beans, garbanzos (chick peas), and lentils are deficient in tryptophan, isoleucine, and lysine. The biological value of plant proteins can be improved by combining them so that their amino acids complement each other—for example by having corn and beans at the same meal.

MINERALS

Adolescents must include all of the elements and inorganic compounds essential for normal metabolism and growth in their diets; of particular significance during adolescence are the needs for calcium and iron. Individual growth variability influences calcium requirements; higher intakes are recommended during periods of rapid growth, reaching a maximum of 1,200 mg/day for males and females 11 to 18 years of age.

Iron needs are increased with the expansion of blood volume, muscle mass, respiratory enzymes, and storage. Adolescents are predisposed to iron deficiency because of increased losses during menstruation in females and higher muscle mass in males. Diets in North America have been estimated to provide 6 mg iron/1,000 kcal. The RDA for iron in adolescence are 18 mg/day, assuming a 10% absorption rate. Organ meats, dried legumes, meats, and beans are the most usable sources. Whole grains, green vegetables, eggs, and peanut butter contribute some iron to the diet. Special attention in food selection with regard to iron sources is necessary if iron needs are to be met.

IODINE

Because of increased thyroid activity associated with growth, iodine intake should be ensured, especially in areas where the iodine content of food is low. Iodine in food varies from region to region depending upon the amount of iodine in the soil or the availability of seafoods. Iodized salt should be highly recommended in areas of scarcity.

VITAMINS

Vitamin needs are more likely to be met when a variety of foods are included in the diet. Milk, green and yellow vegetables, and fruits all provide Vitamin A. Intake of fortified milk will ensure an adequate intake of Vitamin D. Good quality protein foods provide an important source of B vitamins; legumes contribute significant amounts of B-1, B-6, niacin, and folacin. Many vitamins are destroyed or lost by improper cooking methods, such as boiling too long or in large amounts of water. Overcooking of meats also contributes to vitamin loss. Vitamin C and folacin are particularly labile in cooking and storage; Vitamin C and folacin intake may be improved if certain quantities of fresh fruits and vegetables are eaten daily. (For RDA of different vitamins and other nutrients see Table 4–1.)

TABLE 4–1. *Recommended Dietary Allowances for Adolescents*

		MALE			FEMALE			Pregnant	Lactating
		11–14 Years	15–18 Years	19–22 Years	11–14 Years	15–18 Years	19–22 Years		
Weight	kg	44	61	67	44	54	58		
Height	cm	158	172	172	155	162	162		
Energy	kcal	2800	3000	3000	2400	2100	2100	+300	+500
Protein	g	44	54	54	44	48	46	+30	+20
Vitamin A activity	IU	5000	5000	5000	4000	4000	4000	5000	6000
Vitamin D	IU	400	400	400	400	400	400	400	400
Vitamin E activity	IU	12	15	15	12	12	12	15	15
Ascorbic Acid	mg	45	45	45	45	45	45	60	80
Folacin	μg	400	400	400	400	400	400	800	600
Niacin	mg	18	20	20	16	14	14	+2	+4
Riboflavin	mg	1.5	1.8	1.8	1.3	1.4	1.4	+.3	+.5
Thiamine	mg	1.4	1.5	1.5	1.2	1.1	1.1	+.3	+.3
Vitamin B_6	mg	1.6	2.0	2.0	1.6	2.0	2.0	2.5	2.5
Vitamin B_{12}	μg	3.0	3.0	3.0	3.0	3.0	3.0	4.0	4.0
Calcium	mg	1200	1200	800	1200	1200	800	1200	1200
Phosphorus	mg	1200	1200	800	1200	1200	800	1200	1200
Iodine	μg	130	150	140	115	115	100	125	150
Iron	mg	18	18	10	18	18	18	18+	18
Magnesium	mg	350	400	350	300	300	300	450	450
Zinc	mg	15	15	15	15	15	15	20	25

Source: Adapted by Carolyn T. Torre, R.N., M.A., from *Food and Nutrition Board Recommended Dietary Allowances*, 8th rev. ed. National Academy of Sciences, Nutritional Research Council, Washington, D.C., 1974. Copyright March/April 1977, American Journal of Nursing Co. Reproduced with permission from *MCN, The American Journal of Maternal Child Nursing*, Vol. 2, No. 2.

FOOD GUIDES

Knowing the amounts of the various nutrients needed during adolescence is of little help if one is unable to interpret the RDA in terms of foods, size and number of servings, and adolescent daily food practices. Food guides have been designed to aid in simplifying and interpreting the principle of an adequate diet. Most foods contain more than one nutrient, but no single food contains all the nutrients in the amounts needed for individuals; therefore, foods have been arranged in groups, each of which makes a major contribution to the diet. A well-known food guideline is the Basic Four Food Groups. Since the Basic Four Food Groups concept was developed in 1953, many changes have been recommended to keep up with research discoveries and newer prepared foods and food preparation methods.

New guidelines for the Basic Four Food Groups have been proposed. Pennington's food guide,[5] developed in 1976, is based on seven "index nutrients." According to this Dietary Nutrient Guide, if the diet selected provides the recommended intake of the suggested index nutrients, it should be adequate in approximately all of the 45 essentials. The index nutrients are: Vitamin B-6, magnesium, Vitamin A, pantothenic acid, iron, folacin, and calcium. Excellent tables of food composition in relation to these nutrients are included in Pennington's guide.

King and associates,[6] in their analysis and modification of the Basic Four Food Guide, consider that a simple guide based on food groups is the most practical. The revised food group guide proposed is essentially an addition of subgroups to the original Basic Four Food Groups. These subgroups improve the intake of food sources of the nutrients that had been added and/or changed to meet the requirements of the 1974 RDA.

Daily Food Guide for Adolescents: The Daily Food Guide for Adolescents was adapted by the author from the food groups recommended for women during pregnancy and lactation by the California Department of Health.[7,8] (See Table 4–2.) The guide is intended to provide a quick and easy way of checking the adolescent's intake of protein, vitamins, and minerals. Since the calorie content of any diet varies considerably according to the foods selected and their method of preparation, the calorie content of a representative diet should be calculated, especially if weight is a problem. An easily obtained calorie counter or food composition book is required for this.

The suggested number of servings from each food group on the Food Guide provide an *average* of 2,400 calories. This is adequate for the 11- to 14-year-old female. The 15- to 16-year-old female requires 2,100 calories, a decrease of approximately 300 calories. Adolescent females following the food guide can consume few, if any, additional foods without gaining weight. Adolescent females requiring less than 2,400 calories should be advised to choose lower calorie foods within the Food Guide, to use low-calorie methods of food preparation, and/or to increase their physical activity.

Males 11 to 14 years old require 2,800 calories, an increase of approximately 400 calories over the average calories provided by the Food Guide. For the 15- to 19-year-old males, 600 additional calories are needed.

The Food Guide supplies the RDA for all of the nutrients except iron. Using the

TABLE 4–2. *Daily Food Guide for Adolescents**

FOOD GROUPS	NO. OF SERVINGS	NUTRIENTS
I. PROTEIN FOODS	4	
A. **Animal Protein.** A serving is 2–3 oz (60–90 gm) cooked and boneless, unless otherwise noted. Beef, lamb, pork (including ears, feet, ribs), veal, poultry (including duck), rabbit. *All organ meats:* liver, kidney, heart, tongue, liverwurst, chitterlings, tripe. *Seafoods:* fish fillet, steak, or sticks; crab; lobster; canned tuna (1/2 can); clams (4 large or 9 small); shrimps, scallops (5–6) large); oysters (10–15 medium). Luncheon meat (2 slices). Frankfurters (2). Sausage links (4). Bacon (6 slices). Eggs (2).	2	Protein (complete), Fe, riboflavin, Vitamin B-6, niacin, Vitamin B-12, Zn, I, P.
B. **Vegetable Protein.** A serving is 1 cup cooked, unless noted. 1) *Beans:* soybeans, black, kidney, pinto, garbanzo (chick peas), lima, navy, blackeyed peas, lentils, tofu (soybean curd), etc. 2) *Nuts:* walnuts, pecans, peanuts, Brazil nuts, almonds, cashews, filberts (1/2 cup). Nut butter (1/4 cup). 3) *Seeds:* sesame, sunflower, pumpkin, squash, etc. (1/2 cup).	2	Protein (incomplete), Fe, thiamin, folacin, Vitamin B-6, riboflavin, niacin, Vitamin E, P, Mg, Zn, and fiber (roughage).
II. MILK AND MILK PRODUCTS. A serving is 8 oz. (1 cup, or 240 cc), unless noted. *Cow's milk:* whole, nonfat, low fat, nonfat dry, chocolate milk, buttermilk, cocoa made with milk. *Cheese:* hard and semisoft—except blue, Camembert, and cream—(1 1/2 oz); cheese spread (2 oz); cottage cheese (1 1/3 cups). Goat's milk (low B-12 and folic acid). Soybean milk (low B-12). Ice cream (1 1/2 cups). Ice milk, milkshakes (when prepared with 12 oz milk or 1 1/2 c. ice cream). Puddings, custard (flan). Yogurt (1 cup). Tofu (soybean curd) is also a source of calcium.	4 or more	Calcium, Vitamin D, riboflavin, Vitamin A, protein, P, Vitamins E, B-6, and B-12, Mg, Zn.

* Adapted from "Food Groups" in *Nutrition During Pregnancy and Lactation,* California State Department of Health, revised, 1975, pp. 37–41.

TABLE 4–2. (*continued*)

FOOD GROUPS	NO. OF SERVINGS	NUTRIENTS
III. BREADS AND CEREALS. A serving is 1/2 cup unless noted. A. **Grain Products (Whole Grains)** Wheat, oats, rice, corn, barley, millet. Cereals, ready-to-eat: corn and wheat flakes, shredded wheat, puffed oats, Granola (3/4 cup). Cracked and whole wheat bread (1 slice). Wheat germ (1 Tbsp). B. **Enriched Breads, Cereals, and Pastas** Breads, rolls, bagels, cornbread, muffins, biscuits, dumplings, etc. (1 slice or 1 piece). Pancake (1 medium). Waffle (1 large). Cereals, hot: cream of wheat, cream of rice, farina, cornmeal, grits. Cereals, ready-to-eat (3/4 cup). Pasta: macaroni, spaghetti, noodles (cooked, 1/2 cup). Tortilla, corn (2). Tortilla, flour (1 large).	4	Protein (incomplete). Whole grain items have Vitamins E, B-6, and folacin; Mg, Zn, and fiber; refined cereals and breads lose these in milling. "Enriched" and whole grain products have thiamine, riboflavin, niacin, Fe, and protein.
IV. VITAMIN C RICH FRUITS AND VEGETABLES A. **Fruits** Orange (1), grapefruit (1/2). Orange or grapefruit juice, (4 oz), fruit juices (6 oz). Cantaloupe (1/2), guava (1/4), strawberries (3/4 cup), tangerines (2), papaya (1/2), mango (1). B. **Vegetables** Bok choy (3/4 cup), cabbage (raw 3/4 cup, cooked 1 1/3 cup), chili peppers, watercress (3/4 cup). Greens: collard, kale, mustard, turnip greens, Swiss chard (3/4 cup). Broccoli (1 stalk), cauliflower (raw or cooked, 1 cup), brussels sprouts (3-4), pepper (red or green, 1/2), tomatoes (2 medium). Fresh, frozen, or canned forms may be used; Vitamin C is lower in canned products.	1 of either A or B	Specifically for Vitamin C. In addition, these foods contribute varying amounts of B-Complex vitamins and minerals.
V. DARK GREEN VEGETABLES. A serving is 1 cup raw or 3/4 cup cooked. Asparagus, bok choy, broccoli, brussels sprouts, cabbage, dark green lettuces such as chicory, endive, escarole, romaine, and red leaf. Greens: beets, collard, kale, mustard, spinach, Swiss chard, turnip, scallions, and watercress.	1	Specifically for folacin. In addition, these foods supply Vitamins A, E, B-6, and riboflavin; Fe, Mg.

TABLE 4–2. (*continued*)

FOOD GROUPS	NO. OF SERVINGS	NUTRIENTS
VI. OTHER FRUITS AND VEGETABLES. A serving is 1/2 cup, unless otherwise noted. Fresh, frozen, or canned may be used. Artichokes, bamboo shoots, carrots, celery, corn, cucumbers, eggplant, mushrooms, onions, parsnips, peas, pea pods, potatoes, radishes, avocados. Squash, sweet potatoes, yams, etc. Apricot (fresh, 1 large), peach (1 medium), prunes (4), pumpkin (1/4 cup), apple (1 medium), banana (1 small), berries, cherries, dates (5), figs (2 large), grapes, pears (1 medium), watermelons, plums (2 medium), raisins.	1–2	Yellow fruits and vegetables supply significant amounts of Vitamin A. They also contribute varying amounts of B complex vitamins and Vitamin E, Mg, Zn, P.
VII. FATS AND OILS Margarine, oils (preferably vegetable oils), mayonnaise, salad dressings.	3 Tbsp	Calories, Vitamin E, lineoleic acid (an essential polyunsaturated fatty acid).

typical adolescent's food selection, the Food Guide provides an average of 12–15 mg of iron. Consequently, in order to meet the recommended iron needs, foods rich in iron should be selected *frequently*. Foods particularly high in iron content include organ meats such as liver, kidney, heart, or liverwurst; lean meats such as beef, veal, or lamb; dark green vegetables; eggs; dried beans; dried apricots; raisins; enriched or whole grain cereals; raisin bran and bran flakes. These foods also furnish valuable amounts of the daily allowances of other nutrients.

The ideal diet for adolescents is one that provides a wide variety of foods. The ideal diet does not fall below the RDA for an extended period of time, and thus avoids the increased risks of developing a nutrient deficiency. The nutritional content of the ideal diet must not only fulfill the RDA but also respond to the adolescent's unique individual variations under specific conditions. The Daily Food Guide may be readily adapted to meet both ethnic food patterns and individual food styles.

Dietary Habits of Adolescents

Most of the nutritional problems of adolescents in the United States are associated both with food practices learned in infancy and childhood and with the physical and psychosocial characteristics of this age period. The formation of food habits begins at birth, and the family, particularly the mother, is the primary influence. The method or pattern which the mother follows in selecting, preparing, and consuming food varies according to many factors, such as family background and economic status, geographical location, cultural and religious influences, and educational level. The various factors that influence individual food habits are important determinants of an individual's acceptance of food and attitudes toward eating.

FACTORS INFLUENCING DIETARY HABITS

A like or dislike for certain foods is learned from the parents' likes or dislikes, and is affected by the mother's willingness to spend time and effort in preparing certain foods. In this sense, parents transfer their own food prejudices to the child. Likewise, children learn to control concerned parents by the foods they accept or reject. Parents, anxious about their children's nutrient intake, sometimes urge, nag, or bribe children to eat, and children often assume control of the feeding situation. Parents respond to their children according to the reinforcement they receive from them, and may use food to control the child's behavior, either as a punishment or as a reward.

Food habits develop along with other aspects of growth; as the child grows older and enters school, he is allowed greater freedom of choice in deciding what he shall or shall not eat. His choices are then influenced by: the food's taste, look, and smell; the peer group's response to a particular food; the food's promotion through advertising; and the psychological or symbolic meaning the food may have for him. Even if the individual had good dietary habits prior to adolescence, it is probable that he will adopt faddish or bizarre diets during the teen years because of the many internal and external pressures to which he is exposed. Teenagers are subject to peer group pressures to conform to norms, to manipulate their physical appearance, and to experiment with different living patterns and diets. Because of the accelerated pace of urban life in North America and the busy schedules which result, much time is spent outside the home, allowing for even more freedom in food choices and less time for regular, balanced meals. In spite of all these factors, surveys indicate that, compared with people in much of the world, most North Americans are relatively well-nourished from the viewpoint of getting enough of the essential nutrients. However, nutritional deficiencies do occur.

The Ten State Nutrition Survey 1968–1970[9] reported that adolescents from 10 to 16 years of age had an unsatisfactory nutritional status compared with all other age groups. Iron-deficiency anemia among teenage females was the only deficiency found consistently. Other nutrients commonly lacking in adolescent diets are Vitamin A, calcium, and, to a lesser extent, Vitamin C, riboflavin, and thiamine.[9,10,11] This survey assessed the nutritional status of about 40,000 individuals in ten states of the United States. The survey was conducted in low income areas and reflects the nutritional problems related to specific ethnic groups and income levels. Although all of the subjects studied had low incomes, those who lived in Texas, Louisiana, South Carolina, Kentucky, and West Virginia had a median Poverty Income Ratio below the overall median for the ten states. Those who resided in Massachusetts, New York, Michigan, Washington, and California had a median Poverty Income Ratio above the overall median.

Adolescent males are considered to be consistently better nourished than females. Although their caloric needs are higher for a longer period of time, they are more likely to meet their needs for nutrients with additional food intake. Females at this age frequently have finicky appetites and, if they develop phobias about remaining slender, it is difficult to get them to take all of the protective foods they need.

One of the dietary practices that apparently contributes to nutritional inadequacies is skipping meals. Documented studies and clinical investigations reported that breakfast and lunch are the meals most likely to be missed.[12,13] School, work, and social activities take teenagers away from home during some of the family meals. The effect of omitting meals is reflected in the efficiency with which some mental or physical work is performed. An additional problem that occurs with the pattern of skipping meals is the tendency toward increased snacking. Snacks then become an important factor in the teenager's nutrient intake and food habits and as such should be considered a normal practice among teenagers. The pattern of snacking seems to be preferred and physiologically desirable. However, nibbling is a good practice *only* if all the food forms part of a well-balanced diet.

Experimental research on both animals and humans indicates that more than three meals daily are desirable. When an individual eats more than five or six meals a day which are appropriately balanced in protein, fat, and carbohydrates, the metabolic load at a given time is less, and the nutrients can be more effectively utilized. For example, protein is more efficiently used if it is distributed throughout the day's meals rather than concentrated in one meal. It has been demonstrated that when large amounts of carbohydrates are consumed at a given meal, alternate metabolic pathways which favor the deposition of fat are required.

Although adolescents are increasing in their self-sufficiency, they still need help in planning their diets so that their nutritional needs will be met. They are presented with confusing, conflicting information about nutrition via beauty magazines, television, newspapers, teachers, parents, food faddists, and health professionals. They express their confusion with statements such as "So many things are said about vitamins and health foods that I don't know what to believe or what to do," and "Are snacks really bad?" With exposure to so many different sources of advice adolescents have difficulty distinguishing between misinformation and fact and often lack the educational background and judgment to discriminate. In addition, adolescents are frequently dissatisfied with or anxious about their changing body configurations. This leads to dietary manipulations in an effort to conceal or modify their body changes.

Some of the most common nontraditional eating practices adopted by many young people in North America include vegetarianism, diets based on organically grown health foods, and the Zen macrobiotic regimen. These dietary practices may not be nutritionally sound, especially if the adolescent has little basic knowledge of nutrition. A knowledge of these food preferences and attention to them will help health practitioners to understand and to offer valuable nutritional counseling to the adolescent and family in need of assistance.

VEGETARIAN DIETS

A vegetarian diet excludes meat, poultry, and fish. At present, vegetarianism includes a wide array of dietary practices. The most common type of vegetarian diet is the "lacto-ovo-vegetarian" diet, which includes both dairy products and eggs in addition to the traditional, or strict, vegetarian diet of fruits, vegetables, and grains. The "fruitarian" diet is mainly composed of raw or dried fruits and nuts.[14]

The lacto-ovo-vegetarian diet provides adequate nutrition for the adolescent since milk, which is one of the critical food items in the diet, supplies calcium and other essential nutrients, and complements the vegetable proteins. The more restrictive the food choices in a diet the more difficult it is for the adolescent to meet his nutritional needs.

On a very strict vegetarian diet, especially those which eliminate eggs and dairy products, supplies of Vitamin D, calcium, riboflavin, zinc, iron, and niacin, in addition to protein, are likely to be marginal. B-12 is totally absent; therefore supplementation is advised. In addition, vegetarian diets tend to be low in calories, which may present a concern in view of the high calorie demands of adolescents.

Most of the young vegetarians believe that exclusion of meat is healthier. They believe that animal foods contain toxins and too much uric acid or are infected with salmonella.[15]

For others, the main reason for adopting a vegetarian diet is ecology—the efficient use of land and protection of animals and natural resources. Very few teenagers cite religious beliefs as their rationale; instead, their concern is based on economic considerations. Adolescents living "on their own" express their economic concerns by statements such as "I can afford meat only once a week or so," "I heard that if a vegetarian drinks milk it is easy to get the complete proteins. Is powdered milk the same nutritionally as whole milk?"

ORGANICALLY GROWN FOODS AND HEALTH FOOD ADVOCATES

The "organically grown" foods and "natural" foods advocated by many adolescents today indicate their concern for and interest in food ecology, pollution, and the natural way of life. The rise in the number of health stores and health food restaurants throughout the country indicates the popularity of these foods.

By definition, "organically grown" foods are "foods grown without the use of any agricultural chemicals and processed without the use of food chemicals or additives."[16] Because of inadequate surveillance, the claims made by natural food producers may be misleading and inaccurate.[17] Unless the young teenager and her/his family grow their own food, as in a vegetable garden, there will be no guarantee of the standards used in raising different crops. Experiments failed to show any superiority in either nutritional value or taste of "organically grown" crops over crops grown under standard agricultural conditions.[18] In addition to claims about the nutritional superiority of "natural foods," claims are made that the traditional food supply is poisoned with pesticides and food additives, and this creates distrust about its adequacy and safety.[19] The use of additives and pesticides is regulated by law. The objectives of the Food and Drug Administration's law have been summarized as "safe, effective drugs and cosmetics; pure, wholesome foods; honest labeling and packaging."[19]

The higher cost of the "natural" and "organically grown" foods is another factor to consider. In general, these foods cost about twice as much as regular foods. Wholesome foods, such as whole wheat bread, wheat germ, yogurt, honey, and the like, can be purchased at local supermarkets and need not be sought on special shelves or at special prices in health food stores. However, an optimally healthy diet includes primarily foods that are whole and unprocessed. Processing of food removes more nutrients than are ever added to the final product. For example, whole wheat has more nutrients than enriched bread. In addition, potentially dangerous food colorings and chemicals are absent from whole, unprocessed foods.

ZEN MACROBIOTIC DIETS

The most rigorous of the three styles of dietary practices adopted by some teenagers is the Zen Macrobiotic Diet, which is especially favored by the young mystics around Berkeley, California, and Cambridge, Massachusetts. To these young people the term ''macrobiotic'' means ''the way of life.'' The major claims of this diet are that it cures all varieties of disease and that it is believed to be a technique of rejuvenation. According to the macrobiotic system, there are ten diet plans. As the diet advances, it becomes more restrictive in food choices. This diet is grossly inadequate in many of the essential nutrients. For example, one of the diet plans allows only whole grains, usually brown rice, and the ultimate goal is a diet that is 100% cereal.[14]

The dangers of the macrobiotic diet are generally greater for individuals who have adhered to the diet for long periods of time. The diet may lead to the development of anemia, scurvy, or tissue damage because of a deficiency of iron, Vitamin C, and protein. The American Medical Association Council on Foods and Nutrition stated that the macrobiotic diet is one of the most dangerous dietary regimens, posing not only serious hazards to the health of the individual, but even to life itself.[20]

Erhard[21] worked with counterculture groups in the San Francisco Bay Area. She stated that in order to work with an individual who adheres to the dietary practice of the Zen Macrobiotics, it is necessary to understand both the group's and the individual's cultism and religious and philosophical beliefs, and the individual's work within the value system of the group.

Adolescent Obesity

The obese adolescent presents special and difficult problems to health professionals. Changes in body composition occur not only in height and weight during growth, but also in the components of body fat (adipose tissue), lean body mass, hydration, and skeletal maturation. Sex differences in body composition begin in infancy, but they are most dramatic in adolescence. Commonly, just before puberty, both males and females have an increased amount of subcutaneous fat. Fat content is higher in the female after approximately 12 years of age. By late adolescence, it is one and a half to two times the male value, resulting in approximately 22.8% body fat in the female and about 7.9% body fat in the male.[22] Consequently, the female has a lower percentage of body water and a lower percentage of lean body mass than the male. In addition, adolescents present other variables which are not present in younger children or adults, such as rate of sexual maturation, rate of growth (in height), and increased muscular development.

Dramatic physical changes coupled with simultaneous psychosocial, environmental, and emotional changes may lead to adolescents' anxiety and dissatisfaction with body image, whether or not they are in reality obese. Studies[23,24] indicate that teenage males wish to have larger biceps, shoulders, chest, and forearms. Females desire smaller hips, thighs, and waists. One study[25] demonstrated typical dissatisfaction with body images; 70% of adolescent females wanted to lose weight, but no more than approximately 15% were actually obese. On the other hand, 59% of the males wanted to gain weight, but only 25% were lower than average weight.

Studies are in agreement that the incidence of obesity is higher in females than in males at all ages.[25] Accurate figures on the number of obese adolescents are not available, although the incidence of obesity is estimated to be fairly high, reportedly affecting from 10 to 35% of the adolescent population.[26] This represents approximately 10 million or more adolescents in the United States.

Obesity usually occurs before adolescence; overweight infants tend to become overweight children and adolescents.[27,28] Research in the mid-seventies showed that obesity during the first six months of life leads to the formation of a permanent increase in the number of fat cells in the body. To lose weight, these patients can only reduce the size of the fat cells, not the number.[29] This may have implications for the individual's ease or difficulty in losing weight later in life.

It has been estimated that for obese 12-year-olds, the odds against having normal weight as adults are 4 to 1, and if weight loss is not accomplished by the end of adolescence, the odds rise to 28 to 1.[26] These important facts are essential in helping the obese adolescent set realistic goals. The nonobese teenagers who are dissatisfied with their body builds also need help in learning to accept their body size.

Since nutritional needs during adolescence are high for the obese as well as the nonobese, obese adolescents are even more vulnerable to malnutrition because of restricted calorie intake in attempts to lose weight. The complexity of the problem is further intensified by the multiplicity of etiological factors involved in the development of obesity that are not yet fully understood. For teenagers as well as for adults, the problem of obesity is a combination of social and psychologic difficulties; but, especially for the adolescent, the psychological implications can be overwhelming.

Obese teenagers are especially affected by social rejection by peers, parents, and other persons important to them. The pervasive attitudes in our culture—the constant emphasis on being slim and on small model sizes as being normal—reinforce feelings of rejection. These factors lead many a teenager to develop a fetish about remaining slender at any cost. This accounts for the popularity of every new fad diet that comes along. Fad diets that emphasize a single food item such as bananas, grapefruit, eggs, or cottage cheese invariably lead to failure if followed for any length of time. Such unbalanced diets can result in malnutrition and serious harm. Most important, fad diets fail to teach food habits that maintain weight loss permanently. In all probability, the obese adolescent who loses weight on a fad diet will regain the lost weight and be faced with another failure that will deflate self-esteem.

Obesity results from an imbalance between energy intake and energy expenditure; the amount consumed exceeds the amount needed for growth, maintenance, and activity. Most studies suggest that the primary cause of adolescent obesity is inactivity. Obese adolescents tend to exercise less than normal weight adolescents.[30] One study which used motion pictures to observe adolescent females playing in various competitive sports discovered that even when engaged in the same activity, the obese females both stood still more and moved less energetically than nonobese females.[31] No study has yet determined whether the obesity predisposes to less activity, or whether the reverse is true.

Adolescents face special nutritional problems whether or not their obesity is real or imaginary; they are in need of care, help, and support. Teenagers may diet because it is the desired thing to do in their peer group, or because of the non-acceptance of the "puppy" or chubby stage of the pubertal growth spurt, in the absence of true obesity.

The first step in treating adolescent obesity is to define it. One criterion that has been used in defining obesity is weight that is greater than 20% of normal. This classification is more appropriate for evaluating populations than it is for individual adolescents. Research in body composition has developed different methods of defining criteria for obesity. In general these studies on body composition are directed to identifying the nonfat components of the body in order to estimate the amount of body fat. This involves such measurements as body density, total body water, or total body potassium to estimate lean body mass. At present these techniques are not adaptable to routine clinical use.

For the adolescent age group, the height-weight chart is one of the best guides in arriving at a diagnosis of obesity. Available tables provide a convenient guide to desirable body weight for height. Because the concern in obesity, from the clinical point of view, is the excessive amount of adipose tissue (fat) rather than overweight per se, it is imperative that the diagnosis be based on excessive fat deposits and not on well-developed musculature. For example, a football player with a well-developed musculature could be overweight according to the usual height-weight tables.

According to the Ten State Survey,[9] skinfold measurements seem to be the simplest and the most practical single determination of adiposity. This clinical procedure requires the use of the *caliper,* an instrument that measures the thickness of skin and subcutaneous fat. Heald and Khan[22] describe the use of the caliper in detail. Skinfold thickness may be used to judge total body fat, simply by referral to appropriate tables.[32,33,34] The obesity standards developed by Seltzer and Mayer[33] suggest that for a 16-year-old female the criterion for obesity is 25 mm minimum triceps skinfold thickness. For a 16-year-old male the minimum triceps skinfold thickness indicating obesity is 15 mm.

Several approaches to treating obesity have been used; they include calorie restriction, anorexic drugs, physical exercise, therapeutic starvation, bypass surgery, behavior modification, and hormonal treatment. The majority of studies are not conclusive as to their effects in long-term weight reduction because of inadequate follow-up data, and studies have been limited in number and poorly defined.[35] In addition, all of the approaches used in obesity treatment are not safe for the adolescent because of the possible adverse effects on body function and growth.

In considering the food practices and activity patterns of obese adolescents, the best approach for treatment should be the one that provides realistic goals and expectations. Many factors must be taken into account in setting realistic goals: age; motivation to lose weight; emotional stability; hereditary body build; history of obesity; degree of overweight or obesity; values and attitudes toward food; the circumstances in which the adolescent lives that may make it impossible to change eating habits and/or activity patterns; physiologic state (weight reduction contraindicated during pregnancy); and consideration of consequences of weight reduction for the individual.

A realistic goal is a slow weight loss of no more than one to two pounds a week, plus the establishment of a healthy meal and activity lifetime regime. The most satisfactory way of achieving weight reduction is to cut down on the concentrated energy foods—fats, alcohol, sugars, and starches—while maintaining a well-balanced, adequate diet. Because of the reduction of calories the carbohydrates and fats must be chosen with considerable care in order that proteins, calcium, iron, and vitamins may be included in optimal amounts. It has been suggested that the fat intake might be reduced to 30% of the total calories, carbohydrates to 58% of total calories, and proteins to 12% of total calories. Part of the fat might be obtained from the vegetable oils that are rich in polyunsaturated fatty acids. To reduce intake of fat, limit intake of lard and hardened animal fats, and avoid fried foods. To reduce intake of carbohydrates, especially simple ones such as sucrose that contribute to both obesity and dental caries, reduce intake of table sugar, candy, carbonated beverages, cakes, pies, pastries, cookies, and syrups. A 500 calorie daily deficit will result in a loss of about one pound per week. The minimum calorie level for the obese adolescent compatible with nutritional needs should be around 1500–1800 calories per day. More drastic reduction of energy intake is not recommended because it will severely limit the sources of essential nutrients.

Further, a cycle of gaining-losing-gaining weight may be more detrimental to health in the long run than the maintenance of a slight to moderate degree of overweight. Physical activity is essential for the proper functioning of the body and its various organs and systems, and this proper functioning in turn is essential for normal growth. Regular activities which require use of the large muscles of the body are particularly important for optimum muscular growth and maintenance of ideal body weight. Thus, the essential components of a sound treatment of obesity are: diet, activity, adequate nutrition counseling, psychological support, and continuous follow-up.

Adequate nutrition counseling requires assessment of and intervention in three critical environments of the client: the physical environment, or the setting in which the client functions; the social environment, or other persons with whom the client comes in contact; and the private environment, which includes the thoughts, emotions, and basic physiological systems.[36] These environments influence and control behavior and should be considered in counseling obese adolescents about nutrition.

In summary, the treatment for obesity does not just imply eating less and exercising more. The adolescence must *want* to lose weight, he must know *what to do,* and he must know *how to do it.* Therefore, a great deal of motivation, education, and supportive counseling by the health professional, family, and significant others is required.

Iron-Deficiency Anemia

Adolescence is a period of increased risk for iron deficiency in both females and males. Dietary iron deficiency is the most common cause of anemia in the world today and is probably the most common nutritional deficiency in the United States.

In adolescence, the risk factors to be considered in iron nutrition are the amount and availability of iron ingested, rate of body growth, and iron losses. The deficiency may be mild or severe, chronic or acute. The speed with which the deficiency syndrome develops and the degree of manifestation depend on the relative severity of the dietary inadequacy, the body stores, and the capacity of the body to adapt successfully to lower intakes. Usually, a nutritional deficiency develops in progressive steps. Although the speed of progress varies greatly, the general pattern involves (1) exhaustion of nutrient reserves; (2) tissue depletion; (3) biochemical lesion (blood tests) or abnormal metabolic pathways; (4) clinical lesions (client complaints) observed by physical examination.

Symptoms of anemia include fatigue, anorexia, pallor, inability to concentrate, listlessness, and irritability. Iron deficiency is diagnosed when transferrin (serum concerned with binding and transportation of iron) saturations fall below 16%.[37] Anemia is diagnosed when hemoglobin concentrations fall below 11.0 gm/100 ml and hematocrits fall below 33%.[38] This hemoglobin value is applicable equally for males and females until the sexual changes of puberty occur. At this point, the testosterone production by males is associated with rising levels of hemoglobin concentration. Thus, after puberty for males, the lower limit of normal generally accepted is 12.0 gm per 100 ml of blood.[39]

Data from the Ten State Nutrition Survey[9] indicated widespread iron deficiency based on dietary intakes and biochemical data. The incidence is generally high in preschool children, adolescents, and women in the childbearing years, and is higher among black and Spanish-speaking populations than among white populations. Even though it is more common among low-income groups, it is not limited to this socioeconomic level.

Despite numerous attempts to establish the exact incidence of anemia in adolescence, the figure remains rather elusive. Surveys differ with respect to age of subjects, social and nutritional status, the specific parameters measured, and definitions of normal. Although the criterion in most surveys has been the hematocrit or hemoglobin concentrations, others have determined that the state of iron stores or the response to administration of iron are better criteria. Some surveys have included only adolescent females, others have involved both females and males. Nevertheless, in a careful review of surveys made before 1960,[40] 17% of adolescent girls were found to have hemoglobin values of less than 12 gm/100 ml and 5% were found to have values below 11 gm/100 ml. In these surveys, the incidence of anemia was usually found to be at least 50% lower in adolescent males than in adolescent females. Similar data were obtained by later research.[41] The RDA for iron during adolescence is 18 mg/day, for both males and females. Studies indicate clearly that adolescents rarely achieve the RDA for iron in their diets. About 80% of females and 75% of males consume less than the recommended allowance.[39]

There are several possible causes for this low iron intake. The major cause is the quality of foods the adolescent eats between meals; these tend to be "fast," convenient foods that are generally low in iron. It has been estimated that almost one fourth of the recommended calorie intake for adolescents is obtained from foods eaten between meals.[42,43,44] Fad diets such as vegetarianism and others based on rice, grapefruit, etc., limit one of the easily absorbed sources of iron, red meat. Iron absorption from vegetable and cereal foods can also be enhanced when the food is eaten with meat.

There are other factors that may contribute to the incidence of iron-deficiency anemia in some population groups. In addition to the poor iron content of snack foods eaten between meals, the practice of pica is commonly associated with the occurrence of anemia. Such nonfood substances as clay, starch, dust, ashes, or ice are the more commonly craved items. Even though the etiology of pica is still unknown, several factors seem to be responsible for its practice: custom and culture, hunger, low economic status, preference for the substance's odor and taste, super-stition, and habit. Certain cultures believe that these substances will relieve such symptoms associated with pregnancy as nausea, dizziness, vomiting, swollen legs, and headaches, and that they will ensure beautiful children.[45] Others believe that if pregnant women fail to eat a particular substance, the baby will be born with skin marks and discolorations.

Because the encouragement of the practice of pica is frequently passed on to teenagers from family and relatives, especially during such critical situations as pregnancy, it is important to know that this practice, especially clay ingestion, has a negative effect on nutritional status because: (1) the clay replaces other foods; and (2) clay may interfere directly with iron absorption by binding iron and making it unavailable for absorption.[46,47] It has been demonstrated that black, low-income women turn to eating starch when their favorite clay is not available. Anemia in starch eaters is caused by a lack of dietary iron and may be complicated by a decrease in the absorption of iron.[48]

Whereas several studies seem to support the theory that pica causes iron deficiency, many others seem to indicate the reverse—i.e., that iron deficiency may lead to the practice of pica. Lanzkowsky[49] found that 12 children in his study who chronically ingested such substances as sand, soil, and clay, had iron-deficiency anemia. When these children were treated with intramuscular injections of iron, the habit disappeared. Whether pica is the cause or the consequence of iron deficiency, it appears that a relationship between this practice and the nutritional status of iron exists.

If we consider the dietary practices of adolescents and the factors conducive to iron deficiency, it is clear that nutrition education is vital. It is imperative that the adolescent learn the importance of iron for the functioning of his body so that he can be motivated to eat iron-enriched foods. The most effective way to decrease the prevalence of iron deficiency among adolescents is to motivate the adolescent to increase dietary iron intake. Food sources of iron were discussed earlier in the chapter.

Adolescents with Unique Nutritional Needs

The adolescent has the greatest nutritional needs at a time when it is most difficult to meet them. Teenagers are not only forming their own values but are also practicing their newly acquired independence; these factors have long-lasting effects on their dietary practices and food choices. In addition, adolescents are often exposed to conditions of stress that alter their normal nutritional needs. These conditions require an adjustment in their RDA. It should be emphasized that the RDA are intended for healthy normal individuals and that more research is needed to establish specific dietary recommendations for adjustments during illness.

PREGNANCY

An adolescent is particularly at nutritional risk if she becomes pregnant and lactates before her own growth is completed. There has been extensive research on nutrition during pregnancy. It is evident that nutrition is one of the major environmental factors affecting the health and well-being of the pregnant woman and her unborn baby. The pregnant teenager is especially vulnerable to the emotional stresses of pregnancy and to the biological strains that accompany the altered physiological processes and the increased nutritional demands of the body.

The increase in nutritional needs during pregnancy corresponds to the growth patterns of the deposition of fetal and maternal tissue, the additional metabolism created for the synthesis of these new tissues, and the increased energy required to move the extra weight gained when performing physical activity.

The nutritional needs of a pregnant adolescent will depend on her stage of physical growth. Thus, if the teenager becomes pregnant before linear growth is completed, she must meet both her own nutrient needs for growth as well as the added needs of pregnancy. This puts her at high biological risk. Generally the adolescent girl does not complete linear growth until about four years post menarche.[52]

The RDA for pregnant teenagers represents the additional RDA for adult pregnant women added to the RDA of nonpregnant teenagers (see Table 4–1). At the present time these approximate estimations are the best available in determining nutritional needs.

As with nonpregnant adolescents, calorie requirements are difficult to predict and vary widely among pregnant adolescents according to daily activity levels and timing of growth rate. If the adolescent's physical activity remains constant during the second and third trimesters of pregnancy, that is, if she continues to attend school, work, participate in social events, and engage in moderate physical activity, her energy needs may be as much as 50 kcal/kg.[51] The RDA estimation for the pregnant adolescent is about 45 kcal/kg; an additional 300 kcal daily is suggested to meet the gross energy cost of pregnancy.

The best indication of an adequate amount of calories is a satisfactory, steady weight gain. An average of 24 to 30 pounds weight gain is recommended during pregnancy for both nonobese and obese adolescents. Usually a total of 2 to 4 pounds during the first trimester (1–2 kg) and approximately 0.9 pounds per week (0.4 kg) during the second and third trimesters are desirable.[8]

Protein is essential for both normal adolescent growth and for maintenance of maternal and fetal tissue. To allow for optimum protein retention, pregnant adolescents must consume at least 75 gm/day when caloric needs stand at 2,700. The 75 gm of protein for a teenager of 58 kg is equivalent to 1.3 gm of protein per kg of body weight.[52]

The accelerated energy and protein metabolism requires an increase in the amounts of several other nutrients which are needed in the metabolic pathways of tissue synthesis and energy production. Thiamin, riboflavin, niacin, and Vitamin B-6 are also involved in energy production, functioning as enzymes and coenzymes, and should be increased in the pregnant adolescent's diet.

Fetal skeletal development accounts for the increased requirements for calcium. If the teenager has completed her growth, 1.2 gm of calcium daily are recommended. If the adolescent is still growing, her calcium needs will be higher, on the order of 1.6 gm/day.[52] It is important to note that Vitamin D on the order of 400 I.U. is needed to aid in the absorption of calcium.

Because both dietary sources of iron and maternal iron stores of the pregnant woman are limited, it is recommended that all pregnant women receive a supplement of iron. They should receive 30 to 60 mg of elemental iron daily to meet the increased need for iron and to protect iron stores.[8]

Folacin is also likely to be inadequately supplied by dietary sources, and a daily supplement of 400–800 mg is recommended. Folacin requirements correlate with the increased maternal blood volume and the rapid cell division that occurs in growth.[8]

SPORTS AND ACTIVITY

Adolescents who become involved in competitive physical activity need to make adjustments in their nutritional intakes. Adolescent athletes have increased energy requirements due to greater energy expenditure. There is no rationale to support a theory that these additional calories should be supplied by specific kinds of foods or food groups; rather, the diet must be adequate in all essential nutrients.

The energy expenditure for various activities varies from one individual to another, depending on the athlete's body size and the energy demands of the particular sport as well as variations in the intensity of effort expended. The more strenuous types of activity likely to be performed by adolescents include swimming, tennis, running, bicycling, dancing, skiing, football, soccer, and other active team sports.

Some representative calorie expenditures associated with these activities, measured by the oxygen consumption method (indirect calorimetry) for a man weighing 70 kg, range from 450 to 600 kcal/hour.[53] It may be inferred that the minimum level of calories for the adolescent athlete should be around 3,450 kcal/day, and up to 5,000 calories or more per day during seasonal events. The calorie intake should be great enough to allow for what would constitute a continuation of adequate weight gain for his or her age.

Scientific evidence indicates that protein is not consumed by the working muscle. The requirement for protein does not increase with exercise, except to a slight degree when muscle mass increases. There is no scientific evidence to demonstrate that high protein diets and increased muscle mass are beneficial in improving work capacity.[54]

It is important to note that higher protein intake necessitates additional water intake for metabolism and excretion of the end metabolic products; otherwise, dehydration may result.

Carbohydrates appear to be the preferred energy source for the working muscle; muscle glycogen stores can be altered by changes in the diet. A dietary manipulation, known as carbohydrate loading, has been reported to increase glycogen stores in the muscles, which improves performance during endurance events that last longer than 30 to 60 minutes.[55,56,57] It appears that excessive amounts of high carbohydrates taken near the time of the sports event may present a possible risk of water retention in the muscle, to such an extent that a feeling of heaviness and stiffness is experienced. This glycogen water retention may reduce the athlete's capacity for maximal intake of oxygen.[58,59]

Fat intake should be moderate in adolescence and should be accompanied by proportionate increases in carbohydrates. The optimum diet can be obtained when calories are distributed in a proportion of 10 to 15% from protein, 30 to 35% from fat, and the remainder from carbohydrates.

Because of the important role of the many biochemical reactions which make energy available for muscular work, several reviews cite an increased demand for B-complex vitamins. This additional need will be supplied when the total calorie content of a nutritionally balanced diet is increased. Supplements are not usually advocated because the water soluble vitamins cannot be stored in the body and once the tissue levels are saturated, excesses are excreted in the urine. In addition, recent investigations report that Vitamin C supplementation may increase biochemical reactions in the body that destroy Vitamin B-12.[59] The fat soluble vitamins can be stored, and daily supplements of large quantities of Vitamin A have been known to be toxic in some cases.

Sodium loss in perspiration will vary according to temperature and among individuals. This need can be met adequately by salting foods at meals and using salted crackers and nuts as snacks. It is important that water losses from perspiration be replaced; failure to do this leads to fatigue, lower efficiency, higher body temperatures, and eventually heat stroke. Water deprivation can be extremely dangerous since it could result in the formation of crystals in the urine and eventually cause kidney damage and death.[54] Water is the most essential of all the nutrients. The water lost in perspiration due to increased activity is more easily replaced when a salty food increases thirst.

In view of the increased competition and training by women athletes in recent years, especially among adolescents, the physiological adaptations and nutritional aspects of female athletes are just now being explored. When the additional nutritional requirements are adjusted for her body size, the principles suggested for the male athlete are to be followed for the female.

It is important to note that iron therapy may be recommended for women who are engaged in endurance sports.[62] Strenuous exercise causes an increase in red cell destruction and places an additional demand upon iron stores. At the same time, the adolescent girl experiences higher demands for iron due to menstrual losses. Some studies suggest that iron-deficiency anemia exists in 5% and low iron stores occur in 15 to 25% of women athletes.[61]

Both male and female adolescent athletes are constantly exposed to widespread misconceptions about high-protein diets, mega-vitamins, food supplements, and commercial products available as replacements for food or drinks to improve athletic performance. Coaches often impose rigorous dietary regimes upon athletes. Often these rules may be based upon their own experiences rather than upon sound nutrition information. There is no scientific evidence that any of these beliefs improve performance. There is no proven evidence that the so-called isotonic solution or electrolyte "ades" that basically contain sodium, potassium, and carbohydrate, have any physiological advantage over water, saline solutions, or glucose syrup drinks in improving athletic performance.

Food faddism and ignorance are more prominent in the area of athletics than in any other sphere of nutrition. Specifically detrimental to health are the nutritionally unsound practices of the frequently drastic weight-loss regimens undertaken by sports competitors prior to a weigh-in before a match in order to qualify for the lowest weight class. These unsound regimens often include starvation and extreme water deprivation. Starvation depletes protein, glycogen, vitamins, minerals, and enzyme stores which are essential for optimum adolescent growth and optimum athletic performance.[62]

The tension and nervousness experienced by a young athlete just before competition may alter the digestion of food and an upset stomach may occur. Common symptoms of nervous tension, such as nausea, vomiting, abdominal cramps, and diarrhea are not only experienced by the adolescent athlete, but often by their coaches and trainers as well. A sound recommendation is to eat a light, balanced meal high in carbohydrates. Liquid foods are preferred because they seem to be easier to digest; a few hours of rest before participation should be allowed. There is general agreement that high protein meals are undesirable just before athletic competition.

ORAL CONTRACEPTIVES

The normal nutritional needs of adolescent females are altered by the widespread use of oral contraceptives. Upwards of four million United States female teenagers are estimated to be at risk for pregnancy due to sexual activity, and the highly effective "Pill" is a contraceptive method of choice for a great number.

Recent advances of research on metabolism, drugs, and nutrition have provided a better understanding of the effects of oral contraceptives on the nutritional status of users. There are medical indications against the use of oral contraceptives by women of all ages who have vascular or clotting problems, diabetes, liver disorders, cancer, and multiple other conditions, and who smoke. Adverse reactions have been reported concerning the Pill's influence on the hormonal system. The metabolism of females taking oral contraceptive agents (OCA) is similar in many respects to that of pregnant women. The estrogen component of hormonal contraceptive therapy has associated symptoms similar to those of early pregnancy: nausea, vomiting, breast engorgement, weight gain, headaches, and dizziness. Changes in carbohydrate metabolism and vitamin deficiencies are among the side effects seen in women.[63]

Very few clinical signs of nutrient depletions have been seen in OCA users.

Among the nutrients found to be depressed in circulating blood levels of OCA users are folic acid, Vitamin C, riboflavin, Vitamin B-6, and zinc.[63,64,65] Clear-cut clinical deficiencies of vitamins other than folic acid have not been well established and only about 24 cases of megaloblastic anemia have been observed. The OCA increases serum/plasma levels for Vitamins A and K, copper, and iron.[63,64,65]

The recommendation for increased Vitamin B-6 has been studied specifically because of its association with tryptophan metabolism (an essential amino acid). Pyridoxine (Vitamin B-6) is essential as a coenzyme in many reactions of protein and carbohydrate metabolism. Findings of increased urinary xanthurenic acid (tryptophan metabolite) excretion after a test dose of tryptophan in OCA users imply Vitamin B-6 depletion.[66]

Depression, mood changes, and altered sleep patterns in women taking OCA have been corrected with 30 mg of pyridoxine daily, about 10 to 15 times the RDA, if their plasma B-6 levels were also low.[63] At this point it seems reasonable to explore the value of supplementation of this vitamin in women with tendencies toward pessimism, dissatisfaction, crying, and tension that are very clearly related to oral contraceptive use.[67]

Because of the complexity of the mechanisms involved, the effects of the Pill on folic acid, as well as on several other nutrients, are still open to much debate; consequently, to properly advise specific increases is not yet possible. However, present evidence of alterations of metabolism does assist us in helping the young woman to reduce the nutritionally related complications from oral contraceptives. It is particularly important to consider these alterations of normal nutrient requirements with regard to the teenager, since her nutritional status before becoming pregnant, and between pregnancies, influences the health of her unborn children as well as her own health.

Iron needs may be slightly reduced in oral contraceptive users since there is a diminution of menstrual blood loss, and there are indications that iron serum levels and iron-binding capacity are increased.[67] In contrast, the use of the intrauterine device (IUD) is well known to cause increased blood and iron loss. The supplementation of absorbable iron salts, such as ferrous sulfate or ferrous gluconate, is then advised.

CHRONIC ILLNESS

All kinds of acute or chronic infection, disease processes that cause decreased gastrointestinal function, or diseases that upset the mechanisms controlling the metabolism of essential nutrients, will alter the normal requirements of nutrients in the adolescent because of the impairment of ingestion or digestion and the greatly increased metabolic demand imposed by the pathology.

During the period of illness, nutritional intakes have to be adequate to provide for the needs of growth as well as for the metabolic demands imposed by the stress of illness. Special factors that should be considered are the stage of physical, social, and emotional development of the adolescent and the presence of physical handicaps. Factors such as anorexia, emotional adjustments during illness, and the disease process itself, which may affect appetite and food acceptance, must be evaluated.

Illnesses that involve gastrointestinal malabsorption will increase the requirements for all nutrients. Trauma, anxiety, fear, and other common factors of stress associated with illness have an even more pronounced effect in altering protein requirements because of hormonal responses that increase the rate of synthesis of cells.

In kidney and liver diseases, for example, the normal utilization of vitamins is compromised. The conversion of Vitamin D to its active metabolic forms depends upon the liver and kidneys. Individuals suffering from kidney disease may show skeletal abnormalities similar to those seen in rickets, a disease of Vitamin D deficiency. When patients are given synthetic forms of the active vitamin they show a marked improvement in health.

Dietary therapeutics are based upon the principles of good nutrition. If any modification is required, it should be based upon the requirements of normal adolescent nutrition and adapted to the specific needs of the individual at that time. For example, if the pathologic condition requires modification of sodium intake to maintain water balance, this nutrient should be adjusted and all other nutrients should be kept at optimum levels to maintain good nutritional status.

It is essential that calorie intake be adequate to maintain desirable weight and allow proteins to function for tissue synthesis and recovery. In the nutritional care of patients unable to take food by mouth, all nutrients must be given by parenteral route (usually intravenous). In prolonged illnesses caloric inadequacies usually become a major problem. New commercial products and alternative methods have been developed to improve parental nutrition.

The nutritional care of the chronically ill adolescent presents many obstacles: the strange environment, absence of typical teenage snack foods, fatigue, drugs, pain, and anorexia caused by the illness itself. All of these factors make it difficult to ensure an adequate diet. Health care professionals need to be sensitive and understanding of each adolescent's unique needs. The team approach, provision of an adolescent unit, parental support, group meals with peers, and provision of certain teenage snack foods usually help the chronically ill adolescent to eat better.

Nutrition Counseling

The National Dairy Council has published some helpful tips for more effective nutrition counseling of adolescents. These "Starting Pointers"* are:

1. *Review basic nutrition information.* Even though you probably know a good deal on the subject, it is wise to review current nutrition information so that you are more secure in your knowledge as questions come to you. . . .
2. *Check up on yourself.* How are your own food habits? It is important to practice the principles of nutrition which you are trying to get across to others. . . .

*Reprinted by courtesy of the National Dairy Council, 6300 North River, Rosemont, Ill. 60018, from the *Nutrition Source Book,* 1971, p. 3.

3. *Know your resources.* . . . You will also want to learn the names of nutritionists and other resource people you can turn to if you meet special nutrition problems.
4. *Understand your audience.* You will be counseling a wide variety of families from many cultural and economic backgrounds, from different geographic origins and ethnic groups. You need to know something of the social characteristics and food patterns of these groups. However, an individual or family does not necessarily have all the habits of the group. Get to know each family, gain confidence, and establish rapport before giving them advice.
5. *Experiment with new approaches.* You'll doubtless find varied responses as you help . . . [adolescents] check up on their food practices. An approach which works with one may not work with another. But if you recognize the good points in the present food practice, you'll usually win an interest on which you can proceed *gradually* with suggestions. Some ideas for improvement may be adopted immediately; others may take longer to be accepted.

Adolescents fall into two major categories according to their nutritional needs: (1) the well adolescent, and (2) the adolescent whose diet requires therapeutic modification. Nutrition counseling of these two categories of adolescents can be offered in a wide variety of settings and situations, on a group or individual basis. Counseling, one of the essentials of good nutrition health care, can be given with or without complete nutritional assessment.

The general procedure in beginning the counseling is to assess the client's current status; one needs to gather the pertinent data about the individual that gives the necessary information for determining the basis for the kind of counseling needed. This assessment process requires the multidisciplinary approach of the whole health team. The determination of the individual's nutritional status—a process which may occasionally be complex, expensive, and hard to interpret, is too often neglected.

NUTRITIONAL ASSESSMENT

Nutritional assessment is the process of defining the health status of the individual as it is influenced by dietary intake and the utilization of essential food nutrients. It commonly consists of four types of data:

1. Initial or past health history.
2. Physical examination. Clinical signs of nutritional status are assessed.
3. Laboratory tests—usually blood and urine analysis.
4. Dietary history.

The information presented in the patient's general health care record is usually a good beginning for a nutritional assessment. Combining this information with data from the physical examination and laboratory findings will help to identify those teenagers most vulnerable to nutritional problems or identifiable as belonging in nutritional risk categories. The history alone will reveal many adolescents at nutritional risk:

- •Adolescents from low-income situations; poverty among minority groups is probably the most easily identifiable risk category
- •Adolescents with unique nutritional needs, such as the pregnant adolescent or the young athlete
- •Adolescents with history of anemia, obesity, underweight
- •Adolescents with unusual nutritional problems, such as food faddists, those on macrobiotic diets, constant dieters, those who have anorexia nervosa
- •Adolescents with chronic illness, diabetes, chronic infections, drug abuse or addiction, alcoholism, malabsorption syndromes
- •Adolescents with severe emotional and psychological problems

The physical examination in which the clinical signs of nutritional status are assessed also includes height and weight measurements. Weight is a very critical factor in the assessment of nutritional status. Attained weight, growth rate, and weight changes are all indicative of food intake. Any causes of undesirable weight changes should be pursued and corrected. General examination of the adolescent's skin, mucous membranes, tongue, eyes, and hair condition provides useful information in assessing the nutritional status.

Laboratory testing is valuable because marginal deficiencies can be detected before they appear clinically. Blood and urine samples are commonly analyzed. Hemoglobin, hematocrit, serum proteins, serum vitamins, serum lipids, and serum enzymes are measured in the blood. Urinalysis determines nutrients normally excreted (soluble vitamins and metabolites such as creatine, creatinine, and urea) and also the excretion of nutrients not normally excreted (glucose, albumin).

The fourth component, the dietary history, is the most useful tool for defining nutritional needs and providing the base for counseling. The dietary history should include the following information:

1. Cultural background of the adolescent
2. Economic factors in food selection
3. Preparation of food (Who is responsible? Living alone? Parents cook?)
4. Food allergies or lactose intolerance
5. Recent or ongoing special diets
6. Medication taken (drugs, vitamins, contraceptive pill)

Once this information is elicited, the next step is to obtain a 24-hour dietary recall. This is an attempt to record and assess the usual dietary habits of the teenager by determining the exact intake for the previous 24 hours. The interview will enable the practitioner to learn about the teenager's food habits, likes and dislikes, emotions, frequency of food intake, attitudes about food, settings in which foods are eaten, and, most important, the teenager's schedule and activities. The 24-hour dietary recall has the advantage of being practical, and quickly enables one to start counseling based on the immediate needs of the adolescent.

Another tool used in identifying dietary habits is the Three Day Food Record. The teenager is required to keep a diary of foods eaten for 72 consecutive hours. In some cases the combination of the two tools is required for a more comprehensive evaluation of the teenager's dietary practices.

EVALUATION OF DIETARY ADEQUACY

The foregoing process established the quantity and quality of food intake. The most common method of evaluation is to compare the food intake with a standard guide for dietary adequacy. This evaluation may be based on food groups or individual nutrients:

1. Food Group guides (servings of food by groups)
2. Recommended Daily Allowances (amounts of specific nutrients using food composition tables)

The more practical method is the evaluation of food intake based on the Daily Food Guide for Adolescents. (See Table 4–2.) For this evaluation the foods eaten are first classified according to food groups. This classification is then compared with servings recommended for adolescents. This process will show the strong points of the diet, which should be pointed out to the adolescent as well as the weak areas, deficiencies, or marginal intakes of specific nutrients. Next, priorities of remedy should be set. The energy needs of the body always take priority over other needs, and if the diet does not provide sufficient calories from carbohydrates and fat, proteins will be used for energy.

In order to help the adolescent identify and work on his nutritional problems, the health care practitioner must explore with him the environmental, cultural, and social influences which have contributed to the nutritional problems presented. Exploration of these many influences requires a discussion of the following with the adolescent:

1. The adolescent's nutritional knowledge: has he had nutrition counseling before? Has he taken nutrition courses at school? Has he read nutrition books? If so, which books? What does he know about nutrition?
2. Available resources:
   a. Economics: does he receive an allowance that allows him to spend money for snacks? Are financial restraints such that his family cannot afford enough food?
   b. Equipment available for food preparation: refrigeration, stove, storage, cooking utensils, hot water, electricity.
   c. Time schedules that make it difficult for him to plan, to shop for, and to cook food.
   d. Places where food may be purchased.

Often, by exploring these environmental factors with the collaboration of the entire health team, solutions may be obtained.

It is impossible to present possible solutions to all of the problems that may be seen in the clinical setting. However, nutritional counseling should focus on the preventive aspects of health care and the problems associated with malnutrition as well as overnutrition of the adolescent. Health educators must recognize that the adolescent as well as the general public is exposed to risk factors that are associated with nutrition-related diseases, i.e., obesity, hypertension, cardiovascular disease, and cancer of the colon.

The health educator can be more effective in counseling by posing hypothetical situations that lead adolescents to think about altering dietary practices. Unless the adolescent alters such habits as going to school without breakfast and then eating potato chips, a candy bar, and a carbonated beverage for lunch, his protein will be inadequate and will not be distributed optimally throughout the day.

CULTURAL BACKGROUND

The adolescent's ethnic or cultural background should receive special attention during the counseling process. Because of limited space, only the outstanding dietary characteristics of the three ethnic groups presented in Chapter 3 will be briefly discussed here.

Teenagers from ethnic groups have dietary practices common to all American teenagers but are also strongly influenced in the home by their cultural heritage. Some are subjected to strong pressures by their elders in the family (especially more recent immigrants) to eat special foods and herbs to ensure good health. This may be especially true in the case of a mother or mother-in-law, who often exerts pressure on an adolescent to eat certain foods and to avoid others, or not to combine foods because of specific ill effects on health. Adolescent males are exposed to the highest pressures from families at the time when their voices start to change, body hair develops, and they become sexually active. Adolescent females are exposed to these pressures particularly during menstruation, pregnancy, and lactation. Both males and females may experience such pressures during an illness.

Each particular ethnic group is identified by predominant food habits, but uniformity in food practices is unlikely within a specific group. In general, it may be said that new immigrants will probably maintain their own food habits until they become involved with school, work, or English classes and adapt somewhat to their new schedules and activities within this culture. Usually, the most festive dishes of each culture are elaborate dishes that require much time in preparation, and are saved for special occasions and holidays. What is often featured at typical ethnic restaurants may not reflect the usual dietary habits of a particular ethnic group. For example, tacos, enchiladas, tamales, and other well-known Mexican foods may not be prepared frequently at home once the family moves into the accelerated pace of life of the United States.

In considering an ethnic teenager's food habits, one must examine his activities and schedules and the places where most of his time is spent. He will probably be involved in many of the same activities and have the same concerns about body image as his peers.

MEXICAN AMERICANS

Mexican Americans comprise one of the major cultural groups in the United States, particularly in the Southwest. Most Mexican Americans eat one "good" meal daily at noon; this is a hot meal including soup, vegetables, beans, tortillas, and meat. Usually breakfast and supper are light: sweet coffee or milk and tortillas. Milk is not a common beverage among Mexicans. Since adolescents cannot be home for their usual noon meal, they adopt food habits similar to those of their peers; they adopt the worst practices of empty-calorie snacks, fast foods, and high consumption of sugary carbonated beverages. Cold sandwiches cannot substitute for the nutritious traditional noon meal. Also, to avoid being labeled Mexicans or Chicanos, these teenagers may particularly avoid their usual nutritious foods such as beans and tortillas.

Not surprisingly, the major nutrients lacking in their diets are Vitamin A, Vitamin C, iron, and calcium. Vitamin A deficiency has been reported as the most prevalent nutritional problem of Mexican American children.[68] The National Nutrition Survey in the Southwest showed that a high proportion of Mexican Americans had low blood levels of riboflavin and hemoglobin. Deficiencies of thiamin, ascorbic acid, and protein were less frequent, but of a magnitude great enough to constitute a problem.[69]

Economic limitations, cultural isolation, language, and educational barriers also make Mexican American adolescents highly vulnerable to nutritional problems. Frequently, they do not seek health care—and then only in extreme crisis situations, when it is almost too late.

In working with Mexican American adolescents a most helpful approach to use is that of including other family members. The Mexican American looks to his family to meet his needs. Family comes first, the self is second. Very few decisions are made without the family.

The Mexican American adolescent female often experiences pressures from relatives to eat or to avoid certain foods. Citrus fruits are especially avoided during menstruation and pregnancy. Many have said to the author, "Are lemons bad? Why? I've been told they are too acid and my Mom wouldn't let me eat anything acid while I was pregnant; they will thin my blood. But, I have cravings for lemons, limes, and acid things; can I eat them?"

Oftentimes teenagers do not follow their parents' advice to eat or not to eat certain foods. Once good rapport is established with a health care practitioner, young people become more open and less resistant to adults, and they ask questions to clarify concerns, providing an excellent opportunity for nutrition education.

CHINESE AMERICANS

The largest Chinese American communities in the United States are in New York and San Franscisco. The Chinese have definite food preferences based upon the eating habits of their culture.

Food plays an important role in preventing and treating disease. Foods are divided into groups: Yang (hot)—meat, eggs, ginger, etc., and Yin (cold)—winter melon, watermelon, bananas, cold fruit juice, etc.—and they must be balanced in every meal. Vegetables constitute the major part of their diet; they are consumed quite often but seldom eaten raw. Calcium is the nutrient of concern since milk intake is minimal. Chinese teenagers prefer eating ice cream, custard, or cheese to drinking milk. Health professionals need to know about high calcium substitutions for a Chinese diet. Part of the milk group for a Chinese adolescent could be tofu (a soybean curd made by precipitating protein of soybean milk with calcium or magnesium salts), which is usually liked. It is a good source of calcium, protein, and iron. A two-inch cube portion of tofu can substitute for a protein equivalent of two to three ounces of hamburger or two eggs. Also, green vegetables will contribute a large part of the required calcium in their diets. Meat intake is moderate; fish is used often, and white rice and noodles form the staples of the diet.

Folk medicine practices during pregnancy are encouraged in many families. Shellfish is avoided during the first trimester to prevent development of allergies later in life. Some young women refuse to take iron supplements because they think that the iron will harden their bones and make delivery of the child more difficult.[70]

BLACK AMERICANS

The outstanding characteristics of the black American diet are that it may furnish too much pork fat, fried food, sweets, and starches, too few green salads and eggs, and too little milk. "Soul food" has always been popular and is enjoyed by the black community. "Soul food" for the black American culture, especially in the South, represents feelings and emotions. The traditional breakfast in the South consists of fried meat, rice grits, biscuits, gravy, fried sweet or Irish potatoes, and coffee or milk. In the north it consists of eggs, bacon or sausage, biscuits, and coffee.[71] For many black Americans in the South poverty is extreme, and the diet is quite restricted. As the income improves, black Americans spend increasing amounts of money for meat. Too little emphasis is placed on vegetables, fruits, and milk.[71] Since large amounts of fats and carbohydrates are consumed, more than enough calories are provided. However, in working with the black teenager, one commonly finds two extremes of caloric imbalance—the obese teenager and the underweight teenager. Because many have poor living conditions, poor nutrition, and crowded homes, black adolescents may face serious problems with respect to nutritional status. Often when they seek health care they are reluctant to take advantage of nutrition counseling at the clinic and seek to meet their appointment only. If nutrition counseling does not take into account their food habits and the food available to them, it can be a waste of time for both the adolescent and the counselor. It has been this author's experience that the best way to gain rapport with black teenagers is to offer nutrition counseling in a group. Peer pressure is one of the strongest influences on food choices among teenagers. For example, when a pregnant 14-year-old was observed by a group of peers at school eating candy and drinking carbonated beverages frequently during the day and omitting meat, fruits, and vegetables provided by the school at lunchtime, her peers chided, "You are starving your baby; he is going to be skinny." The use of films, slides, or food demonstrations seems to be effective. The reinforcement of the importance of proper nutrients by the doctor, nurse, or other health professional can be of great help in assisting the adolescent to understand her nutritional needs.

Special Approaches to Improve Adolescents' Diets

This section of special approaches is based on some of the author's case examples and experiences, taken from everyday situations, which resulted in successful solutions to the difficulties inherent in improving adolescents' food habits. From observations in working with teenagers of different ethnic backgrounds and a variety of socioeconomic statuses, one special approach that is both valuable and successful is personal enthusiasm about nutritional care. Unfortunately, nutritionists have not found any magic formula that will motivate teenagers to select good diets; however, a positive attitude and enthusiasm greatly contribute to the success of counseling, and it is possible to bring about change and improvements in food habits.

Because of both increased emphasis on science in schools and greater knowledge provided by the mass media, adolescents in the United States are generally more sophisticated, more philosophical, and even more politically oriented than teenagers were in the past. Young people, as well as their adult models, are concerned about ecologic balance, world food issues, and hunger. They are more aware of the importance of staying healthy; they are concerned about chemicals in food and cosmetics, chemicals and pollutants in their environment, cholesterol, fiber, and carcinogens. They seek nutrition information and are capable of understanding more advanced information than simply the four food groups. They expect scientific responses and meaningful answers to their inquiries, and one must be prepared to deal with these adolescents' nutritional concerns by providing them with substantial facts and thorough explanations to correct misinformation.

Adolescents usually know what kinds of foods are most nutritious and what kinds are not. Their interest in diet and nutrition has given them a general familiarity with nutrients and their functions. Unfortunately, they frequently are misinformed by unreliable, unscientific sources. Nevertheless, they do have the interest and a basis on which to begin sound nutrition education.

The following approaches can be helpful in improving adolescent diets and in promoting lasting and beneficial nutritional habits:

1. The nutrition counselor must be enthusiastic in what he is doing as well as patient, alert, sensitive, and supportive.
2. The counselor must be honest and realistic in the type of suggestions he or she offers for change. Adolescents must understand that the ultimate decisions to change and to adopt new practices lie with themselves. All efforts exercised by others will be for naught if they choose not to cooperate.
3. The counselor must listen. A very common adolescent expression is "But you don't listen!" Teenagers need somebody to listen to what they are trying to express as well as to what they actually express. This is a very valuable quality in health care professionals, and, because of pressures of time and work, major points that can be the targets for changes are often missed. By listening, much is learned about the teenager's problems of communication and his conflicts with dominant parents; the counselor becomes aware of whether the teenager is isolated, emotionally depressed, anorexic, or a

frustrated eater. Among adolescents there will be found those who enjoy cooking and eating good food, as well as those who like to be disciplined because discipline is lacking at home. It is important to "listen" not only to the words but to the tone of voice, facial expressions, and body language, to help identify their attitudes toward foods.

4. The counselor must actively involve the adolescent. Adolescents should be instructed to evaluate their own dietary records. The health professional and the teenager must work together and the adolescent should be encouraged to participate. The teaching-learning process is aimed at bringing positive results which will reinforce what teenagers have already learned and practiced. Share with them the available charts of weight and height—show where they stand and explain variables. If an adolescent is pregnant, she should have a copy of her own weight gain curve to use in keeping track of her gradual and steady gain during pregnancy.

5. The counselor can demonstrate food preparation. Many adolescents who are faced with food preparation are inexperienced in basic cooking. The preparation of food may be to them time-consuming, monotonous, and boring—they may just not like to cook or not know what to cook. Food demonstrations are very successful. Preparing and eating food adds interest to the counseling sessions. This is a convincing method of introducing foods that are not customarily consumed. Recipes using squash, potatoes, and even liver sauté sticks dipped in catsup are very successful when they have been demonstrated and prepared alongside the adolescent. Some expressions that reinforced the author's belief in this approach are "You converted me. I may like liver now." "I've made squash sticks dipped in catsup at home and everybody liked it."

6. The counselor involves the family in nutrition when possible. The role of the family will vary from case to case. Sometimes family support can be enlisted either to provide, or to assist the adolescent in choosing, nutritious snacks. At other times, adults might be advised to leave the teenager alone and not overemphasize what must be eaten.

   Mothers select and prepare foods they believe their families will enjoy. Bryan and Lowenberg[72] found that 89% of mothers served infrequently or eliminated from the family menu foods that their husbands disliked. Eppright and associates[73] demonstrated that 80% of the mothers planned meals on the basis of their husbands' likes and dislikes, 72% chose foods on the basis of likes and dislikes of other family members, and that 58% considered likes and dislikes of children. The father has much influence on what foods go on the table and on what the children learn to like or dislike. It is important to identify the persons in the family who are most influential and responsible for the food choices of adolescents.

7. The counselor provides continuity and reinforcement in nutrition counseling. In order to be successful, nutrition counseling must be a continuous process. It is not realistic to try to improve diets within one session of 10 to 15 minutes. Follow-up sessions allow for continued evaluation of progress;

problems encountered may be communicated at such times. Further support and encouragement should be given. A phone call or a personal note will help to maintain motivation or to remotivate when lapses or failures occur. Communication of assistance to the young teenager should convey interest and care.

8. The counselor considers special foods likes and dislikes. Everybody naturally has food likes and dislikes, but sometimes adolescents completely dislike an entire food group, such as vegetables. This particular attitude deserves special attention if our concern is to improve adolescent diets. When this real life situation occurs, there are several alternatives available for arriving at a good solution. The person responsible for the food preparation in the home may need counseling, since the educational level and nutritional knowledge of the mother influence the quality of the diet.

9. The counselor provides positive feedback to the adolescent that emphasizes what he has done right, no matter how small the progress. Effective and permanent changes in eating habits are likely to be achieved through gradual and comfortable alterations. Emphasizing the fact that the adolescent can change his life style helps to stimulate and motivate him to continue his change in behavior.

10. The counselor gets to know the adolescent's cultural customs and cultural values. The need to understand the adolescent's culture, beliefs, attitudes, emotions, and why he acts as he does in terms of dietary practices is essential for effective counseling.

Summary

The adolescent presents a unique set of nutritional needs which are not easily fulfilled. Careful consideration must be given not only to the general characteristics of this group, but also to individual requirements dictated by a particular rate of growth, physiologic state, and pattern of activity.

The most notorious nutritional problems among adolescents—obesity and iron-deficiency anemia—are conditioned by their food practices. In addition, factors based on the emotional, physiological, psychological, and socioeconomic aspects of health put the adolescent in a special category of nutritional risk. The implications of this high risk classification in adolescence create an urgent need for in-depth and continuous nutritional assessment and counseling. Adolescents have the freedom and responsibility of making individual food choices that are important to them. Because of their unique health demands they cannot afford nutritionally to miss regular meals and snack on empty-calorie foods. Therefore, it is incumbent upon health care professionals to provide adolescents and their families with the necessary nutritional information to ensure the maintenance of optimum nutritional practices which will indeed influence their futures.

REFERENCES

1. National Academy of Sciences, National Research Council, Food and Nutrition Board. *Recommended Dietary Allowances,* rev. ed. Washington, D.C.: National Academy of Sciences, 1974.
2. Williams, S. ed. *Nutrition and Diet Therapy,* 3rd ed. St. Louis: C. V. Mosby Co., 1977, p. 414.
3. Heald, F. P., Remmell, P. S., and Mayer, J. "Caloric, Protein and Fat Intakes in Children and Adolescents." In Heald, F. P., ed. *Adolescent Nutrition and Growth.* New York: Meredith Corp., 1969.
4. Hampton, M. C., et al. "Caloric and Nutrient Intake of Teenagers." *J. Am. Diet. Assoc.* 50:385, 1967.
5. Pennington, J. *Dietary Nutrient Guide.* Westport, Conn. Avi Publishing Co., Inc., 1976.
6. King, C. J., et al. "Evaluation and Modification of the Basic Four Food Guide." *J. Nutrition Ed.* 10(1):27–29, 1978.
7. Maternal and Child Health Branch, California Department of Health. "Food Guides: Their Development, Use, and Specific Changes Suggested for Nutrition During Pregnancy and Lactation." June 1977, pp. 2–3.
8. Maternal and Child Health Unit, California Department of Health. *Nutrition During Pregnancy and Lactation—For Professional Use.* 1975.
9. U.S. Center for Disease Control. *Ten State Nutrition Survey, 1968–1970.* DHEW Publication No. (HSM) 72–8134; 72–8133. Washington, D.C.: U.S. Government Printing Office, 1972. Vol. 1, pp. 1–13; Vol. 5, pp. 181–185.
10. Hampton, M., et al. "Caloric and Nutrient Intakes of Teenagers." *J. Am. Diet. Assoc.* 50:385–395, May 1967.
11. U.S. Health Services. *First Health and Nutrition Examination Survey, U.S. 1971–1972.* Rockville, Md.: U.S. Health Services. DHEW Publication No. (HRA) 74–1219, 1974.
12. Hodges, R. E., and Krehl, W. A. "Nutrition Status of Teenagers in Iowa." *Am. J. Clin. Nutrition* 17:200, 1965.
13. Huenemann, R. L., et al. "Food and Eating Practices of Teenagers." *J. Am. Diet. Assoc.* 53:17, 1968.
14. Frankle, T., et al. "Food Zealotry and Youth: New Dilemmas for the Professionals." *Am. J. Pub. Health* 64(1):11–18, 1974.
15. Dwyer, J. T., et al. "The New Vegetarians: The Natural High?" *J. Am. Diet. Assoc.* 65:529–536, 1974.
16. White, H. S. "What It is and What the Food Industry Should Do About It." *Food Tech.* 26:29, 1972.
17. Kamil, A. "How Natural are Those Natural Vitamins?" *J. Nutrition Ed.* 4:92, 1972.
18. Mitchell, S., et al. *Nutrition in Health and Disease,* 16th ed. Philadelphia: J. B. Lippincott Co., 1976, p. 208.
19. Larrick, G. P. "The Role of the Food and Drug Administration in Nutrition." *Am. J. Clin. Nutrition* 8:377–382, 1960.
20. Sherlock, P., and Rothchild, E. O. "Scurvy Produced by a Zen Macrobiotic Diet." *JAMA* 199:794–798, 1967.
21. Erhard, D. "The New Vegetarians. 1. Vegetarianism and Its Medical Consequences." *Nutrition Today* 8:4–12, 1973.
22. Heald, F., and Khan, M. "Disorders of Adipose Tissue." In Gallagher, J., et al., *Medical Care of the Adolescent.* 3rd ed. New York: Appleton-Century-Crofts, Prentice Hall 1976, pp. 125–138.
23. Huenemann, R. L., et al. "A Longitudinal Study of Gross Body Composition and Body Conformation and Their Association with Food Activity in a Teenage Population: Views of Teenage Subjects on Body Conformation, Food and Activity." *Am. J. Clin. Nutrition* 18:325, 1966.
24. Dwyer, J., et al. "Adolescents' Attitudes Toward Weight and Appearance." *J. Nutrition Ed.* 1(2):14, 1969.
25. Abraham, S., et al. "Preliminary Findings of the First Health and Nutrition Examination Survey United States, 1971–1972: Anthropometric and Clinical Findings." Rockville, Md.: U.S. Dept. Health, Education, and Welfare. DHEW Pub. No. (HRA) 75–1229, 1975.
26. Gifft, Helen. *Nutrition Behavior and Change.* Englewood Cliffs, N.J.: Prentice Hall, Inc., 1972, pp. 222, 241.

27. Heald, F. P., and Hollander, R. J. "The Relationship Between Obesity in Early Adolescence and Early Growth." *J. Pediat.* 67:35, 1975.
28. Asher, P. "Fat Babies and Fat Children: The Prognosis of Obesity in the Very Young." *Arch. Dis. Child.* 41:672–673, 1966.
29. Knittle, J. L. "Basic Concepts in the Control of Childhood Obesity." In Winick, M., ed. *Childhood Obesity.* New York: John Wiley & Sons, Inc., 1975.
30. Hampton, M. C., et al. "Caloric Intakes of Teenagers." *J. Am. Diet. Assoc.* 50:385, 1967.
31. Butten, B. A., et al. "Physical Activity of Obese and Non-Obese Adolescent Girls Appraised by a Motion Picture Sampling." *Am. J. Clin. Nutrition* 14:211, 1964.
32. Mayer, J. *Overweight: Causes, Cost, and Control.* Englewood Cliffs, N.J.: Prentice Hall, Inc., 1968, p. 33.
33. Seltzer, C. C., and Mayer, J. "A Simple Criterion of Obesity." *Postgrad. Med.* 38:101–107, 1965.
34. Durnin, J. V. G. A., and Womersley, J. "Body Fat Assessed from Total Body Density and Its Estimation from Skinfold Thickness: Measurements on 481 Men and Women Aged 16 to 72 Years." *Brit. J. Nutrition* 32:77–97, 1974.
35. Coates, T. J., and Thoresen, C. E. "Treating Obesity in Children and Adolescents: A Review." *Am. J. Pub. Health* 68(2):143–150, 1976.
36. Mahoney, M. J., and Caggiula, W. A. "Applying Behavioral Methods to Nutritional Counseling." *J. Am. Diet. Assoc.* 72:372, 1978.
37. Smith, N. J., and Rios, E. "Iron Metabolism and Iron Deficiency." In Schulman, I., ed. *Advances in Pediatrics.* Chicago: Year Book Medical Pubs., Inc., 1974.
38. World Health Organization. *Nutritional Anemias.* Report of World Health Organization Scientific Group. Technical Report Series No. 405, Geneva, 1968.
39. U.S. Dept. Health, Education, and Welfare. "Iron Nutrition in Adolescence." Washington, D.C.: National Academy of Sciences. DHEW Pub. No. (HSA) 77–5100, 1976, pp. 5, 7.
40. Kuo, B., Daino, E., and Roginsky, M. S. "Endocrine Function in Thalassemia Major." *J. Clin. Endocr. Metab.* 28:805, 1968.
41. Cividally, G., et al. "Relation of Beta and Gamma Synthesis During the First Trimester: An Approach to Prenatal Diagnosis of Thalassemia." *Pediat. Res.* 8:553–560, 1974.
42. Hampton, M. C., et al. "Caloric and Nutrient Intake of Teenagers." *J. Am. Diet. Assoc.* 50:385, 1967.
43. Wharton, M. A. "Nutritive Intake of Adolescents." *J. Am. Diet. Assoc.* 42:306, 1963.
44. Thomas, J. A., and Call, D. L. "Eating Between Meals—A Nutrition Problem Among Teenagers?" *Nutrition Rev.* 31:137, 1973.
45. Luke, B. "Understanding Pica in Pregnant Women." *MCN: Am. J. Mat. Child Nurs.* 2(2):97, 1977.
46. Minnick, V. A., et al. "Pica in Turkey: 2. Effect of Clay Upon Iron Absorption." *Am. J. Clin. Nutrition* 21:78, 1968.
47. Mengel, C. E., Carter, W. A., and Horton, E. S. "Geophasia with Iron Deficiency and Hypokalemia." *Arch. Int. Med.* 114:470, 1964.
48. Roselle, H. A. "Association of Laundry Starch and Clay Ingestion with Anemia in New York City." *Arch. Int. Med.* 125:57, 1970.
49. Lanzkowsky, P. "Investigation into the Aetiology and Treatment of Pica." *Arch. Dis. of Child.* 34:140–148, 1959.
50. Committee on Maternal Nutrition, Food and Nutrition Board, National Research Council. *Maternal Nutrition and the Course of Pregnancy.* Washington, D.C.: National Academy of Sciences, 1970.
51. Blackburn, M. L., and Calloway, D. H. "Energy Expenditure and Pregnant Adolescents." In *Protein Requirements of Pregnant Teenagers,* Final Report of National Institutes of Health, Division of Research Grants, Grant No. HD 05 246, 1973.
52. King, C., and Jacobson, H. N. "Nutrition and Pregnancy in Adolescence." In Zackler, J., and Brandstadt, W., eds. *The Teenage Pregnant Girl.* Springfield, Ill.: Charles C Thomas Pub., 1975, pp. 142, 144.
53. Guyton, A. C. *Textbook of Medical Physiology,* 3rd ed. Philadelphia: W. B. Saunders Co., 1966, p. 980.
54. Consalaziom, C. Summary of Presentation on *Nutrition and Performance.* "Proteins, Carbohydrates, Vitamins and Water." Trends in Nutrition: A Symposium, January 15, 1977. Palo Alto, Calif.

55. Astrand, P. O. "Diet and Athletic Performance." *Fed. Proc.* 26:1772–1777, 1967.
56. Astrand, P. O. "Diet and Athletic Performance." *Nutrition Today* 3(2):9, 1968.
57. Bergstrom, J., and Hultman, E. "Nutrition for Maximal Sports Performance." *JAMA* 221:999–1006, 1972.
58. Karlston, J., and Saltin, B. "Diet, Muscle Glycogen, and Endurance Performance." *J. App. Physiol.* 31:203–206, 1971.
59. Herbert, V., and Jacob, E. "Destruction of Vitamin B-12 by Ascorbic Acid." *JAMA* 230(2):241–242, 1974.
60. Brown, H. "Nutritional Aspects of Women Athletes." Presented at Trends in Nutrition: A Symposium, January 15, 1977, Palo Alto, Calif.
61. Yoshimura, H. "Anemia During Physical Training (Sports Anemia)." *Nutrition Rev.* 28:251, 1970.
62. "Nutrition and Athletic Performance." *Dairy Counc. Dig.* 46:7–10, 1975.
63. Luke, B. "Think Nutrition if She's on the Pill." *RN* 39(3):33–34, 1976.
64. Thener, C. "Effect of Oral Contraceptive Agents on Vitamin and Mineral Needs: A Review." *J. Reproductive Med.* 8(1), 1972.
65. Briggs, M., and Briggs, M. "Vitamin C Requirements and Oral Contraceptives." *Nature* 238:277, 1972.
66. Luhby, A. L., et al. "Vitamin B-6 Metabolism in Users of Oral Contraceptive Agents. 1. Abnormal Urinary Xanthurenic Acid Excretion and Its Correction by Pyridoxine." *Am. J. Clin. Nutrition* 24:684, 1971.
67. Worthington, S., and Roscius, N. D. "Nutrition and Family Planning: Effect of Specific Birth Control Methods on Maternal Nutrition Status." *Nutrition in Pregnancy and Lactation.* St. Louis: C. V. Mosby Co., 1977, pp. 186, 188.
68. Larson, L. B., et al. "Nutritional Status of Children of Mexican-American migrant families." *J. Am. Diet. Assoc.* 64:29–35, 1974.
69. Barley, M. A. "Nutrition Eucation and the Spanish Speaking American." *J. Nutrition Ed.* 2:50–54, 1970.
70. Campbell, T., and Chang, B. "Health Care of the Chinese in America." *Nurs. Outlook* 21(4):245–248, 1973.
71. Jerome, N. W. "Changing Meal Patterns Among Southern-Born Negroes in a Midwest City." *Nutr. News,* National Dairy Council, Chicago, October 1968.
72. Bryan, M. S., and Lowenberg, M. E. "The Father's Influence on Young Children's Food Preferences." *J. Am. Diet. Assoc.* 34:30, 1958.
73. Eppright, E. S., et al. "Eating Behavior of Preschool Children." *J. Nutrition Ed.* 1:16, 1969.

5

Contraceptive Counseling and Care

Diana Taylor, R.N., M.S.

Theresa, a 16-year-old high school student, is visiting a teen contraceptive clinic for the first time. She tells the counselor, "I think I might be pregnant." After talking with Theresa, the counselor discovers that Theresa and her boyfriend have been dating for about one year and have recently become sexually active, "because my boyfriend wanted to, and I didn't think I could get pregnant." The counselor asks Theresa if she wanted to be sexually active, and she replies, "I didn't at first, but everybody else is doing it."

Theresa is typical of many young women attending family planning clinics: sexually active, afraid they are pregnant, and uncertain about their developing sexual identities. These sexually active teenagers are in a period of transition. They are incorporating new sexual behaviors into an identity which is also in a process of development. The integration of a sexual identity becomes even more difficult when the teenager adheres to a parental moral or behavioral code which prohibits non-marital sexual activity.

When asked, many teenagers will state that nonmarital sexual activity is not acceptable, yet national studies report an increase of sexual activity among unmarried adolescents.[1] In a study of 400 black teenage mothers, only 25% thought sexual activity before 18 years was acceptable.[2] However, 42% of teenagers are sexually active by age 19.[3] This discrepancy between words and deeds shows that teenagers are accepting a morality to which they are unable to adhere. This moral code has often been mandated by parents or other influential adults and accepted unquestioningly by the teenager.

It is not so surprising that teenagers are sexually active but are not utilizing methods of contraception consistently or at all. Using a method of contraception means that the teen is acknowledging that he or she is sexually active—which is often not acceptable behavior. For the teenager, the immediate costs of contraception may be higher than the more distant costs of pregnancy. Most sexually active teenagers do not desire to be pregnant, yet they risk pregnancy because they are more concerned with the immediate risks of using birth control—such as parental awareness, disapproval, and punishment; acknowledgment of their sexuality by planning for continued sexual activity; or the unavailability of contraceptive methods.

It is apparent that teenagers need assistance in developing their sexual identities and value systems. Many communities nationwide have seen the need for separate family planning services for teenagers and have instituted individualized programs in order to meet their special contraceptive needs. In 1971, a Teen Center in New York City made changes in the clinic setting to individualize contraceptive care for the 215 adolescent women who attended.[4] They began seeing the teen client more frequently (every three months) and a "rap" group was initiated to pick up possible problems. At the end of 18 months, this Teen Center described a low dropout rate (8%) and attributed it to the accepting and caring attitude of the clinic professional as well as the individualized services.

As early as 1967, Planned Parenthood Teen Clinic in San Francisco began focusing on teenagers' special contraceptive needs. It was at this center that specially trained staff and professionals initiated a program prepared to provide family planning services to teenagers. One popular aspect of this "after-school" clinic was the group discussion in which a range of topics in the area of sexuality, venereal disease, and contraception were covered. In the two years between 1967 and 1969, 476 young women were seen in the clinic for contraception while approximately another 150 were seen only in the discussion group. Their 11% dropout rate compared favorably with those of other contraceptive clinics.[5]

Even though a few contraceptive programs have specially designed services for their adolescent clients, patient education and counseling have not been developed to the same extent as other services. Contraceptive care for the adolescent client is an aspect of adolescent preventive health care which demands a closer and more creative investigation.

This chapter focuses on the comprehensive area of adolescent contraceptive care. Two teaching-learning strategies are described for use in a group session. A format is outlined for structuring a contraceptive care clinic which incorporates education and counseling specific to the adolescent. An overview of contraceptive methods follows. Special considerations influencing the care given to adolescents, such as confidentiality, legal aspects, and partner participation are discussed. For advanced clinicians a section on the pelvic examination of the adolescent is included.

Teaching-Learning Strategies

It has been suggested that the negative results of teenage sexual activity can be solved by providing education in the area of sexuality and contraception. Many contraceptive services have attempted to incorporate an educational component into the clinic visit. However, "education" has usually meant a lecture about birth control methods combined with a question and answer session. In a study of teen clinics, 67% of the programs provided an educational session for their teen clients, but "most of the sessions were conducted as lectures and entailed little, if any, group discussion.''[6] However, when asked how they would like to learn about contraception, 62% of the teenagers in the study indicated ''rap'' sessions would be preferable, whereas only 9% preferred the lecture format.[6]

The ''methods'' lecture emphasizes only one aspect of learning, the acquisition of methodology knowledge, and is based upon the assumption that people are rational and will make satisfying reproductive decisions when given appropriate information. Fischman[7] criticizes this method of patient education on the basis that the assumption is faulty. Fischman emphasizes that the chief determinant of sexual behavior is not factual information but the general feeling of satisfaction and worth that the individual has been able to develop about himself as a person.

Studies of teaching-learning strategies show the lecture method to be an inferior strategy when the objective is to promote conceptual knowledge, problem-solving skills, and patient participation. It is also an inadequate method for allowing for individual differences of learners. All of these factors are important considerations in teaching teenagers about sexuality and birth control.

A review of educational theories, as they relate to patient teaching, reports that the acquisition of knowledge is the lower level of learning.[8] The lecture method of teaching does not allow for higher levels of learning, such as comprehension and application of knowledge. Taba[9] suggests that if, in learning, the learner can discover relationships for himself and can apply the principles, the learning of new tasks and concepts will be better. Understanding the concepts surrounding sexuality and contraception is equally as important as learning specific facts. For example, understanding a process of sexual decision making may be more useful to teenagers than learning specific contraceptive facts.[10]

There is experimental evidence that when problem solving is the goal, active participation on the part of the learner is more effective than passive listening and observing. Since clients typically have few opportunities to make responses during a lecture on contraception, they seldom receive feedback on their efforts to learn. Auerbach[11] reports that when traditional or formal teaching methods are utilized, the teenager's ''impulsiveness, emotionalism or lack of concentration'' (p. 207) often make it difficult to learn specific content or tasks. She found that teenagers learn better in discussion groups where they are allowed to practice or obtain feedback about what is presented. When content, practice, and feedback are present in the learning episode, there is more likelihood that behavior change will occur in the learner.[12]

Although knowledge of contraceptive technology is necessary, it is not sufficient to solve the problems of poor contraceptive utilization by teenagers. Because reproductive behavior is determined by one's norms and culture, people make reproductive decisions based upon past customs, cultural values, and personality factors. Knowledge is a tool the individual will use only when he recognizes the tool as a means of satisfying needs and providing rewards.

Assessment of the adolescent's developmental and learning needs indicates that an educational approach different from the lecture method is needed. An educational method must recognize the adolescent's need for independence and a separate identity. It is during the adolescent years that a person clarifies who she is, what her role in the world will be, and to what group she belongs. It is a time of turmoil, when biological, social, psychological, and sexual forces are being integrated toward maturity. While struggling with a changing self-concept and new sexual identity, the adolescent needs to plan her own life and course of action in collaboration with others and in light of her sociocultural traditions. Knowledge and understanding about contraception and sexuality are not sufficient to promote problem solving; a climate that actively facilitates growth—one in which the adolescent examines options, accountability, and responsibility—is important.

Few situations we face in adult life are black and white and contain no decisional conflicts. Usually we face obstacles and alternatives, none of which is clearly better than others. Nor are intuitive or passive decisions always successful. Because the ultimate measure of education is its power to bring about more effective thinking and action, an educational process which promotes problem solving should provide for satisfactory and positive decisions.

As described, the group educational session employed in most contraceptive clinics was developed merely to provide information about birth control methods and clinic procedures. However, there are better and more efficient ways of providing teenagers with contraceptive information and concepts. Toward this goal the following two teaching-learning strategies are effective models which can be used for client education at teen contraceptive clinics: the decision-making strategy and the values clarification strategy.

Although a few young men accompany their partners to a contraceptive clinic, the majority of teen clients are women. Since the most effective birth control methods require little participation from the male partner, the young man may feel useless in the clinic setting. In any event, he is an infrequent visitor. It is for this reason that female examples are used primarily throughout this chapter. This does not imply that young men should not be encouraged to participate in all aspects of the clinic. The young man's understanding of contraceptive methods and participation in choosing a method can contribute to his enthusiasm for assuming responsibility in following through with its use. It is certainly the responsibility of clinic personnel to include partners during all phases of the clinic and perhaps to establish special programs for men. Decision-making and values-clarification strategies can be of equal benefit to the young man and the young woman.

DECISION-MAKING STRATEGY*

The decision-making model as a teaching strategy is based on concepts of decision making: teaching and learning, role modeling, and adolescent development. The decision-making model provides a framework within which discussion and learning can take place. Also, the decision-making model focuses on the process of choosing contraception rather than merely providing information about what to choose. This teaching strategy emphasizes a cooperative approach between learner

*This section of the chapter includes almost all of the article "A New Way to Teach Teens about Contraceptives," by the author. Copyright Nov./Dec. 1976, The American Journal of Nursing Company. Reproduced with permission from *MCN, The American Journal of Maternal Child Nursing* Vol. 1, No. 6, 378–383.

and teacher, in which the learner plays an active role in the educational process.

Decision making is defined as a process of developing a plan for a proposed course of action toward some end or goal. It involves (1) identifying the goal to be attained, (2) considering the alternatives and the consequences of various courses of action, and (3) selecting the alternative which carries the greatest probability of attaining the goal. The following is an example of how this process applies to adolescents in a teen clinic.

First, a tentative decision is made by a young woman to avoid pregnancy and focus on a particular method of birth control. Alternatives to the initial decision are then considered. Perhaps she will think about other possible choices such as pregnancy, abstinence from intercourse, or another method of contraception. Then, conflict may arise as the young woman considers the consequences or barriers to her initial choice. She may consider as obstacles the side effects of various methods, such as weight gain with the Pill, or "messiness" with the diaphragm. The next step is to reevaluate her alternatives in light of the consequences and barriers. The final step is to make a commitment to one decision.

The decision-making process is taught by two group leaders: the teen clinic nurse or counselor, and a teen or male volunteer. The nurse and co-leader promote the process of participatory learning by moving from simple to complex concepts. Decision-making concepts are introduced in a general manner by using a nonthreatening or familiar example, such as the selection of a pair of blue jeans. The nurse and co-leader pose questions to the group as a way of encouraging the teenagers to become actively involved in the decision-making process. They are asked to look at motivating and inhibiting factors, alternatives, and consequences to their decision regarding "jeans":

> Suppose you decide that you need a new pair of jeans. Your present pair is nearly in shreds. You say to youself, "I need a new pair of jeans." At this point you have made a decision—the decision to get a new pair. Then you must decide where to buy them.

A question is then posed to the group: "Where might you go to buy a pair of jeans?" In this way, the leaders encourage the teens to become actively involved in learning about decision making. After some exchanges in answer to this question, the hypothetical story resumes.

> So, after making the decision to buy new jeans you now have decided where to buy them. Your next step is to make some other decision on the style, the price, the length, and so on. Then you take a number of jeans into the dressing room. After you try them all on, you narrow the selection down to three or four pairs. Now you have come to the final decision, and it is at this stage that you may meet some obstacles.

To encourage the teens to recognize barriers to decision making, another question is asked: "What factors will keep you from fulfilling your first decision to buy a pair of jeans?" Responses might be "too expensive," "wrong style," ''poor fit,'' or ''lack of quality construction.'' The leaders then ask the teens to find alternatives to their decisions for each of the obstacles they mention. They then point out just how vital and pervasive the process of decision making is in a person's everday functioning.

> Let's say you find a pair which is just right for your pocketbook. You decide, ''These are for me,'' buy them, and take them home. But the decision doesn't end there. You have to decide if the jeans are too long and need hemming, or if they might look better with a belt, and so on. So you see, decision making never ends. We are constantly making decisions in our lives; often we aren't even aware we are making a decision. Some decisions are more important than others. It's the important decisions which we need to be aware of and to make with good information and thought.

At this point the teens are told that sexual decision making is a process similar to the one used in choosing jeans. The group leaders acknowledge, however, that choosing to be sexually active, to be a parent, or to avoid pregnancy is more personal and more important than choosing a pair of jeans. Acting as role models, they demonstrate through personal or other experiences how a sexual decision is made. As a role model, the leader not only serves as a dynamic educator, but by sharing her own sexual decision making, gives the teens implicit permission to discuss their own feelings and values regarding sexuality and contraception.

This part of the teaching strategy uses the general concepts of decision making to look at the more specific process of sexual and contraceptive decision making. The concept of role modeling is an integral part of the teaching strategy. Kramer[13] described modeling as ''behavior that takes place in response to modeling stimuli'' (p. 50). It is a type of vicarious learning phenomenon in which the teacher provides an example that can be imitated by the learner. Bevis[12] described role modeling as ''self-experienced'' learning. While teens are in the process of developing their new self-concepts, they need a safe environment in which they can ''try on'' and experience new behaviors. This is a step in directing their own learning and another step towards independence.

The role-model exercise involves both leaders: one presents a sexual decision-making example while the other clarifies the process by paraphrasing, reflecting, or asking the first leader questions. The focus is on feelings, values, and the decision-making process rather than on any specific incident. The role modeling might proceed as follows:

Leader 1: My partner and I had sex a few times before we talked about pregnancy or birth control. It was then that I realized how confused my feelings were about continuing to have sex with him, and I made the decision not to have sex again until I was less confused.

Leader 2: Abstinence—or no sex at all—that's the best method of birth control! So, you started out making a decision not about intercourse but about birth control. Then you realized having sexual intercourse was in conflict with your values, attitudes, and feelings about yourself.

Leader 1: Yes. In a sense I had already made a decision to have sex. But when I came against the obstacles of my feelings and personal values, I had to choose an alternative so that I could feel good about myself.

Leader 2: That doesn't happen to everybody, although you made a right decision for you. I made a different decision, a very conscious decision to have sex. But I knew that I didn't want to become pregnant. My obstacle was communication. It took me awhile to be able to talk with my boyfriend about birth control. Then when we did talk about contraception, neither of us knew where to go for it.

Leader 1: So you made the decision about sexual intercourse and pregnancy, but met some barriers in the area of communication and contraception. It was hard to talk about birth control with your partner and you didn't know about available services.

In this way, the group leaders were able to introduce factors which inhibit and motivate people in making decisions about sexual intercourse, parenting, and contraception.

The leaders may want to go on to list some specific examples of obstacles and motivators in seeking and using contraception. Among the obstacles are fear of reprisal by authority figures, lack of knowledge about birth control methods, embarrassment about their new self-concept as sexually active people, fear of side effects of birth control methods, lack of planning to have sex, and the belief that conception is not in the realm of reality for them. Motivating factors include increased awareness of self as a sexually active person, support from partner and significant others, knowledge of services, peer knowledge of services, peer acceptance of birth control methods, and fear of pregnancy.

The time necessary for introducing the decision-making process and putting it into context with the sexual role-model excercise is approximately 15 to 20 minutes. The teens are usually comfortable during the "jeans" presentation, freely contributing to the discussion. But when the information about sexual decision making is introduced, the group almost always becomes silent and fidgety. Upon being reassured that they are not required to participate, however, they once again become attentive, and one can perceive much nonverbal response. Heads nod, there are smiles and frowns, and occasionally someone even says, "Yeah, I've felt that way, too!"

At this point the leaders must assess the adolescents' understanding of decision making and their ability to share feelings and questions about their own choices. Some groups immediately begin focusing on what led them to seek contraceptive care and proceed to discuss obstacles and alternatives to that decision. Others are more reticent or are confused about the decision-making process. With groups such as the latter in mind, a third exercise has been developed which is directed specifically to the individual's own private sexual and contraceptive situation.

The group is encouraged to arrange themselves comfortably on their cushions or chairs and to lean back and close their eyes. To dispel any suspicion that the teenagers will be called upon to reveal private information, the leaders reassure the group, saying, "We are going to ask you just to *think* about your own decision-making process." They then proceed to guide the teenagers' thoughts in the appropriate direction.

Think about a sexual relationship, or if you have never been sexually active, imagine such an experience. We are going to review the decision you had to or would have had to make in that new situation.

Focus on who you were with and where you were . . . how did you feel? Who made the decision to have intercourse, one or both of you? Do you remember thinking about pregnancy? If you did, do you remember if you talked about your feelings? What did your partner say? Did you think about birth control? Did you think about a particular method? How did you make the decision whether or not to use birth control?

Once you chose a method, where did you go to get what you needed? What were the obstacles or barriers to getting it? Were you afraid of side effects? Were you afraid your parents would find out? Were you afraid of asking someone for birth control and admitting you were sexually active?

Did your partner help you overcome any barriers? Did you talk about alternatives to the method you chose? Then once you obtained a method, what were the barriers to using it consistently? Was it messy or did you forget to use it? What were the factors which prompted you to use that method?

The exercise lasts five to ten minutes, after which the group leaders invite the teens to share any of their thoughts or feelings about their own decision-making processes or on birth control in general. Reassurance of privacy is once again important; the focus is on the process through which they reached a decision and not the content of that choice or any personal facts which influenced it. Direct and clarifying questioning often is helpful, for the group may have initial difficulty sharing feelings and ideas due to the sensitive nature of the subject matter.

Adolescents are in the process of developing a new adult identity, which often produces physical, social and psychological instability. The sexual self is certainly part of that new identity. Questions can therefore assist by helping teens focus on their new sexual identity and behavior; by providing a framework for organizing their feelings, values, and behavior; and, once again, by eliciting feedback about their understanding of how a decision is made.

The following is an example of an interchange between a group of adolescents and its leaders:

Leader 1: After thinking through your own decision-making process, what do you think is the most important decision for you to make now?

Teen 1: Not to get pregnant.

Leader 1: So you have decided you want to continue sexual activity, but you don't want to get pregnant?

Teen 1: Right.

Leader 2: Then what is your next step in the decision-making process?

Teen 1: To use birth control!

Leader 1: (To the group) Now that she has made that decision, what does she have to think about?

Teen 2: The kind of birth control that she wants.

Leader 2: Remember when we talked about choosing jeans? I mentioned some obstacles to a decision. What are some factors that might keep her from using birth control pills?

Teen 3: They might make her fat.

Leader 1: So side effects can be an obstacle.

Teen 4: Her mother might find them and throw them out.

Leader 2: Pressure from parents is another obstacle. (Specific problems with parents often are mentioned and a discussion usually ensues about parents' versus teens' values.)

Teen 2: What about blood clots . . . or cancer from the Pill?

Leader 2: [Blood clots are a possible side effect of the Pill. Currently no research has shown an increased risk for cancer.] (To the group) What do you know about side effects to the Pill? (Another discussion begins regarding thromboembolism and [side effects] as related to oral contraceptives.)

Leader 1: What are the alternatives to the Pill if she is unable to use it?

Teen 5: She could use a diaphragm—but how effective is it?

The above conversation is typical for the remainder of the session. Depending on the group's interests and concerns, discussions may focus on communication between partners about sexuality and contraception or attitudes toward pregnancy and abortion rather than on parents' reactions. But questions relating to specific contraceptive use—side effects, effectiveness, safety, and partner responsibility—always arise during the session.

The remainder of the "rap" is utilized to answer individual questions. These questions are placed in the context of decision making. If the adolescent is concerned about side effects, the leaders help them to see that side effects are an inhibiting factor in the decision-making process. The teenager can then move on to look at alternative solutions, should the side effects become a problem. Such a teaching strategy can provide a safe environment for the teen to explore alternatives and solutions. The teenager is challenged to participate actively in affirming a plan of action best suited to her values.

This teaching strategy has proved effective for integrating contraceptive information with a process of decision making. It encourages group participation, maintains an active interest, and allows teens to formulate their own ideas and questions. Furthermore, subjective responses from participating teens indicate that the method is accepted and generally successful.

With this strategy, the adolescent is offered a safe environment in which to explore the decision-making process and is challenged to participate actively in affirming a plan of action best suited to his or her individual values. The role of the leader (and other clinic personnel) is to be an ally in decision making, not the decision maker. The teaching strategy therefore not only conveys the necessary information about contraception but helps teens to put the facts to good use. It teaches them to make an informed decision and thus promotes the achievement of an important developmental task—independence and value clarity.

VALUES CLARIFICATION STRATEGY

In addition to making satisfying decisions, developing values and ideals that give meaning to life is an important part of our existence. The teenager who is in the process of making decisions about pregnancy, sexual activity, and birth control must consider many other factors. Factors such as future life goals, self-image, or parental expectations must be considered along with reproductive values and goals. Values which surround reproductive issues influence the teenager's choices and decisions. Every decision that is made and every course of action that is taken is based on consciously or unconsciously held beliefs, attitudes, and values, many of which are in a state of flux for the adolescent. Ideally, these choices are made on the basis of the values a person holds, but frequently people are not clear about their values. Everyone, at one time or another, becomes confused about personal values. But for young people these value conflicts are more acute since they are in the process of developing a personal value system for adulthood.

One method which attempts to help people think through values issues for themselves is the Values Clarification model. This method, developed by Raths, Harmin, and Simon,[14] does not aim at instilling any particular set of values. Rather, the goal of this approach is to encourage people to discover their own values. Like the decision-making approach, the values-clarification method is concerned with the process people use in developing their values.

Kirschenbaum[15] defines the valuing process as "a process by which we increase the likelihood that our living, in general, or a decision, in particular, will have a positive value for us—and second, be constructive in the social context" (p. 102).

It is predicted that the values clarification process will help to bring a person's thoughts and actions into congruence. Through the use of value-clarification activities, the individual is encouraged to explore his own valuing process in order to unify thoughts, feelings, and actions. It has been hypothesized that the valuing process can produce change within the individual. Rokeach[16] found that this process tends to cause conflict within the individual because of contradictions in his personal value system. When the conflict occurs, the individual seeks to realign his values to coincide with his new self-concept. Rokeach concludes that a person will change in order to eliminate the inevitable dissatisfaction.

Miller[17] in a study of unwanted pregnancies discovered periods of vulnerability in a woman's reproductive cycle. He describes one stage as occurring when a woman first becomes sexually active. She finds herself developing new feelings about herself and others. The teenager who is sexually active may therefore experience acute value confusion, for she must explore not only her new sexual indentity but also other factors in her adolescent growth and development.

As part of the normal growth and development process, the teenager begins to adopt independent values which will take the place of values that she once unquestioningly accepted from parents, teachers, or extended family. The formation of personal values which are uniquely her own requires the adolescent to consciously and unconsciously explore and question the values taken from others. The teen needs to be allowed to choose freely those values which are important to her rather than adopt a set of values only to maintain a relationship or to please someone else.

The methodology of values clarification is composed of active exercises to be utilized in a group setting. This method of teaching is specifically applicable to an adolescent birth control clinic, since values confusion is common in the area of teenage sexuality. Teens are constantly bombarded by different sets of shoulds and should nots. Parents offer one set; the church suggests another. The peer group offers a third view of values, and popular magazines present a fourth view. The young person is ultimately left to make his own choice about whose advice or values to follow. Too often, teens have not learned a process for selecting the best and rejecting the worst elements contained in the various value systems which others have been urging them to follow. Therefore, the important choices in life are made on the basis of peer pressure, unthinking submission to authority, or the power of propaganda.

The values clarification method was developed in the traditional classroom, but can easily be adapted to the clinic setting where teens are particularly concerned with sexual and contraceptive values. With this method, the leader introduces specific exercises in the area of contraceptive knowledge and sexuality. The goal is to involve the group in considering practical experiences, giving them permission to become aware of their own sexual feelings, their own ideas, their own beliefs, so that choices and decisions they make are conscious and deliberate, based on their own value systems. The important point to remember regarding the values clarification process is that it does not seek to develop a particular set of values, but rather desires to help teens better perceive the values they already possess.

The following exercises have been adapted from Simon, Kirschenbaum, and Morrisson. They are presented in a sequential fashion, as they might be used in a clinic session. Two or three can be used in a 30-minute session. These value clarification activities can be adapted to fit other situations and target populations.

VALUES CLARIFICATION EXERCISES

Group Building Activity*

Building trust among participants is important to effective group functioning. This is especially important when discussion centers around controversial topics such as sexuality and reproduction. Starting the group interaction with an exercise in which members learn one another's names is a first step to decreasing anxiety and promoting participation by each individual.

PROCEDURE:

1. Form a circle.
2. Give the following directions:
   We will be talking about all sorts of things which concern us personally. When I talk to people, I like to be identified as (first name), not as some nameless person who happens to be speaking. It is important to me that people know and remember my name and use it when they are talking to me. You may not feel as strongly about this, but it probably makes you feel good when other people remember your name and use it.

   To help us remember each other's names, I will start by saying my name. Then the person to my right will give the name that he or she prefers being called, and will repeat my name. We will continue around the circle with each person in turn giving his or her name and repeating the names of those who went before.
3. After all have introduced themselves, an option is to change the seating arrangement and practice again. (Usually there is not enough time to allow for this option.)

What We Know and What We Want to Know†

In order to individualize the content provided to the teenage client, it is necessary to determine what the group already knows. This strategy provides a creative and active method for determining the level of knowledge among the participants and also generates group interest in the area of sexuality and birth control. In addition, this exercise teaches a method which may be helpful with future decisions and values questions.

PROCEDURE:

1. At the beginning of the class on contraception, the leader says, "There are many things you probably already know about this topic, and even may have studied it formally in school. Let's see what you know about birth control."
2. Two group members are picked to be board secretaries to record items of information on a chalk board. No judgment is made about any item. If a teen

---

*From *Values In Sexuality: A New Approach to Sex Education* by Eleanor S. Morrison and Mila Underhill Price, copyright 1974 Hart Publishing Co., Inc., p. 15.

† Adapted from *Values Clarification: A Practical Handbook of Practical Strategies for Teachers and Students* by Sidney B. Simon, Leland W. Howe, and Howard Kirschenbaum, copyright 1972 Hart Publishing Co., Inc., p. 335.

contributes it, it goes up on the board. (Later on, either the group will discover or the leader can point out any factual errors.)

3. When all the things the group knows about birth control are up on the board, the leader says, "OK, now what don't you know about birth control? Let's organize another list of all the things we want to find out about this topic."

4. Again, the board secretaries record all of the ideas. The leader can and should contribute items to both lists.

Strongly Agree—Strongly Disagree*

Many reproductive decisions do not allow intermediate reactions or "maybe's"—one is either pregnant or not. This strategy forces teens to examine the strength of their feelings about a given series of issues surrounding sexuality and contraceptive values.

PROCEDURE:

The leader provides the teens with a worksheet containing a series of belief statements. The worksheet is completed individually. Then the leader breaks the group into groups of three to share and discuss their responses. (In a small group, this will not be necessary.)

Worksheet:

Instructions: Circle the response which most closely indicates the way you feel about each item:

SA   Strongly Agree
AS   Agree Somewhat
DS   Disagree Somewhat
SD   Strongly Disagree

ITEM	RESPONSE
1. I would encourage nonmarital sex for everyone.	SA AS DS SD
2. I think the Pill is the best method of birth control.	
3. I want to be pregnant before I am married.	SA AS DS SD
4. I think the diaphragm is an easy method of birth control to use.	SA AS DS SD
5. Most men like to use rubbers.	SA AS DS SD
6. My partner doesn't want to take responsibility for birth control.	SA AS DS SD
7. Sex should be spontaneous and birth control takes all the spontaneity out of sex.	SA AS DS SD
8. The easiest time to get pregnant is right after my period.	SA AS DS SD
9. I would like to talk to my parents about sex and birth control.	SA AS DS SD
10. If I had a choice, I would rather not have sex at all.	SA AS DS SD

*Adapted from *Values Clarification: A Practical Handbook of Practical Strategies for Teachers and Students* by Sidney B. Simon, Leland W. Howe, and Howard Kirschenbaum, copyright 1972 Hart Publishing Co., Inc., p. 252.

Values Choice Exercise*

In order to choose one alternative and reject others, the teens have to examine their feelings and their values. This process helps the individuals to clarify what is really important to them. Having to justify a choice forces a person to look carefully at the decision and evaluate it clearly.

PROCEDURE:

1. Introduce the excercise to the entire group: We are going to do an exercise called values choice, and in the process we will break into small groups. I will read a set of statements. Each of you is to choose which of the statements is the most important in your life and which is least important. Then we will discuss the reasons for your choice.
2. It is important that individuals do not take a great deal of time to make their decisions, but rather trust their initial response. After discussing their choices with the group, they may discover that they would have chosen differently if they had taken other factors into account, or they may find they can trust their initial reactions.
3. Read the first set of statements:
   The method of birth control I would choose would be:
   . . . no sex
   . . . the Pill
   . . . diaphragm
   . . . IUD
   . . . foam and rubbers
   . . . other
   Of the possible side effects of the Pill, which one would keep me from choosing it as a birth control method?
   . . . weight gain
   . . . breakthrough bleeding
   . . . skipped periods
   . . . moodiness
   The worst thing I could find out about my boyfriend—girlfriend is that he/she:
   . . . has VD
   . . . is sterile
   . . . is having sex with another person
   If my parents discovered that I was using birth control, I would:
   . . . feel good that we could be more honest with each other
   . . . stop using birth control
   . . . be afraid of being punished
4. Give five to ten minutes for sharing each time you present a set of statements. Encourage the group to think about questions such as, "What made me choose this statement rather than one of the others? What does that tell me

*From *Values In Sexuality: A New Approach to Sex Education* by Eleanor S. Morrison and Mila Underhill Price, copyright 1974 Hart Publishing Co., Inc., p. 95.

about myself?'' Suggest that they not be judgmental toward those who have different reasons for their choices and try to understand what others are trying to communicate.

Alternative Action Search*

Decisions which are made without consideration of alternatives and consequences may later be regretted by the teenager. This strategy enables the teenager to consider alternatives for action in various situations. The goal is to help the teenager act in a way that is consistent with his or her feelings and beliefs.

PROCEDURE:

The leader introduces this activity by initiating a discussion about things that we did that we later regretted (e.g., buying a pair of shoes that looked good but were uncomfortable, or forgetting to tell someone special how much you appreciate them). Then the teens are presented with a specific situation or vignette which calls for some proposed action. (See sample vignettes which follow.) The leader then asks, ''Now, given all your beliefs, feelings, and values related to this example, ideally, what would you want to do in this situation?'' If the group is large, separate into smaller groups of three or four.

Sample Vignettes:

1. Sandra has been going out with Steve, on and off for a few months. He starts pushing her to have sex. Sandra says no, because she doesn't love him. He keeps hassling her. Finally she says, ''Well, I guess so.''
2. John and Barbara have been seeing each other regularly. When they started having sex, both of them went to a birth control clinic where Barbara was fitted for a diaphragm. She uses it every time they make love, but tonight she forgot to put it in before they went out. Barbara and John make love anyway.
3. Sue got a birth control method from a clinic without her parents' knowledge. She has been using it consistently and is sure she doesn't want to become pregnant. One day she discovers that her mother has found her birth control method.

Removing Barriers to Action†

Teenagers may be willing to take a stand, to articulate a value, to affirm it publicly, and to choose freely from alternatives with knowledge of the consequences, but they may be unwilling or unable to act upon a decision because of perceived or real barriers to action. This strategy is designed to help teens identify and remove barriers to action which often block their values development.

---

* Adapted from *Values Clarification: A Practical Handbook of Practical Strategies for Teachers and Students* by Sidney B. Simon, Leland W. Howe, and Howard Kirschenbaum, copyright 1972 Hart Publishing Co., Inc., p. 198.

† Adapted from *Values Clarification: A Practical Handbook of Practical Strategies for Teachers and Students* by Sidney B. Simon, Leland W. Howe, and Howard Kirschenbaum, copyright 1972 Hart Publishing Co., Inc., p. 209.

PROCEDURE:

The leader asks one member of the group to write at the top of the blackboard the decision she would like to make regarding contraception. For example, 'I have chosen _____ as a method of preventing pregnancy.'' Then she draws a line lengthwise down the middle of the blackboard. On the right-hand side of the line she is to list all of the perceived or real barriers, both within and outside herself, which seem to keep her from acting on the decision. On the left-hand side of the line she is to list steps she could take which might help remove or reduce each of the barriers. Finally, on the back of the board or leaving space at the bottom, she is to develop a plan of action for actually removing the barriers. This exercise can be repeated using the example of another contraceptive method.

Other examples might be:

I am pregnant and wish to keep the baby.
My boyfriend and I are eighteen and want to get married.

Role-Play: Parental Attitudes Toward Sexual Behavior

Research and experience seem to indicate that the liberal attitudes toward sex expressed by young people are often in sharp contrast to what their attitudes would be as parents. This is demonstrated by their responses when they place themselves in a parenting role and respond to specific hypothetical situations. This exercise was designed by the writer to make individuals aware of that inconsistency.

Usually, the exploration of options and alternatives stimulates new ideas and triggers a rethinking of customary responses.

Situation:

Now let's do a future projection. It is years from now. You are married and have children. Your 15-year-old daughter has been going out with a 19-year-old man, much against your better judgment. One day you discover her leaving her bedroom with an old pack of birth control pills which you had forgotten to throw away when you switched to a different formula. What do you say or do?

Discussion Questions:

1. Does what you would like to do match how you feel now about the situation?
2. How do the actions you would like to take differ from your feelings?
3. Do you find yourself being less ''liberal'' when people younger than you are involved?
4. How do you think the daughter might feel?

(Another situation would be to follow this up by changing the age of the daughter to 12 or 13.)

ASSURING SUCCESS OF TEACHING STRATEGIES

Certain factors are important to the success of both the decision-making and the values-clarification teaching strategies.

Leadership is an essential component for a successful group activity. If possible, co-leading should be considered. A good combination is a man and a woman or a professional and a teen volunteer. The strategy of two leaders reflects an interdisciplinary approach to human sexuality, contraception, and values, especially when the team shares the planning and teaching responsibilities. Having an equal representation of sexes also provides a positive role model for male-female communication. The values clarification process can be exciting and stimulating for the group leaders: they can directly witness the process of human growth and discovery. Rather than promote their own values, the leaders can create an environment where teenagers can develop and explore the values they want to live by.

Other factors influencing the effective use of the teaching strategies are time and continuity. It is difficult enough to establish rapport with one person. How do we do it with a group of people, within a reasonable length of time, so that they can get started on a problem? This factor is clearly dependent on the leadership component. The leader's patience and awareness of the difficulties involved in establishing trust, interest, and openness in a group situation are prerequisites to getting started. The active exercises of the two strategies also help to stimulate interest and create openness. The leader must then encourage the teens to feel free to differ and to express their feeling toward the group work and each other as the work progresses.

An important aspect of these strategies is that the group discussion approach utilizes the motivation of peer support. Messanotte[18] has utilized group education and found that in a group of preoperative patients, individuals have a tendency to identify with others having the same goals or problems and thus gain moral support and encouragement through this identification. In Messanotte's study, 20 of 24 patients preferred the group session to an individualized session.

Ohlsen[19] points out that group education can facilitate an adolescent's self-understanding, the development of ego strength, the search for identity, and the development of broader interpersonal relation skills. Marram[20] wrote, "The group approach tends to be an effective means of meeting an array of needs and problems . . . [and] can offer a number of advantages to persons that other approaches cannot" (p. 3). Groups can offer a source of support and guidance, a sense of identification, sound advice, and help to members in understanding the consequences of choosing one behavior over another. In addition, the group process can enhance the adolescent's awareness of new role expectations and his confidence and skill in assuming those new roles. This is especially important for sexually active adolescents who find dramatic changes occurring in their self-concepts.

EVALUATION OF TEACHING STRATEGIES

Finally, the factor of evaluation must be integrated into the teaching strategy. In order for the model to remain relevant to the educational needs of the teenagers, the content should have a built-in evaluation component which will measure both the process and the outcome. According to Meleis and Benner,[21] outcome evaluation ascertains how effective the strategy is, and process evaluation provides feedback which enables educators to change and develop the content and strategy of the model while it is still in progress. They describe outcome evaluation as a scientific approach to determining the effectiveness of programs. Process evaluation facilitates decision making aimed at effecting important changes in the objectives and strategies of an innovative teaching program.

Process evaluation that could lead to necessary changes in a contraceptive program for teens might include measures of teen satisfaction, participation, or comprehension of the decision-making or values-clarification process. After the education programs have stabilized, then outcome evaluation would be appropriate. Such an evaluation could determine whether the programs were effective in reducing unwanted teen pregnancy rates, improving return visits to the teen clinic, or increasing consistent contraceptive use.

In addition, a teen advisory committee could be developed to evaluate and improve educational models. This seems simplistic, but who can be more knowledgeable about what teenagers want to learn than teens themselves? To include a group of teens in the evaluation process of client education strategies would increase the credibility of such a program immensely.

Additional Learning Experiences During the Clinic Visit

A comprehensive, well planned educational component of the teen clinic provides for learning experiences throughout the clinic visit. A comprehensive approach to clinic education attempts to introduce practice, feedback, and reinforcement along with information. Opportunities for teaching and learning can be planned for the waiting periods and the interview session.

When the adolescent first enters the clinic, written materials can be given to be read during waiting periods. These brochures might describe various contraceptive methods, clinic procedures, or information on health topics of concern to teenagers. Audiovisual materials may be developed or purchased for explaining procedures such as the pelvic examination and laboratory tests. Since these procedures produce much anxiety for the teen attending a clinic for the first time, a thorough explanation and visual description may decrease anxiety enough to allow greater learning to occur.

The interviewing session, usually reserved for the medical and social histories, can provide an individualized aspect to the teaching-learning situation. Using the decision-making process also, the interviewer reinforces the teenager's own decision and valuing process which was presented in the group session. During the private session, the interviewer can present any additional content necessary in choosing and using birth control.

One objective of the interview session is to help the teenager explore decision making and valuing in a confidential setting. Not all people feel comfortable participating in a group setting; many can learn better in a one-to-one situation. For the teenager who needs the support of an empathetic person, who is unclear about the decision-making process, or who is uncomfortable in a group, the interview session is an acceptable educational alternative.

The interviewer may use questioning to lead the adolescent through the contraceptive decision-making process. Questioning is one way of obtaining feedback from teenagers and determining if they understand or can apply concepts. Questions which the interviewer might use to lead an adolescent through the decision making process are: What method of birth control have you chosen? What are the reasons for choosing this method? (motivating factors). What might keep you from choosing this method? (inhibiting factors). What can you do to overcome these problems? (alternatives).

The answers which the teen gives to these questions will lead the interviewer to teach content specific to sexuality and contraception. The nature of her responses will point out what that teenager is interested in learning, which is essential to any teaching-learning situation. For example, if the teen says that her choice of birth control is the diaphragm, then the interviewer will focus on that method, leaving questions about other methods until later. Perhaps the teen states that an inhibiting factor associated with using the diaphragm is that one has to use it with every coital experience. The interviewer can help the teen find ways to overcome the problem or provide her with information about a method which requires less preparation. In addition, content which the teen has learned through other sources can be clarified or corrected. Using this model allows teenagers to answer many of their own questions and promotes active participation in the learning process.

The interview session provides an opportunity to teach skills necessary to effective contraceptive use. Again, the teaching and practice of these skills fits into the decision-making format. Should the adolescent say that one of the inhibiting factors associated with using the "Pill" might be that she would forget to take it, the interviewer may respond by asking the question, "How would you overcome this obstacle?" which helps the teen develop "Pill-taking" skills.

While the decision-making model provides for the teen's active participation in the teaching-learning situation, the interviewer-teen relationship is facilitated through a more equal interchange. The interviewer allows the adolescent to verbalize about any unique variables which affect the learning situation. When given this kind of personalized instruction, the teenager is better prepared to respond to questions needed in a medical and social history. If trust is established, the teen will be more apt to give honest responses regarding reproductive and social background.

Planning learning situations throughout the clinic visit provides more educational opportunities than does the traditional lecture model limited to the group session. In addition, using a model for education provides the learner with a conceptual framework for action rather than isolated pieces of information.

Individualizing the Clinic Experience for the Teen Client

In addition to education, there are other factors which are important in individualizing the clinic experience for the teen client. Three of these factors—confidentiality, privacy, and partner involvement—will be discussed.

Confidentiality is a very important factor in a teen contraceptive clinic. According to the URSA (Urban and Rural Systems Associates) study,[6] "fear of parents finding out" was the barrier to attending a clinic mentioned more often than any other deterrent (p. 32). The areas in which confidentiality is most likely to break down are the handling of client information, the location of the clinic, or the requirements for parental consent.

Clinics must protect their client records, and, more important, they must let the teenagers know this. Releasing information to the teen client only, and not to parents or friends, is one form of protection. Another way might be to use code names when contacting the adolescent by telephone. During the initial clinic visit, the teen client and the counselor decide on a code name for the clinic which is written in the chart. If called by the clinic, the teenager is alerted to call back to the clinic. Some clinics contact teens through a school nurse or counselor.

Clinic location is an important factor when planning teen contraceptive services. According to URSA, teens find it difficult to get to clinics that are located far away, and will not use a clinic which parents or peers might see them enter.[6] This same study suggests that the ideal clinic site, in terms of confidentiality and convenience, is in a large, nearby facility which houses many different programs.

Other reasons for possible breach of confidentiality are local or state requirements for parental consent to obtain contraceptives. However, with increased liberalization of legal statutes regarding adolescent health care, the need for parental consent will not deter teenagers from attending family planning clinics. Some state laws require a minor to obtain parental consent prior to care. Many states are changing such laws, and in some instances clinic staff do not police these regulations. However, young teenagers will continue to encounter difficulty in consenting for their own contraceptive care.

Including boyfriends in the clinic process was considered important by the majority of teenagers participating in the URSA study.[6] When questioned, less than half of the young men "felt completely comfortable being in a clinic, partly out of general embarrassment and a sense that they didn't belong there" (p. 57). Most teenage males need information about birth control, but rarely do they attend the clinic sessions with their partners.[22] Because of prevailing attitudes of male participation in the birth control process, it may be difficult to include adolescent males in the clinic visit. But, as discussed earlier, encouraging partners to participate in the contraceptive decision making is vital to effective contraceptive behavior on the part of the young woman. The availability of male counselors and co-leaders for groups in the clinic may attract more young men.

Privacy is important to the teenager and needs to be maintained during the clinic process. The need for privacy involves the teenager's concerns about anonymity, modesty, and self-disclosure. Privacy during all phases of the clinic experience is important. At the reception desk, speaking quietly and directly to the teen rather than calling out names in a crowded waiting room can ease the young woman's fears. During the interview, privacy can be maintained by closing doors, protecting the chart information, and conducting interviews in a private space.

The physical examination is the event that causes most young women to feel most uncomfortable and exposed. Often, this is the teenager's first pelvic examination, and removing clothes in the presence of strangers can be an embarrassing and anxious experience. Protection of privacy is most important at this point in the clinic visit. Providing gowns and private dressing facilities can help to ease the teenager's anxiety. By these seemingly minor efforts made during the clinic procedure, the staff is demonstrating to the young woman that her privacy is respected; this approach can also make it easier for her to return to the clinic at another time.

Many factors both affect the adolescent's ability to learn during the clinic visit and influence her willingness to continue with future clinic visits. Other aspects of a teen contraceptive clinic, specific to local communities, must be considered. For example, appointment schedules, fees, staff attitudes, and community constraints must be carefully explored so that they do not act as barriers to clinic attendance. Possible barriers to adolescent health care are discussed in Section 4.

Helping the Teenager Choose a Method of Contraception

Thus far, the emphasis has been on the role of the professional as a facilitator in the contraceptive care of the adolescent. The decision making lies with the individual adolescent, whereas the professional's responsibility is essentially to clarify, reflect, support, and promote decision making for the teenager who is confronted with problems of potential pregnancy, contraception, or sexual relationships. However, the professional in a contraceptive clinic also has the responsibility of providing information about specific contraceptive methods. Helping the teenager to find a satisfactory method of birth control is an important aspect of total comprehensive contraceptive care.

Although there is a large body of knowledge about the advantages and disadvantages of various methods of contraception, there is a limited amount of information about individualizing contraceptive methods for the adolescent. It is the professional's responsibility to inform the teenager that one method may be better suited to her physiology and sexual activity. In addition, there are certain factors to consider about contraceptive choice for the adolescent client which differ from those associated with counseling of the adult. The following section will describe each contraceptive method and special considerations for counseling the adolescent.

The professional who first counsels the teenager prior to her physical examination is in an influential position. He or she is providing an environment in which the adolescent can explore her values and focus on her reproductive decisions. The professional is also individualizing the contraceptive information that is necessary for a "teen" contraceptive decision—a contraceptive decision that will fit the developing young woman's individual life style.

ORAL CONTRACEPTION

On her initial visit to a contraceptive clinic, the typical teenager who is sexually active will have inconsistently used poor methods of birth control. However, when asked prior to any counseling which method of contraception she will choose, the response will most often be "The Pill." Most teenagers choose oral contraception as their birth control method for these reasons: "It is the most effective." "It is the best-known method of birth control." "I don't have to think about using it during sex." "My friends use it."

General medical contraindications to oral contraceptive use are widely discussed in contraceptive literature. However, there are also a few specific considerations to bear in mind when recommending oral contraception for the adolescent client.

One theory advanced against prescribing hormonal contraception for the young woman is that it may suppress her hypothalamus, making it incapable of stimulating ovulation when the Pill is discontinued. In addition, it has been suggested that administration of hormones may close her epiphyses prematurely, precluding growth of her long bones. However, this argument has been refuted by several authors and in fact there is evidence to show that should the adolescent become pregnant, her increased estrogen level would certainly limit her long bone growth more than would the dosage received from the Pill.[4] More important, by the time of menarche, which is occurring at younger ages (at approximately 12½ years) most physiological growth has been completed.[23]

Even though a young woman under 20 years of age is at less risk than older women for other side effects from the Pill, such as thromboembolism, it is recommended that a low estrogen dose Pill (less than 50 micrograms) be prescribed.[24,25] Stolley[26] found that the risk of thromboembolism was decreased by 28% with the use of a Pill with lower estrogen content. Shearin,[25] in a three-year study of contraceptive use by teenagers, reported that less serious side effects such as nervousness, crying, depression, irritability, fatigue, and "feeling of being fat" were a nuisance to most teenagers and influenced Pill continuation. Although not proven, a low estrogen Pill may reduce these "nuisance" side effects and promote consistent contraceptive use by the teen client.

However, the low estrogen dose Pill is not without side effects of its own—primarily breakthrough bleeding and amenorrhea. The teenager must be carefully counseled about these possible ocurrences and must be assured that the symptoms can be alleviated. The young woman should be told that Pill-amenorrhea (when it is not pregnancy) is not an irreversible side effect. Because the amenorrhea is due to a shallow atrophic endometrium, the teen should be reassured that once the Pill is discontinued, normal endometrial growth and function will resume. When breakthrough bleeding occurs, Speroff[27] recommends a short course of exogenous estrogen rather than changing to a higher dose pill. He suggests that Premarin 2.5 mg or ethinyl estradiol 20 μg be administered for seven days in order to stop the bleeding episode.

These clinical factors are important for the safe prescription of oral contraceptives for the adolescent client. In addition, factors specific to contraceptive use and continuation must be considered. Professional counseling for the teenager who desires the Pill as her method of birth control should include the following topics in the counseling session:

1. Forgetting to take a Pill: this may occur because of infrequent sexual activity or not being accustomed to taking medications on a regular basis. A young woman who is ambivalent about pregnancy may also neglect to take her Pill properly.
2. Parents' knowledge of birth control use: the teenager may find it difficult to take the Pills consistently if she must hide her method from her parents.
3. Peer group or partner's acceptance of birth control method: teenagers are influenced by their friends' information about contraceptive use. Many young women, when asked where they obtained inaccurate information about oral

contraceptives, say, "My friend told me." Also, teenagers tend to adhere to traditional sex roles while in the process of developing their own unique sexual identity. It is not unusual for a young woman to defer to her boyfriend's decision about birth control. If the young man has heard rumors of problems with oral contraception, he may forbid his partner to use this method.

4. Inability to cope with side effects which occur (e.g., weight gain, nausea, breakthrough bleeding, amenorrhea). The adolescent who has experienced any irregularities in her menstrual or endocrine system is often alarmed by such symptoms brought on by the Pill. Counseling about possible side effects is very important for continued use of this method. If the young woman has no plan of action for dealing with side effects due to the Pill, she may discontinue its use.

Equally important, the teenager should understand the relationship of the Pill to the functioning of her menstrual cycle. Teenagers commonly discontinue Pill use mid-cycle and thereby cause irregular bleeding or amenorrhea. Also, the adolescent client may not understand that she must take a Pill every day and not just on the day she engages in intercourse.

The teenager may also find it difficult to remember to consider birth control if she has not incorporated sexual activity into her repertoire of behaviors—she may not feel comfortable with her new sexual identity and may therefore use contraception erratically or not at all. In addition, if intercourse is occurring infrequently, the young woman may want to consider another method which would not affect her endocrine system on a continuous basis. Counseling and providing information about mechanical methods might be appropriate at this time.

INTRAUTERINE CONTRACEPTION

In the past, the intrauterine device (IUD) was considered the method of choice for the young woman who, for medical reasons, or because of her fears or dislike of oral contraception, needed a method other than the Pill. Currently, though, there is much concern over an increase in pelvic infections, especially in the young, never-pregnant population, and some clinicians are reluctant to use IUDs unless the patient has been pregnant and has no history of serious vaginal infection or salpingitis. There is recent evidence that never-pregnant IUD wearers have a greater incidence of pelvic infections which could possibly limit future fertility. Swedish investigators reported that the incidence of acute salpingitis was increased sevenfold in the never-pregnant IUD user, whereas there was only a twofold increase in the sometime pregnant IUD user.[28]

Based on this research, it is suggested that the teenager who is sexually active with multiple partners (which increases her risk of infection) or who has a history of pelvic infection should be counseled to use some other form of contraception rather than risk the immediate or future complications of infections.

However, there are situations where the IUD may be indicated for the occasional adolescent client who is multiparous or exceptionally mature. The most commonly used IUDs are the plastic devices (e.g., Lippes Loop, Saf-T-Coil) and the copper-bearing device (e.g., Cu–7). The smaller copper-bearing devices are more suitable for nulliparous and adolescent women because there is less pain associated with insertion. There is no significant difference in pregnancy rates among users of the various IUDs, although the rate of expulsion is increased with the smaller IUDs. Intermenstrual bleeding and dysmenorrhea are often a problem in the nulliparous woman but are not restricted to a particular IUD.[29]

It is important that a discussion of IUD use, insertion, and side effects occur in a personal dialogue between counselor and adolescent. The following are special considerations for counseling the young woman who chooses the IUD as her method of contraception:

1. Preparation of the young woman for insertion and use of the IUD should include a thorough discussion of where it is to be placed. Adolescent women are frequently confused about the anatomy of their reproductive organs and a model of the uterus and vagina, as well as pictures, is essential in helping them to visualize the position of the device.
2. If the adolescent has a stable relationship with one partner, it would be helpful to involve him also in the teaching and counseling about the IUD. The adolescent male is often not knowledgeable about the anatomy and physiology of the female reproductive system and may have fears about where this device is placed and whether it might injure his penis. He may not be able to voice this concern, but if he has a clear picture of the location and function of the IUD, he may be helpful and supportive in the continued use of the device. Many IUDs are removed because of complaints of the partner stemming from fears for himself.
3. The adolescent needs concrete and sensitive instruction about checking the IUD string monthly so that she is continually reassured that the device remains in place. For many young women, touching the genital area is difficult because of childhood prohibitions. Again, visual aids are an important teaching tool so that the teen can see that the IUD cannot get ''lost'' and that she will not injure herself by placing fingers in her vagina. For young couples who are comfortable with the idea, the partner can check for the string as part of sexual foreplay.
4. The possible side effects of the use of the IUD, such as increased or mid-cycle bleeding, longer duration of menstruation, dysmenorrhea, and leukorrhea, should be discussed, and reassurance should be given that if these symptoms continue, or if they are too severe, the device can be removed. The teenager who chooses the IUD needs help in understanding the possible consequences involved with use of the IUD and her personal responsibility in caring for her reproductive health. Although these topics are important for all of the birth control methods, they are of special concern with the IUD because possible side effects could seriously affect the young woman's future pregnancy plans.
   It is important to emphasize the possibility of pelvic infection with the IUD and to carefully explain the symptoms to watch for. The teen should be

counseled to contact the clinic if unusual cramping or bleeding occurs intermenstrually, if she experiences dyspareunia, or if she becomes febrile with no other known cause. To prevent future complications, it is wise to impress upon the teenager that she should consult the clinic whenever she has questions about the IUD or symptomatology indicating a pelvic infection. Too often, young women will refrain from calling their clinicians with what they consider to be minor complaints. They should be made to feel the reassurance that no question is too simple; also, these questions and inquiries can be productively utilized as informal teaching situations.

5. The young woman needs to know that the IUD, just as other contraceptive methods, can fail to prevent pregnancy and that if she suspects pregnancy she should immediately seek professional advice. While the IUD prevents intrauterine conception at a rate of about 98%, it prevents tubal pregnancy at a rate of only 90%.[29] A woman who becomes pregnant with an IUD in situ has about one chance in 20 of having an ectopic pregnancy.[29] Abortion, as a backup to contraception, often seems acceptable to the adolescent who has an IUD in place or who has unknowingly expelled it. The failure is not hers but is rather the fault of the method, which can allay feelings of guilt she may have about being pregnant.

So that a pregnancy may be detected early, the clinician can suggest that the young woman keep a record of her menstrual cycle. The menstrual record is also of benefit in teaching the young woman to become aware of her reproductive cycles, and can be recommended along with any chosen contraceptive method.

DIAPHRAGM

More and more teenagers are choosing the diaphragm as their primary contraceptive method. It is a good method for the young woman who has intercourse infrequently and neither needs nor wishes to put up with some of the side effects or possible complications associated with the Pill or the IUD. In the largest study of diaphragm use in the United States, Lane, Arceo, and Sobrero[30] found that among 2,000 young, mostly never-married, never-pregnant women who chose the diaphragm, only 2% became accidentally pregnant, and more than 80% continued to use the method after the first year.

However, the mechanical barriers to using the diaphragm are often too great for the teenager to overcome. Not only must she be comfortable enough with her body to properly insert and remove the diaphragm, but she must also think about birth control with every act of intercourse. For the young woman who is only beginning to explore and define her sexual identity and anatomy these tasks are often overwhelming.

It is common to hear the teen saying that she "forgot to use the diaphragm," or "It just didn't seem right," or "It was too much trouble." Whatever the reasons, the teen is communicating that she has not fully incorporated birth control behavior into her repertoire of sexual behaviors. Using the diaphragm consistently may be difficult for the teen who is often romantic and idealistic about her new sexuality. Spontaneity and excitement are important qualities in the sexual relationship and interrupting this to insert a diaphragm may be impossible.

Fitting of the diaphragm and subsequent follow-up are critical in the case of the adolescent client. The teenager must know exactly how to use the diaphragm before she leaves the clinic; requiring her to return two weeks after examination will allow a time for experimentation and for questions or problems to be resolved.

The clinician must be assured that the largest diaphragm is chosen—it should rest with its posterior rim behind the cervix and its anterior rim in the groove behind the symphysis pubis—but must make certain that the young woman has no sensation of its being in place. Another important consideration is that the teen be able to manipulate the rim of the diaphragm for easy insertion and removal. The clinician should require the teenager to demonstrate that she is able to place the diaphragm properly as well as to remove it. In order to reduce any embarrassment that the teenager might experience, the clinician or counselor can demonstrate various positions for diaphragm insertion (e.g., squatting, sitting, lying down). Going through the motions of diaphragm insertion and removal involves the clinician with the teen's experience and decreases anxiety in a way that verbal instruction cannot.

Certain points are important to consider when counseling the teen who chooses the diaphragm:

1. A willingness to touch her body is crucial to consistent use of the diaphragm. If the teen is hesitant or repulsed by touching or examining her vagina, the diaphragm will probably be kept in the case. Staying in the examination room to observe, as well as to assist the teen in inserting her diaphragm, can help the clinician assess how willing she is to touch her body. The use of female clinicians is important in order to decrease embarrassment on the part of the teen client.
2. Describing the insertion of the diaphragm at various points during sexual play can assist the teenager to utilize the diaphragm. Advising her to insert the diaphragm prior to intercourse—before she leaves her house on a date, in the bathroom or in a private place—can decrease her anxiety about when to put in the diaphragm during intercourse. According to Lane and associates,[30] the teenager can be encouraged to insert the diaphragm with contraceptive jelly or cream as long as two hours in advance of anticipated need; this can decrease her anxiety about inserting the diaphragm and decreasing spontaneity in the coital act.
3. Based upon studies of intravaginal physiology by Johnson and Masters,[31] the young couple should be counseled that the diaphragm may become malpositioned during the excitement and plateau stages of the sexual cycle. This loss of position could result in a contraceptive failure. Suggestions to the teenager might be to (a) apply spermicidal jelly to the whole diaphragm; (b) check the diaphragm position post-coitally to determine if it has indeed moved off the cervix (avoid those positions during ovulation), or (c) have the male partner use a condom during the ovulation phase of the young woman's menstrual cycle.

FOAM AND CONDOMS

When used together, foam and condoms provide as much protection from pregnancy as does the Pill. Prior to attending a contraceptive clinic, these two methods and withdrawal are used most frequently by the teenage population.[3] However, when able to choose from among all contraceptive methods, teen clients will rarely decide upon foam and condoms as a primary method. It has been suggested by teens that the mechanics of incorporating condoms and foam into lovemaking decrease "spontaneity" and physical pleasure. The "messiness" and "hassle" of this method provide an actual and implied barrier to the young couple's sexual pleasure.

Although the condom and foam are inherently better adapted to sporadic sexual patterns than the Pill or the IUD, and are available in most drugstores, these methods have never achieved more than a limited degree of acceptance among the teenage population.

Yet the barrier methods have advantages which health professionals may be neglecting to emphasize sufficiently. For the teenager who has multiple partners, the condom can protect against venereal disease. Butler[32] in a study of contraceptive foam and cream found that those women who used either the vaginal cream or foam had 25% fewer gonorrhea reinfections than women who did not. This is important to note when statistics show that 1,200 out of every 100,000 women aged 15 to 19 years have had gonorrhea at one time. Also, in the teenage population, since sexual intercourse is usually infrequent or unplanned, these methods are ideal because of their lack of side effects.

It is obvious that counseling the adolescent female about use of the condom must involve her partner. Again, because adolescents often adopt stereotypical sexual roles, they may accept the belief that contraception is the woman's responsibility. It is not uncommon to find a young woman reacting negatively to the use of condoms. In a sense she is preventing her partner from accepting contraceptive responsibility by maintaining the tradition that condoms are unacceptable. This can be a good time to initiate discussion about the male's responsibility in contraceptive use and his reasons for refusing to "use a rubber." The most frequent complaints about the condom are that it reduces penile sensation or that it reduces spontaneous pleasure because the sexual activity must be interrupted in order to apply the device. These problems can be overcome in a variety of ways. Teaching can include information on the different kinds and thicknesses of condoms as well as on the possibility that putting on the condom can be incorporated into the foreplay of intercourse.

Talking about the use of foam and condoms is one way of beginning a discussion about sexuality. Usually young men and women are not very experienced in lovemaking, and sexual activity often means inserting a penis into a vagina and immediately ejaculating, with no consideration of foreplay or the young woman's orgasm. When counseling about the condom, emphasis might be placed on the fact that the condom can slow the rate of ejaculation and thereby create more sexual pleasure for both partners. It has been suggested that spermicidal preparations can interfere with oral lovemaking. However, the couple can be advised to insert the foam after oral sex and therefore avoid the offensive taste of the spermicide.

It is common for young women to complain of discomfort or lack of lubrication during sexual activity. Using a foam, cream, or jelly as a lubricant as well as a contraceptive can minimize the discomfort of vaginal irritation.

Even though the teen may choose another method of contraception, the clinician can introduce the use of foam and condoms as an alternative or "backup" method. Should pills be forgotten or a diaphragm left at home, the condom and foam can be an easily obtained method for preventing pregnancy. Supplying the teen with foam and condoms during the clinic visit is a good practice.

ABSTINENCE

Should the teenager refuse any method of contraception, her decision should be supported. The decision not to be sexually active at that time does not preclude her need for education and counseling for a future time. It is necessary to reassure the young woman that contraceptives and education will always be available to her when she wants them. To be nonjudgmental about her decision to refrain from intercourse is important, for to doubt her sincerity can keep her from returning for contraception at a later time.

Ineffective or Alternative Contraceptive Methods

There are contraceptive methods which do not work very well, such as douching, withdrawal, and rhythm. Although these methods are not recommended as effective contraception, they can be advised as an alternate or "backup" method of birth control. It is important that the teenager know the risks associated with these contraceptive methods.

DOUCHING

Douching after intercourse will wash away some of the semen but the woman cannot really douche fast enough. Sperm have already moved into the upper pelvic tract—enough sperm to fertilize an existing ovum. If the young woman is able to think about douching, perhaps she can be encouraged to plan more effective contraception, e.g., the use of spermicidal foam.

WITHDRAWAL

Withdrawal is another method which is used by the young couple when they have no other means of contraception. The young woman has forgotten to take her Pill or to put in her diaphragm and the young man has no condoms. Or, perhaps the couple are just beginning to experiment with sexual activity and have heard that she cannot get pregnant if he "pulls out" before ejaculation.

The problem with this method is that most men produce a few drops of lubricating fluid on the end of the penis when it becomes erect. Enough sperm exist in this fluid to fertilize an ovum. In addition, the young man is usually unable to control his ejaculations and may fail to "pull out" at the last minute. But, when no other contraceptive is available, withdrawal is better than nothing at all. And for the young person who takes risks and values spontaneity, withdrawal may be the only method available.

RHYTHM

Rhythm includes a number of methods—calendar, cervical mucus change, basal body temperature, astrology, etc.—of determining the woman's fertile period; intercourse is avoided for two days before, during, and for two days after the fertile period. It is difficult for adults and teens to use rhythm consistently. One positive aspect of the rhythm method is that it promotes communication between the young woman and her partner. In addition, the method becomes an educational opportunity to familiarize adolescents with the menstrual cycle and periods of fertility.

The obvious problem with this method is that many young women have irregular menstrual cycles, and it is therefore difficult to predict when they will ovulate from month to month. Another problem is the period of abstinence each month. Most teenagers equate sexual expression with vaginal-penile intercourse and find it difficult to say no for about ten days out of the month. Discussion about alternate ways of lovemaking can be initiated at this time. Masturbation, massage, and oral sex can be ways in which a young couple communicate with each other as well as learn about the range of sexual expression.

The description of the various rhythm methods usually includes very complex and structured directions. These instructions often deter the teenager, who then may not use any method. Rather than emphasize the seemingly inflexible routines, a more casual approach may be advised. Counseling the teen to use a combination of abstinence and mechanical birth control (spermicide or condom) may promote pregnancy prevention.

Encouraging the young couple to graph the woman's menstrual cycle and fertile periods may promote better contraceptive behavior than any method. If both partners are consciously considering their physiology, then perhaps consideration of pregnancy and birth control will also occur.

ABORTION

Abortion is chosen by one third of all pregnant teenagers[1,3] and is often considered as a "backup" to contraceptive failures. Moreover, the risk-taking adolescent may use abortion as a primary birth control method. Whether this practice represents a socially acceptable alternative to contraception is not argued. Rather, the discussion is included because this method has been used to avoid childbirth.

The young woman using abortion as primary birth control has rejected all other methods. It is necessary to understand the basis for this choice before discussing alternative methods. Usually the young woman presents herself at a clinic requesting a pregnancy test. The counselor is alerted when the young woman reveals a past history of one or two pregnancies which also ended in abortion. Many times the counselor is openly disapproving of the behavior and communicates this verbally or nonverbally to the adolescent. It is important to provide a nonjudgmental rationale to the adolescent while supporting her decision to abort should she already be pregnant.

For many teenage women, the first contact with a contraceptive clinic occurs at the time of a suspected pregnancy. The fear or suspicion of pregnancy compels the young woman to seek help—and, at this point, abortion is her only birth control option. This initial contact occurs at a stressful period for the never-pregnant teenager and should be considered a critical learning period. In addition, first impressions are often lasting ones, and the quality of care provided to the teenager considering abortion can become the basis for future reproductive care.

One approach to counseling the young woman choosing abortion might be the use of either the decision-making model or the value-clarification strategies. A structured and positive approach can help to establish a relationship which will encourage the teen to return for further contraceptive care.

Pelvic Examination of the Adolescent Client

The pelvic examination is the procedure most feared by the teenager attending a contraceptive clinic. According to a national study of family planning services for teenagers by Urban and Rural Systems Associates (URSA),[6] "Fear of the pelvic exam was the second most critical obstacle to teenage use of a clinic, second only to their fear of their parents' finding out they were using a clinic" (p. 46). This fear of the pelvic examination often interferes with the adolescent's ability to think clearly and to make a well-informed contraceptive decision.

URSA also found that teenagers wanted an orientation to the clinic, and appreciated being respected as intelligent participants in the clinic visit. The URSA study team concluded that when the adolescent is given the appropriate knowledge and responsibility for her own health care, she will begin to accept responsibility for her own body and sexuality.

Initially, or during the waiting period, a film or verbal description of the clinic procedures, including the pelvic examination, can be presented to the teen clients. Once the adolescent is somewhat prepared for the pelvic examination through the use of audiovisual aids, certain steps should be taken during the actual examination procedure to further reduce her fears, so that learning about her body can occur.

First, an explanation of the procedure should be given. For very young or uneducated adolescents especially, visual aids such as charts or pelvic models are particularly helpful, because the cognitive development of this group often has not yet progressed beyond a concrete level. The teenage client wants to know what is happening to her during the pelvic examination. This explanation or visual aid demonstration is important and should be followed up with a verbal description of the procedure while the examination is in progress.

Johnson's[33] study of intrusive medical procedures found that instructions about the pelvic examination which included relaxation techniques and sensory information significantly reduced the distress associated with the pelvic examination; those women who did not receive the instruction experienced greater distress. Use of the techniques described by Johnson is helpful in the reproductive examination of the adolescent. Because fear of an unknown procedure creates anxiety in the client, full foreknowledge of the informational and sensory aspects of the reproductive examination can help decrease anxiety and therefore reduce the pain and discomfort of the procedure.

The first pelvic examination of an adolescent woman is an important event for both the professional and the young woman. This first reproductive examination is a unique educational experience and it sets the stage for future examinations.

The professional usually reenters the examination room after the adolescent is undressed and draped. Therefore, an assistant will be influential in helping the young woman acquaint herself with the examining table and equipment. Even simple explanations about where to place her clothes and how to arrange the drapes are important to the extremely modest teenager. In the college age group of the seventies, young women are frequently unconcerned with wearing gowns or drapes. But high school and younger teenagers are often very shy about exposing their bodies. Their privacy should be protected by ensuring proper draping and private dressing facilities.

Acknowledging the young woman's anxiety is usually helpful: "Is this your first pelvic exam? . . . I remember how nervous I was during my first exam . . . How are you feeling?" Often, a nod and some nervous giggling are observed, and the clinician can continue: "I know that you must feel tense and I'm going to show you some techniques that can help you to relax. This is not painful, but it can be more uncomfortable than it needs to be when you are tense because your muscles tighten up, even in your pelvis."

The clinician then demonstrates to the teen how to breathe and relax while on the examining table: "I know this position is a bit awkward, but by concentrating on your breathing, you can feel less tense. Now, begin by opening your mouth and take a big, very deep breath. Concentrate on breathing in and out, evenly and deeply. Think about keeping your arms and legs relaxed as you breathe. As long as you are breathing and your body is relaxed then the muscles in your pelvis will be relaxed too."

As the examination begins, a verbal monologue explaining the procedure is helpful. This is where the sensory information is the most beneficial: "I'm touching your labia." "This speculum will be putting pressure on your vagina and making a clicking noise." "You may be feeling pressure on your cervix where I take the Pap smear." "The jelly will feel cold."

Educating the young woman about her body can be the most important part of this first pelvic exam. Using a mirror which the teenager can hold, the clinician can point out the anatomy of her genitals and explain examination procedures. Many teenagers have fears and misconceptions about their vaginal and pelvic space. Actual visualization of the vagina and cervix can not only decrease the teenager's fears, but can also help in teaching placement of the intravaginal contraceptives. Often, young women ignore the changes in their genitourinary tracts that occur with maturation. More often, they may be extremely anxious about some particular development that they fear is a deviation from normal. If they can see their vaginas and orient themselves as to what is normal, adolescents will also become more conscious of physiologic or abnormal changes and will be alerted to health problems early.

Watching the young woman's response to seeing and feeling her body gives the clinician an indicator about the appropriateness of a particular form of contraception. If the teenager is repulsed by looking at or touching her body, then a mechanical method will probably not be used very successfully. Information about genital hygiene can be appropriate at this time: information about normal vaginal physiology, cleansing of the vaginal-vulvar area, and whether or not to douche.

There are certain comfort techniques which should be remembered when examining the adolescent. These measures allow for ease during the examination:

1. Warm the speculum with water or in a drawer with a light bulb.
2. When inserting the speculum, place the speculum on the fourchette and slowly exert downward pressure. This will help to release tension from the hymen and vagina and allow the speculum to slide into the vagina.
3. If possible, raise the head of the examining table to a 60 degree angle. This allows the teen to visualize the examination procedure more easily and is appropriate for teaching.
4. Put covers on the stirrups or have the teen leave her shoes on during the examination. Many teenagers complain about discomfort from the stirrups.

Legal Aspects in Contraceptive Care of the Adolescent

There has been some progress in recent years in changing the legal status usually assigned to teenagers who are consenting for their own health care. Until recently, teenagers have been considered "second class citizens" in terms of their right to consent for health care services. However, this trend is changing in many states because of the lower age of majority. The by-product of this change in the law is that it has encouraged legislatures and courts to affirm the right of young people to consent for their own health care. In fact, state and federal courts have continued to extend a variety of constitutional rights to minors. Two state cases in 1969 and 1970 have instituted safeguards for minors facing disciplinary action by school and juvenile authorities. The state courts maintain that minors are "persons" who possess fundamental rights which the state must respect.[34]

Although tension continues to exist regarding a teenager's right to abortion, "Twenty-six states and the District of Columbia explicitly affirm by statute or court decision the right of young people under age eighteen to consent for contraceptive care" (p. 16).[34] For the first time, the United States Supreme Court considered the adolescents' rights to contraception by striking down a New York statute which prohibited the sale or distribution of nonprescription contraceptives to minors under age 16.[35] State legislatures have been reluctant to recognize the right of minors to consent for their own abortions. In fact, some states have enacted laws requiring parental consent for abortions to teenagers under 18 years of age even though federal and state courts have declared such statutes to be unconstitutional. The trend, nationwide, is toward more controls on abortions to teenagers and less control on contraceptive services. This philosophy, that unmarried minors should not be allowed to consent for abortion without parental consent, reflects a belief that abortion should not be chosen as a method of birth control.

The teenager's right to consent for contraceptive care has been affirmed by many states in a number of key judicial decisions. In 1975, a Utah court struck down a regulation which required parental consent for family planning services to teenagers. They went on to say that the right to privacy for sexually active minors is equal to that of adults. The language in the Utah case requires that federally funded family planning services be made available to teenagers as well as protection of the teenagers' right to consent for their own health care.[34]

The important decision in New York in 1975, that nonprescription contraceptives be made available to minors, supports empirical evidence that restriction on the availability of contraceptives does not deter sexual activity among young persons. In fact, studies have shown that young people rarely seek contraceptive assistance until long after a pattern of sexual behavior has been established.[36,37]

A third milestone was passed in 1975 when California signed into law a bill allowing minors to consent to "medical and surgical care related to the prevention and treatment of pregnancy (including contraception and abortion, but excluding sterilization)" (p. 157).[38]

These decisions and laws have been influential in promoting health care rights for teenagers. Although there is a need in the courts and legislatures to bring about greater equalization, the current status shows progress in the area of medical-legal rights of minors.

In order to provide optimal health care to adolescent clients, professionals should be kept informed of the statutes in their individual states and communities. Statutory decisions which can influence contraceptive care to teenagers may be found by consulting local and state family planning and planned parenthood agencies. Also, juvenile authorities and state maternal-child programs can provide pertinent legal information.

Summary

Contraceptive care for the teenager is a multifaceted component of adolescent health care. In order for this care to be comprehensive and effective, careful consideration of physiological, social, psychological, and educational factors is vital. Effective contraceptive behavior by the sexually active teenager means prevention of unwanted pregnancies, and it can be attained with the establishment of creative and well-planned programs.

REFERENCES

1. Zelnik, M., and Kantner, J. F. "Sexual and Contraceptive Experience of Young Unmarried Women in the U.S., 1976 and 1971." *Fam. Plann. Perspectives* 9(2):55–73, 1977.
2. Furstenberg, F. F., Jr. "The Social Consequences of Teenage Parenthood." *Fam. Plann. Perspectives* 8(4):148–164, 1976.

3. Jaffe, F. S., and Dryfoos, J. G. "Fertility Control Services for Adolescents: Access and Utilization." *Fam. Plann. Perspectives* 8(4):167 (Table 10), 1976.
4. Lane, M. E. "Contraception for Adolescents." *Fam. Plann. Perspectives* 5(1):19–20, 1973.
5. Goldsmith, S. "San Francisco's Teen Clinic: Meeting the Sex Education and Birth Control Needs of the Sexually Active Schoolgirl." *Fam. Plann. Perspectives* 1(2):23–26, 1969.
6. Urban and Rural Systems Associates (URSA). *Improving Family Planning Services for Teenagers*. Final Report submitted to the Assistant Secretary for Planning and Evaluation of Health, Dept. of Health, Education, and Welfare, June 1976.
7. Fischman, S. H. "Change Strategies and the Application to Family Planning Programs." *Am. J. Nurs.* 73(10):1772–1777, 1973.
8. Swezy, R. L., and Swezy, A. M. "Educational Theory as a Basis for Patient Education." *J. Chron. Diseases* 29:417–422, 1976.
9. Taba, H. *Curriculum Development: Theory and Practice*. New York: Harcourt, Brace & World, Inc., 1962.
10. Juhasz, A. M. "A Chain of Sexual Decision Making." *Fam. Coordinator* 24(1):43–49, 1975.
11. Auerbach, A. B. *Parents Learn Through Discussion*. New York: John Wiley & Sons, Inc., 1968, pp. 207–208.
12. Bevis, E. O., and Douglass, L. M. *Nursing Leadership in Action*. St. Louis: C. V. Mosby Co., 1974, p. 47.
13. Kramer, M. "The Concept of Modeling as a Teaching Strategy." *Nurs. Forum* 11:48–70, 1972.
14. Raths, L. E.; Harmin, M.; and Simon, S. *Values and Teaching*. Columbus, Ohio: Charles E. Merrill Pub. Co., 1966.
15. Kirschenbaum, H. "Clarifying Values Clarification: Some Theoretical Issues and Review of Research." *Group & Organizational Studies* 1:99–116, 1976.
16. Rokeach, M. *The Nature of Human Values*. New York: Free Press, 1973.
17. Miller, W. B. "Psychological Vulnerability to Unwanted Pregnancy." *Fam. Plann. Perspectives* 5:199–201, 1973.
18. Messanotte, E. J. "Group Instruction in Preparation for Surgery." *Am. J. Nurs.* 70:89–90, 1970.
19. Ohlsen, M. M. *Group Counseling*. New York: Holt, Rinehart & Winston, Inc., 1970.
20. Marram, G. D. *The Group Approach in Nursing Practice*. St. Louis: C. V. Mosby Co., 1973.
21. Meleis, A. I., and Benner, P. "Process or Product Evaluation?" *Nurs. Outlook* 23:303–307, 1975.
22. Finkel, D. J., and Finkel, M. L. "Sexual and Contraception Knowledge, Attitudes, and Behavior of Male Adolescents." *Fam. Plann. Perspectives* 7(6):256–259, 1975.
23. LeBlanc, A. L. "Teenage Contraception." *Adolescent Gynecology Ross Roundtable on Critical Approaches to Common Pediatric Problems*. Columbus, Ohio: Ross Laboratories, 1977, p. 51.
24. Wouterz, T. B. "Three and One-Half Years' Experience with a Lower-Dose Combination Oral Contraceptive." *J. Reproductive Med.* 16(6):338–351, 1976.
25. Shearin, R. B. "Contraception for Adolescents." *Am. Fam. Phys.* 13(3):117–122, 1976.
26. Stolley, P. D., et al. "Thrombosis with Low-Estrogen Oral Contraceptives." *Am. J. Epidemiol.* 102:197–204, 1975.
27. Speroff, L. "Oral Contraceptives: Low Dose vs. High Dose." (Submitted for publication, 1977.)
28. Westrom, L.; Bengtsson, L. P.; and Mardh, P. A. "The Risk of Pelvic Inflammatory Disease in Women Using Intrauterine Devices as Compared to Non-Users." *Lancet* 2:221–225, 31 July 1976.
29. Mishell, D. R. "Assessing the IUD." *Fam. Plann. Perspectives* 7(3):103–122, 1975.
30. Lane, M. E.; Arceo, R.; and Sobrero, A. J. "Successful Use of the Diaphragm and Jelly by a Young Population." *Fam. Plann. Perspectives* 8(2):81–85, 1976.
31. Johnson, V. E., and Masters, W. H. "Intravaginal Contraception Study, Phase I: Anatomy." *Western J. Surg. OB-Gyn* 70:202–215, 1962.
32. Butler, J. C. "Vaginal Contraceptives as Prophylaxis Against Gonorrhea and Other Sexually Transmissible Diseases." *Adv. in Planned Parenthood* 12:45–47, 1977.
33. Johnson, J. "A Better Way to Calm the Patient Who Fears the Worst." *RN* 40(4): 47–52, 1977.
34. Paul, E. W.; Pilpel, H. F.; and Wechsler, N. F. "Pregnancy, Teenagers and the Law." *Fam. Plann. Perspectives* 8(1):16–21, 1976.

35. *Family Planning Digest Perspectives* 9(4):184–185, 1977.
36. Sorensen, R. C. *Adolescent Sexuality in Contemporary America.* New York: World Publishing Co., 1973.
37. Miller, W. B. "Sexuality, Contraception and Pregnancy in a High School Population." *Calif. Med.* 119:14–19, 1974.
38. *Population Reports.* "Adolescent Fertility." George Washington University Medical Center, Washington, D.C., J(10), 1976, p. 157.

The Adolescent
With a Health Problem

6

Adolescence:
The Clinical Encounter
and Common Health Problems

WILLIAM A. DANIEL, JR., M.D.
ROBERT T. BROWN, M.D.
CAROL L. GARRISON, R.N., M.S.N., P.N.P.

Adolescence is characterized by change. The most visible changes are physical, but growth in cognitive processes and psychosocial attitudes is also part of the change from child to adult. Each of these three areas of change—biologic, cognitive, and psychosocial—can affect the other, and growth in all areas is rarely synchronous. When assessing the health of an adolescent patient and preparing a care plan, all three areas of growth should be kept in mind during the interview, history taking, and physical examination.

Several questions must be answered. Of primary importance is: where along the developmental scale is the adolescent physically, cognitively, and psychosocially? Another consideration is to identify problems in any of the three general areas of growth that demand further investigation or treatment or that will exert a harmful effect (though perhaps only temporarily) in another area. The individual assessing an adolescent's health status should bear in mind that some health problems are more common during puberty, that some disorders or diseases become worse during adolescence, and that a few come to the fore at this time, although they are more typically associated with adults. The objective should be to determine the health status of the adolescent as well as to diagnose and treat medical complaints. Skill is required to reach this objective, and there in no doubt that many persons can more easily relate to adolescents and establish mutual trust with them than can others. But, as is shown in other sections of this book, there are ways to improve, pitfalls to avoid, and considerations to be given that will facilitate the process of health assessment.

The health professional who chooses to work with adolescents must recognize

147

and acknowledge that this period of life marks a separate developmental stage during which special needs, unique stresses, and common experiences and problems are shared. Considered from this vantage point, adolescents tend to present more similarities than differences. They do not, however, form a homogeneous group. For example, the early adolescent differs vastly from the late adolescent, the suburban adolescent cannot be viewed in the same light as the inner city young person, and the male teenager often requires consideration quite unlike that needed by the female.

Faced with such variety and complexity of development, the health professional inexperienced in interacting with adolescents can easily become confused and frustrated. It is often at this point that the neophyte will summarily reject the teenage group as being too difficult or unpleasant. Possession of a firm knowledge base regarding adolescent physiological, psychosocial, and cognitive developmental processes generally forestalls the above situation and thus is an essential prerequisite for anyone endeavoring to deal successfully with adolescents. Furthermore, this knowledge provides a well-defined framework that fosters an expanding awareness of the wide variety of health needs which the adolescent may have.

Interviewing the Adolescent

The interview in a health care setting has a fourfold purpose. First, it provides the opportunity to gather enough data to identify and define problems and/or needs. Next, it indicates the areas in which further data are needed. Third, if handled correctly, the interview, along with the subsequent physical examination, can provide the adolescent with a valuable experience in health education. Last, the interview enables the professional to establish an initial relationship with the teenager. The tone of this relationship is extremely important since it produces the context within which all care will be delivered. The implications for hindering or facilitating future interactions are great.

How does one go about interviewing an adolescent? Unfortunately, there are no guaranteed, clear-cut guidelines. What works well with one adolescent may not necessarily prove fruitful with another. Some general suggestions will be offered, with the caution that they must be adapted to the individual adolescent and to the individual interviewer.

The manner of dealing with an adolescent differs from the approaches used with both adults and children. There is also considerable difference between the early and the late adolescent. Accordingly, teenagers cannot all be talked to, evaluated, or managed in the same way. It is often difficult to remember that the adolescent who is biologically mature may possess thought processes that are still uncertain and confused. In such an instance, expectations for abstract thought and logical reasoning are unrealistic. Conversely, the teenager resents being talked down to as if he or she were a child. The interviewer must be aware of this developmental characteristic and adapt his or her interviewing approach to it.

Setting aside separate times specifically for seeing adolescents is frequently appreciated. Seeing the adolescent first and interviewing him in a private place can also be beneficial. Such actions communicate to the adolescent the assurance that he can freely relate the pertinent features of his problem and that he has the primary responsibility for his health, both now and in the future. It also allows him to pose questions that he would not ask in front of his parents and facilitates the establishment of trust.

Since adolescents are generally skeptical of adults, as well as of adult values and attitudes, it is essential that honesty be employed at all times. If it is necessary to talk with the parents, first inform the adolescent of your plans and of the proposed content of your discussion. Be certain to assure the adolescent of confidentiality and try to have him present, but do not make categorical promises that cannot be kept. Alternately, parents should be reminded that if the visit is confidential, it is more likely to produce results.

Adolescents are often reticent about showing their feelings, thoughts, or worries, and once they do decide to share this information they frequently find it difficult to articulate it clearly and concisely. Thus, sufficient time must be allotted for interviewing them and they should be assured that the language they commonly use is acceptable.

Begin the interview by exploring a nonthreatening and nonsensitive area, allowing time to establish a trusting relationship and for the interviewer to assess a general developmental level. Then give the young person an opportunity to talk and ask questions. Avoid talking more than is necessary. Rather, practice the art of active listening. The adolescent wants you to pay as much attention to him as to his symptoms. He needs you to listen to and to perceive more than just his chief complaint.

Proceed by asking open-ended questions before zeroing in on more specific data. Keep attuned to his body language. How does he react to a particular topic or to a change of topics? Such clues can be of inestimable importance.

The adolescent is often impatient and demands immediate feedback, opinions, or information. A discussion of the problem in order to dispel false assumptions, anxiety, and guilt is generally desired and certainly deserved. Information should be given at the adolescent's level. Indiscriminate use of medical and teenage jargon should be avoided. The adolescent wants to understand, but he also wants competence and skill.

Care must be taken, however, to ascertain the patient's real concern, for nothing will stop an adolescent from expressing his fears more quickly than premature reassurance. This is of paramount importance, since the stated chief complaint is often not the real reason for the visit but just an attempt to give legitimacy to other matters such as a request for birth control information or a discussion of family problems. Furthermore, a large number of young people who are found to have identifiable physical diagnoses also give evidence of problems in psychosocial or cognitive areas. Depression, for instance, is an extremely common, and often overlooked, finding in adolescence.

Care must also be taken not to prejudge an adolescent by his appearance, race, culture, social class, or any other extraneous variable. The interviewer acting on unfounded assumptions often fails to ask pertinent and necessary questions in areas such as sexual relations, pregnancy, and drugs. A nonjudgmental attitude must be maintained throughout the interview. Adolescents demand respect for their points of view and reject persons who moralize or preach to them, but it is not necessary that the interviewer agree with them.

Some clinicians use historical checklists to obtain information regarding past medical history, family history, social history, and the review of systems. The adolescent is given the checklist and is instructed to complete it prior to the initial interview. The advantages of a checklist include: (1) conservation of time, (2) avoidance of omissions, and (3) increased freedom for the adolescent to write down what he would be too embarrassed to say. However, it is the authors' belief that if a checklist is used, it should be employed only as a preparatory step to the formal interview. Time must be spent in reviewing with the adolescent the information contained on the checklist; only then will all four purposes of an interview in a health care setting be realized.

The Health History

A comprehensive health history can be the clinician's most important tool in identifying and defining an adolescent's problems or needs and can be extremely valuable in reaching a diagnosis of illness. If thorough, the history provides the clinician with a picture of the young person's current and past health status and with data about how he is functioning within his unique environment.

The overall components of the health history are standard, regardless of the target population, and include the following: chief complaint, history of present illness, past medical history, family history, review of systems, and personal/social history. Since numerous texts address the basic content and purpose of each of these components, the discussion that follows will focus only on those points that pertain specifically to the adolescent.

The clinician is reminded that caution must be observed when pursuing the chief complaint and history of present illness, since the initially stated reason for the visit is frequently not the most important one. In eliciting this component of the history it is useful to remember that the adolescent has great concerns about his body and that illness can exert a direct impact on his psychosocial development. Thus, specific data in this area should be sought.

Usually the past medical history and the family history cannot be accurately obtained solely from the adolescent. However, an attempt should be made to retrieve this information first from the patient, with later validation from parent or significant other person.

Information about early development, habits, symptoms, illnesses, and family or peer interactions are often erroneously omitted. These should be included, since they have particular relevance to educational, emotional, and/or physical problems that develop in adolescents. The early history should also rule out exposure to diethylstilbestrol (DES) in utero. Females exposed to DES should be followed and watched closely for adenocarcinoma of the vagina. Although there is no history of higher incidence of carcinoma in males exposed to DES in utero, there is an increase in urinary tract abnormality and a higher incidence of infertility.[1,2,3] Semen analysis reveals severe pathological changes in 32% of the males tested. Semen count and average density (which is the count of the number of sperms per ml of the ejaculate) is approximately two times lower in the DES-exposed group than in the normal population. There are also a lower ejaculate volume and a decrease in sperm motility.

A review of immunization is a second component of the past medical history that is frequently omitted. Adolescents usually have no idea of their immunization status, and complete or validating health records are frequently unavailable. Those adolescents with incomplete or undocumented immunizations should be immunized. A summary of immunization follows.

The completely immunized adolescent should receive a tetanus/diphtheria booster every ten years. An adolescent never or incompletely immunized should receive two tetanus/diphtheria doses, eight weeks apart, and a booster in a year. Pertussis vaccine should not be given to anyone over six years of age.

Rubella vaccination is given primarily to prevent the devastating effects of congenital rubella. Girls should be vaccinated before menarche. The postmenarchal female shown to be susceptible to rubella via assessment of serological titers can be immunized, if she agrees to prevent pregnancy for three months after immunization. Determination of a nonpregnant state and contraceptive counseling are required. The clinician must be careful to rule out pregnancy, since many adolescents who are pregnant claim to be sexually inactive and will recount a normal menstrual history. If pregnancy is ruled out, a single dose of the rubella vaccine should be given at the end of the menstrual period.

A single dose of live attenuated measles vaccine should be given to any adolescent who was vaccinated before 12 months of age, vaccinated with killed vaccine, or vaccinated with inactive vaccine. Two doses of trivalent oral poliomyelitis vaccine eight weeks apart and a booster in a year should be given to the adolescent who was never immunized or who was incompletely immunized against polio. A single dose of mumps vaccine should be given to adolescents who have never had mumps or mumps vaccine.

Annual testing for tuberculosis should be included in all adolescent immunization programs. Testing with intradermal purified protein derivative (PPD) is more reliable than utilizing the tine test. However, the tine test is easier to administer and sufficiently reliable for screening purposes. Tuberculin testing must be done prior to or concurrent with the administration of measles and polio vaccine to avoid false negatives.

The family history should include information about the age, occupation, current state of health, significant past illness and/or cause of death of parents and siblings. Information about family life style, income level, geographic mobility, educational levels, and housing is frequently valuable.

Specific attempts should be made to obtain data about the occurrence of sickle cell disease, hypertension, obesity, and cardiovascular disease. A family history of the latter three conditions puts the adolescent at increased risk for developing these problems. The adolescent with a family history of a hereditary disease such as sickle cell disease should receive genetic counseling. Both more careful screening and appropriate counseling are indicated. For example, serum cholesterol and triglyceride levels should be obtained on adolescents with a family history of cardiovascular disease, and preventive dietary and exercise regimens should be discussed.

A determination of the impact of a family member's illness on the adolescent and of the adolescent's perception of the cause and the progression of the illness is another essential component of the family history. Misconceptions are common, and such a determination allows the clinician to clarify and correct misunderstandings.

A review of systems follows the family history. Specific areas crucial to the review of symptoms include: nutrition, dental habits, school progress, pubertal development, contraceptive concerns, menstrual history in females, substance use and/or abuse, emotional problems, and any legal encounters.

A short nutritional history is obtained; it should include what is eaten and also where and when food is eaten. Nutritional intake can then be compared with recommended daily allowances. A determination of weight gain or loss, fad diets, and indications of anemia in the postmenarchal female should be made. Obesity is by far the most common nutritional problem of adolescents, but iron deficiency anemia is not infrequent. See Chapter 4 for further information on the nutritional needs of adolescents.

Tooth decay is prevalent, but teenagers rarely ask for information or advice in this area. It is important for the clinician to ascertain if the adolescent is practicing good dental hygiene and receiving adequate dental care. Accordingly, frequency of dental care, quantity and frequency of high carbohydrate snacks, and utilization of dental floss should be determined. Appropriate instruction and/or referral is instituted if the adolescent is deficient in any one of the above areas.

Progress in school should be covered. Chronic physical diseases or disabilities are often associated with developing school problems during adolescence because of the magnitude of change due to growth. Similarly, a child with mild mental retardation tends to do well in the lower grades but cannot cope with the increased demands for intellectual abilities and abstract thought that are required at the junior and senior high school levels. If a school problem exists, the following questions should be answered. What is the problem? Who is identifying and defining the problem—the parent, the adolescent, or the school? What seems to be the etiology of the problem? What is the adolescent's school history—both past and present?

With both male and female patients a review of the timing and pattern of pubescence is necessary. Additionally, with girls, a review of menstrual history and symptoms is essential. Age and date of menarche, regularity, frequency and character of periods, and presence and timing of intermenstrual bleeding should be recorded. Irregular menses are not uncommon for about two years following menarche. Intermenstrual bleeding may be associated with ovulation but can also indicate pregnancy. Girls who begin menstruating prior to nine years of age should be evaluated for precocious puberty. Similarly, the adolescent female who has not menstruated within five years of starting breast development needs to be further evaluated.

A review of the development of secondary sex characteristics and, in girls, the menstrual history enables the clinician (1) to ascertain any misinformation the patient may have regarding reproductive organs, ovulation, or menstruation, and (2) to provide correction, clarification, and instruction on these points. It also provides for a natural progression to a review and discussion of pregnancy, contraception, masturbation, nocturnal emissions, venereal disease, and sexuality, depending on the stage of sexual development.

Pregnancy, contraception, and venereal disease are common concerns of many adolescents. The clinician is obligated to specifically ask adolescents of both sexes about these areas. It is a grave mistake to assume that a particular adolescent is "too nice" to be questioned or to be given relevant information. Adolescents generally harbor a great deal of uncertainty and doubt about these topics and are reluctant to pursue them with their parents. Thus, the clinician becomes an important source from whom the teenager can obtain accurate information about his body and the prevention of venereal disease and pregnancy.

Tobacco, drug, and alcohol use must be directly and nonjudgmentally pursued. This discussion can serve as an educational experience regarding drugs and related physical problems. If alcohol and/or drug use is confirmed, it is essential to learn the patterns of use and reasons for use, and to make an assessment of how the rest of the adolescent's life is going. Often drug and alcohol use are symptomatic of difficulties in one or a number of other areas in the adolescent's life and are utilized to provide tranquilization, relief from depression, or a sense of belonging. Conversely, many young people experiment with alcohol in a way that is not destructive.

A review of general psychosocial stability is regularly carried out. This area requires great sensitivity since adolescents entering the health care system exhibit a wide range of deviations from the psychosocial norms. Some deviations are judged as slight and/or temporary and are viewed as normal aspects of adolescent growth or as expected manifestations of situational stress. In these cases, helping the adolescent to recognize the problem that is causing the situation and letting him know that it is a common phenomenon is often all that is needed to alleviate the distress. Other problems are more long-standing or pronounced and require referral and intensive follow-up. A general rule of thumb is that chronicity and intensity are associated with severity in adolescents.

Although all behavior must be seen in the framework of the adolescent's age, social situation, developmental history, and present stress index, certain symptoms indicate the need for further investigation. Feelings of anxiety accompanied by palpitations, diarrhea, nausea (unrelated to meals), excessive sweating, chest tightness, and difficulty in getting one's breath, should be investigated. Similarly, changes in affect accompanied by apathy, withdrawal, self-blaming and negative behaviors, anorexia, insomnia, crying, agitated behavior, decreased activity, difficulty in concentrating, lack of interest in grooming, and hopelessness indicate depression and should be followed. Suicide is one of the leading causes of death in adolescents. Thus, the clinician should be particularly attuned to this possibility and should not hesitate to ask about it directly.

By obtaining a psychosocial history the clinician attempts to gain a developmental perspective and to evaluate the adolescent's psychosocial functioning in light of the current knowledge of the various phases of adolescence. This part of the history serves to identify those young people who are having relatively more difficulty with the major developmental tasks of adolescence.

To ascertain how the adolescent is progressing with these tasks one must discuss them with him. Much information relevant to this assessment will have been gained previously in the interview and need not be elicited again. However, upon completion of the interviewing process the following points concerning the adolescent's developmental status should be clear: (1) progress towards independence and self-responsibility, and the family's reaction to this transition; (2) consideration of vocational goals; (3) success in initiating and maintaining appropriate peer relationships, especially with members of the opposite sex, and progress in developing a personal moral code; and (4) progress in constructing a realistic and positive self-identity. If problems or delays are noted in any of the above areas, identification of causative factors is necessary.

Approach to the Physical Examination

A careful physical examination provides a mechanism for assessing the normality of physical development and function. It allows the clinician to further educate the young person regarding his body. The process of the examination can also be a useful way to ease into a discussion of puberty, to reassure the patient about present and future development, and to talk about preventing injuries.

To the self-conscious youngster who is somewhat embarrassed about his body, the specter of a physical examination may represent an unpleasant ordeal. Thus, every effort should be made to minimize stress. To allow time for the establishment of rapport, the history should be taken first, with the adolescent fully clothed. During the actual examination, use of adequate draping preserves the client's modesty. The examiner can put the patient at ease by proceeding slowly, by taking care to explain all procedures prior to implementing them and by explaining what was found. Teenagers want to be found normal.

An adolescent is extremely sensitive about being evaluated by others. He needs to feel that his body is attractive and that his physical development is appropriate. Given this set of circumstances, the examiner must guard carefully against disapproving verbal or nonverbal cues.

Physical Examination

Since numerous texts address the basic procedures and standard outline of the physical examination, the discussion that follows will focus primarily on those aspects unique to the adolescent.

Measurement of height and weight is an essential part of all physical examinations. During adolescence both boys and girls will experience the final 20 to 25% of their linear growth. Adolescent growth generally includes a period of increased growth, a period of maximum growth, or peak height velocity (growth spurt), and a period of decelerating growth. Girls generally experience a growth spurt between 11½ and 13½ years, while boys generally go through a growth spurt between 13 and 15½ years.[4]

Although the velocity, magnitude, onset, and completion of growth are extremely variable within the adolescent population, the pattern of a particular individual's growth should remain constant along a given percentile throughout his life span. Thus, for an accurate evaluation, serial measurements are needed. The third and ninety-seventh percentiles mark the outer limits of normality. Evaluation is necessary for an adolescent who falls outside this range or who deviates from his normal growth pattern of previous years.

Almost half of one's ideal body weight is gained during puberty, and, as with height, the process of weight gain follows a defined sequence of increase, maximum growth, and deceleration. The percentile of an adolescent's height and of his weight should not differ more than 15 points, except during the period of maximum growth. An adolescent whose weight is more than 15 percentile points above his height percentile should be evaluated for obesity. If obesity is suspected, a measurement of subcutaneous skinfold thickness can be estimated at the triceps area. Lacking calipers, measurement is obtained by grasping a pinch of skin from the posterior aspect of the arm between the thumb and forefinger. When more than half an inch separates the examiner's fingers the adolescent is considered to be too fat. Conversely, an adolescent who shows a history of weight loss or plateauing of weight, merits evaluation to rule out chronic or acute disease.

Because normal, healthy adolescents vary widely from one another in the timing, rate, and extent of their growth, chronological age presents a deceptive yardstick against which to measure pubertal changes and biologic values. Many biologic values, however, have been shown to correlate closely with an adolescent's stage of sexual maturation. Sexual maturation is easily determined during physical examination by utilizing standards developed by Tanner (see Table 6–1). Tanner's classification of pubertal development is based on the sequential nature of breast and pubic hair growth in the female and on the sequential nature of genital and pubic hair growth in the male. Although these changes progress in an orderly fashion, they do not necessarily coincide. Thus, it is important to stage each aspect separately.

Rating of pubertal development in both boys and girls allows the examiner to: (1) suspect constitutional delayed puberty or dysfunction of the pituitary gland, hypothalamus and/or gonads, (2) become aware of the beginnings of chronic disease, and (3) counsel the adolescent regarding future expected changes.

In the male adolescent patient the average age of sex maturity rating (SMR) 2 is 11½ years and the first sign is enlargement of the testes. A boy who shows pubescent changes before 9 years or who shows no development by 13½ years needs evaluation for precocious or delayed puberty, respectively. About three quarters of all males will experience their growth spurt while in pubic hair rating 3. The remainder will reach peak height velocity during pubic hair stage 4. Thus, the male adolescent who is concerned about his short stature and has not reached SMR 4 can be assured that he will still grow significantly, although perhaps not as much as he desires. On the other hand, the adolescent who attains SMR 5 without a growth spurt should be evaluated for chronic disease or organ dysfunction.

Any female attaining breast stage 2 or pubic hair stage 2 before 8 years or not attaining them by 13 years requires further evaluation for precocious or delayed puberty. Most girls will evidence their growth spurts in pubic hair stages 2 or 3, with a subsequent deceleration of growth. This information can be useful in alerting the clinician to counsel female patients regarding menstruation, birth control, and pregnancy, since menarche generally occurs during the period of decelerated growth (SMR 4), although often at stage 3. SMR 4 also coincides with the period of most rapid weight gain in the female. An important fact that recent studies indicate is that

TABLE 6–1. *Sex Maturity Ratings**

BOYS

STAGE	PUBIC HAIR	PENIS	TESTES
1	None	Preadolescent	Preadolescent
2	Scanty, long, slightly pigmented	Slight enlargement	Enlarged scrotum, pink texture altered
3	Darker, starts to curl, small amount	Penis longer	Larger
4	Resembles adult type, but less in quantity; coarse, curly	Larger; glans increases in size; breadth increases	Larger, scrotum dark
5	Adult distribution, spread to medial surface of thighs	Adult	Adult

GIRLS

STAGE	PUBIC HAIR	BREASTS
1	Preadolescent	Preadolescent
2	Sparce, lightly pigmented straight, medial border of labia	Breast and papilla elevated as small mound; areolar diameter increased
3	Darker, beginning to curl, increased amount	Breast and areola enlarged, no contour separation
4	Coarse, curly, abundant, but amount less than in adult	Areola and papilla form secondary mound
5	Adult feminine triangle, spread to medial surface of thighs	Mature; nipple projects, areola part of general breast contour

* Source: from William A. Daniel, Jr.: *Adolescents in Health and Disease*, St. Louis: C. V. Mosby Co., 1977; adapted from J. M. Tanner: *Growth at Adolescence*, 2nd ed. Oxford, England: Blackwell Scientific Publications, 1962.

a critical weight of 100 pounds or a total body fat composition greater than or equal to 20% is necessary for the onset and continuation of regular menses in Caucasians and blacks.[5] Any female who has already achieved a peak height velocity and adequate weight for age and who has developed secondary sex characteristics but has not menstruated by age 15 or within five years of starting breast development needs to be evaluated.

Although adolescents are extremely concerned about the development of their secondary sex characteristics, they often will not express this concern. Accordingly, the clinician needs to routinely assure the abolescent that his development is normal. The clinician should also be aware that the definition of delayed puberty for the patient is, "I'm not like my friends." This may or may not be the same as the medical definition, but it always demands careful attention.

Audiometric and visual screening are a routine part of the physical examination. Special consideration should be given to this aspect of the examination if the adolescent is having school problems. Color vision should be ascertained in all males. Questions regarding blurring of vision, eye fatigue, and excessive watering and headaches after reading are included if one suspects visual problems.

Despite the ability of the adolescent to cooperate, the cardiac physical examination may be difficult. Adolescent females, especially, may become embarrassed when this part of the examination is carried out by a male examiner. However, screening for the signs of congenital, rheumatic, or beginning hypertensive or atherosclerotic heart disease is essential. Murmurs in an adolescent with a thin chest wall may appear more prominent than they did when he was younger. Functional murmurs due to anemia and/or pregnancy are not uncommon. A history of chest pain or palpitations requires further investigation. In addition, all adolescents with congenital or acquired heart disease who plan to participate in competitive sports should be evaluated during rest and during active excercise to determine their capacity.

Blood pressure should be taken on all patients because hypertension, a potentially serious disorder, occurs in a significant number of adolescents. Generally, hypertension in this age group is essential in nature; only infrequently are etiologic abnormalities discovered.

In obtaining blood pressure values, the examiner should use a cuff that covers at least two thirds of the width of the upper arm. This is especially important in obese adolescents. Both diastolic sounds, i.e., muffling and disappearance, are recorded. The patient should be relaxed, should not have a full bladder, and should not have exercised recently. A series of readings at separate visits is necessary to compensate for lability. As an adjunctive measure, pulses should be checked in both arms and legs. Blood pressure is measured in all four extremities if a discrepancy in pulses or an elevated pressure is obtained.

The breasts of both males and females should be examined. The areola of the male breast can normally increase in size during early puberty and about a third of all adolescent males will develop some discrete breast tissue. Bilateral nontender enlargement occurs most frequently, but unilateral tender enlargement also occurs. Gynecomastia generally recedes within 18 months.[6] That persisting beyond 24 months is unlikely to resolve. Special care must be taken to reassure the youth that the development of some breast tissue is a normal concomitant of male adolescence.

The breast of the female should be examined to detect masses. Time should be taken to assure the teenage girl that her development is normal, especially if asymmetrical breast size is present. Instructing the adolescent girl in the proper technique for breast self-examination is an essential component of this part of the physical examination. Having her then demonstrate the techniques is the best way of ensuring that proper learning has occurred.

Examination of male and female genitalia should be complete and routine. Ideally, examination of the genitalia would have been done consistently during childhood, so that the teenager would be accustomed to it and would expect it as part of a comprehensive physical examination. This part of the examination provides the opportunity to teach males self-examination of the testes. Good perineal care can be reviewed with both males and females. Females should be counseled against wearing nonventilating clothing and encouraged to wear cotton underwear. Bubble baths and douches should also be discouraged.

Pelvic examinations are not done routinely on all adolescent females, but are performed on any female who is sexually active, who has abdominal symptoms, or who has menstrual problems. The first pelvic examination a girl has should be performed by an experienced examiner, since this examination will sensitize her positively or negatively to all subsequent examinations. A detailed explanation and a slow pace are essential to alleviate fears.

Common orthopedic problems during adolescence include scoliosis, Osgood-Schlatter syndrome, slipped capital femoral epiphysis, and sports injuries to the knees and ankles. The clinician must be on guard when examining an adolescent with a suspected sports injury. Many adolescents will endeavor to cover up or downgrade such an injury because they desire to continue participation in the sport.

Laboratory Evaluation

Specific laboratory tests should be included as part of the adolescent's routine physical examination. Since anemia is not uncommon, annual hematocrits should be obtained. A diagnosis of anemia should be made only after considering the youth's sex, SMR, and race. Although the changes are less evident in girls than in boys, hematocrit percentages increase with increasing SMR.[7] Blacks normally have lower hematocrits than whites.[8] If the hematocrit level falls below the fifteenth percentile

TABLE 6–2. *15th Percentiles of Hematocrits* *

(95% confidence limits in parentheses)
Standards for diagnoses for anemia

		MALES	
		BLACK	WHITE
	1	34.9 (34.3–35.5)	35.6 (35.1–36.1)
	2	36.0 (35.6–36.4)	36.9 (36.5–37.3)
SMR	3	37.1 (36.7–37.5)	38.2 (37.8–38.6)
	4	38.2 (37.8–38.6)	39.6 (39.2–40.0)
	5	39.3 (38.7–39.9)	40.9 (40.3–41.6)

		FEMALES	
		BLACK	WHITE
	1	34.0 (33.4–34.6)	35.8 (35.3–36.2)
	2	35.3 (34.9–35.7)	36.6 (36.2–37.0)
SMR	3	36.0 (35.6–36.4)	37.0 (36.5–37.4)
	4	36.2 (35.8–36.6)	36.7 (36.3–37.1)
	5	35.8 (35.2–36.4)	35.9 (35.3–36.6)

* Source: From William A. Daniel, Jr.: *Adolescents in Health and Disease,* St. Louis: C. V. Mosby Co., 1977; adapted from J. M. Tanner: *Growth at Adolescence,* 2nd ed. Oxford, England: Blackwell Scientific Publications, 1962.

for the individual's sex, race, and maturity level, anemia is present (see Table 6–2) and should be investigated.

A yearly urine specimen should be screened for pH, color, and the presence of sugar, protein, and acetone. Abnormal findings are often the first indication of renal disease or diabetes. Trace protein is considered normal when using a dipstick. Menstrual blood or a heavy vaginal discharge can cause a false positive for protein. Dehydration and recent strenuous physical activity can also cause false positives for protein or red blood cells in the specimen; "crash" or fad dieting may lead to the presence of acetone in the urine.

The black adolescent not previously screened for sickle cell disease should be screened during his teenage years. Counseling of young people exhibiting the trait is necessary but often overlooked.

A yearly venereal disease serology test should also be obtained in all adolescents.

Organic Problems

Adolescence is the only period of extrauterine life during which growth and development accelerate. Any pathological condition that arises de novo in this period, or that is unchanged until pubescence, can be difficult to manage because it is superimposed on a shifting rather than on a stable base. Any abnormal physical condition can have an effect on cognitive and/or psychosocial development. Problems in these areas can sometimes affect organic processes. Therefore in caring for adolescents who have particular problems, one must constantly be aware of the reciprocal effect of changes in physical, cognitive, and psychosocial growth.

In assessing the health of an adolescent, the physical examination can give clues leading to a diagnosis of illness, reveal the presence of one or more handicapping conditions, or indicate the need for additional investigation. Only brief consideration of disease can be given here; detailed information is available in standard texts.[9,10,11]

SKIN

The skin encloses the body parts to form a unique package that functions in the surrounding environment. The skin thus serves as a buffer against external forces, but it can also have diseases peculiar to itself or be a mirror reflecting signs of systemic disease. Sunburn and inflammations caused by poison ivy or certain cosmetics illustrate the reaction of the skin to external agents. The butterfly facial rash of lupus, the blue spots of purpura, and the yellow tinge of liver disease serve to alert the examiner to the possibility of generalized illness. Impetigo, fungus infections, and furuncles occur on and in the skin, but acne is the most common dermatologic condition associated with puberty. Acne can be viewed as a "normality" rather than an abnormality of adolescence. As androgen levels increase in puberty, they cause sebaceous glands to produce a thickened secretion, sebum. Sebum obstructs and distends the pores. Contact with air causes the sebum to become hard and black, and the open comedo is produced. If the epidermal covering is not breached, then a "whitehead," or closed comedo is present. Sebum trapped under the skin can distend the gland and duct to form a sebaceous cyst. If the wall of the cyst ruptures, inflammation occurs secondary to a foreign body type reaction. Comedonal acne occurs commonly in boys and girls, but cystic acne is usually a problem of male adolescents.

Treatment for comedonal acne is primarily topical. Frequent washing and use of drying agents (e.g., benzoyl peroxide) help considerably. Topical retinoic acid and topical antibiotics (e.g., tetracycline or clindamycin) are beneficial in more severe cases. Oral antibiotics (e.g., tetracycline or erythromycin) may be indicated for cystic acne. Intralesional injection of corticosteroids is extremely effective in treating inflamed cystic lesions. Emotional support and encouragement are just as important as drug therapy. Already extremely conscious of every flaw in appearance, the adolescent with acne can become morbidly afraid of social encounters. Counseling should be directed at improving feelings of self-confidence and self-worth. Certainly, successful medical treatment can help. With his or her limited ability to consider the future realistically, it is of little value just to give a pat on the back and tell the adolescent "this too shall pass."

Any noticeable skin lesion assumes much greater significance than it would in a child or an adult because adolescents are obsessed with their appearance. Commonly encountered lesions include: warts, atopic dermatitis, contact dermatitis, keloids, vitiligo, and urticaria, among others. All of these conditions should be considered seriously and treated aggressively, given their amplified importance to this age group.

SUBCUTANEOUS TISSUE

Subcutaneous tissue is of importance to adolescents for many reasons but particularly because of the quantity of fat. Obesity in this age group is extremely difficult to treat. Boys have an advantage in that they tend to lose fat during physical maturation; therefore, nutritional instruction may be more readily acted upon. Girls, however, tend to retain fat and, indeed, increase it if obesity is already present. Many modalities of treatment have been attempted—each with little success. It appears that behavioral modification can be helpful to some obese patients, but long-term results are inconclusive.

Distribution of body fat, especially in females, is still a major source of concern. Breasts that are too large or too small or, worse yet, breasts that are unequal in size, can cause a great deal of psychic trauma. Excessive fat accumulation in the hips and thighs also produces stress. Counseling again is in order. Surgical correction of inequities in breast size can be of help in selected instances, though not all mammary problems are due to excess fat.

Some adolescents are thin or underweight; the most alarming abnormality is anorexia nervosa. Anorexia nervosa is infrequent but serious; it most commonly affects middle-or upper-class adolescent girls. The patient presents with emaciation and is preoccupied with food, calories, and excercise. Victims suffer severe distortion of personal body image, cessation of menstruation, and increased conflict with parents. This condition is very difficult to correct and requires both medical and psychiatric therapy.

SUPPORTING TISSUE

The quantity of muscle tissue they possess—and how to increase its size—are major concerns to many boys. Adolescence is a time of intense physical activity and heated competition, and the size and distribution of "muscles" is considered by many youths to be the "measure of the man." Girls do not have a significant increase in muscle mass after SMR 2. Boys have their growth spurts (peak height velocity) at pubic hair rating 3. It is only after this rapid increase in height that muscle mass in boys begins to increase significantly. This information can be useful in counseling boys so that their expectations do not exceed their bodies' ability to comply with their wishes. Diseases which affect muscles can be serious problems at this period in life. Two examples are muscular dystrophy and myasthenia gravis, but chronic conditions, such as sickle cell disease or diabetes mellitus, also can affect muscle size and function.

Diseases of connective tissue are significant problems during adolescence. This group, known as the collagen vascular diseases, includes: systemic lupus erythematosus, rheumatoid arthritis, dermatomyositis, and other less frequent syndromes. The primary lesion is an inflammation of the small blood vessels in various organs; therefore the effects are systemic. Systemic lupus erythematosus can present with symptoms involving any organ system. Indeed, in recent times it has replaced syphilis as the "great masquerader." Lupus most often affects the skin, the joints, various serous membranes, e.g., the pleura, and, most significantly, the kidneys. It is the severity of kidney involvement that determines ultimate prognosis.

Rheumatoid arthritis is a disease that primarily involves the joints. During adolescence it can present as one of the childhood forms or as the adult type. Joint destruction caused by rheumatoid arthritis can produce severe disability and affect many areas of adolescent growth and development, including the skeletal system.

Orthopedic problems are very common in adolescents. During this period of most rapid growth, preexisting orthopedic problems can worsen and new ones may occur. Scoliosis is common in adolescence as are other epiphyseal and cartilaginous conditions. The incidence of idiopathic scoliosis increases dramatically as pubescence occurs and is most frequent in girls. Any asymmetry of the spine is accentuated during rapid growth. Careful examination of the back of the standing patient with the trunk at a right angle to the legs is mandatory. Any apparent curvature should be confirmed radiographically, and referral to an orthopedist should be made. No scoliosis should be considered benign. It must also be emphasized that scoliosis is not always idiopathic. A spinal curvature can be secondary to spinal column lesions (e.g., hemivertebrae or diastatomyelia) or to muscle or neurologic problems (e.g., polio, muscular dystrophy, and cerebral palsy). Scoliosis is inevitably associated with altered psychosocial development; schooling is frequently interrupted. Early diagnosis and treatment are extremely valuable.

Epiphyses are not all sealed until maturity. An obese young adolescent with a limp and pain in the hip or lower third of the thigh should be thoroughly investigated for a slipped capital femoral epiphysis. Pain and tenderness of the anterior tibial tubercle is caused by chronic trauma to the immature epiphysis by overuse of the quadriceps femoris. This is known as Osgood-Schlatter's syndrome. It is ameliorated by rest and disappears once ephiphyseal closure is achieved. The cartilage of the chest wall is also relatively immature and is subject to tears and pulls by the chest musculature—often brought about by excessive exercise or injury. Adolescents complaining of chest pain should always be examined for tenderness of the rib cartilage.

Adolescence is a time of increased physical activity for both sexes. Competitive, individual, and team sports become significant components of teenagers' lives. Therefore a familiarity with common sports-related trauma and with the methods of a routine orthopedic evaluation is necessary for anyone involved in delivery of health care to adolescents.

BLOOD AND LYMPHATIC SYSTEM

Problems of the hematologic and lymphatic systems are frequently encountered in adolescents. Due to the rapid rate of growth, the demand for red blood cells and quantity of hemoglobin increase. If iron stores are insufficient, iron deficiency anemia can occur. One should be aware that normal hemoglobin and hematocrit values vary directly with sex maturity ratings, sex, and race, particularly in boys. The other major red cell problem in this age group is sickle cell anemia. Typical hemoglobin and hematocrit values in a patient with sickle cell disease are 7 grams and 20% respectively, with a reticulocyte count of 15 to 20%. Sicklers, particularly boys, frequently suffer from delayed onset of puberty and decreased capacity for physical activity. Cerebrovascular accidents are an ever present concern in sickle cell disease and, since this patient is functionally asplenic, pneumococcal infections are also a threat. Patients with sickle cell disease can benefit from pneumococcal vaccine, which can have a preventive value. Liver dysfunction and gall bladder disease are common complications. Abdominal and osteoid crisis are relatively common and the individual patient tends to have either one or the other type of crisis. Hemolytic and aplastic crises are rare but can be life threatening. Repeated hospitalizations for vaso-occlusive crises are usually emotionally, educationally, physically, and financially debilitating.

Neoplasms of hematologic origin, e.g., acute lymphoblastic leukemia, are not as frequent during adolescence as they are in childhood. But infections causing white blood cell abnormalities, specifically infectious mononucleosis, are more common. Mononucleosis, a viral infection associated with atypical lymphocytes found in the peripheral blood smear, should be considered in the differential diagnosis of any adolescent presenting with pharyngitis and lymphadenopathy. Occasionally the pharyngitis is so severe that intravenous administration of corticosteroids is necessary to achieve resolution. An occasional lymph node palpated in the cervical, axillary, or inguinal area is so commonly found in older children and adolescents that, unless of a suspicious texture, size, or location, it should be considered a normal finding.

Lymph nodes that increase in size, that feel matted or rock hard, or that persist in uncommon places, e.g., the supraclavicular area, should make one suspicious of a malignancy—e.g., Hodgkin's disease.

SENSORY ORGANS

Problems of the sensory organs are commonly encountered in adolescents. Acute otitis media is not nearly as frequent as it is in childhood, but acute otitis externa is common, especially in the swimming season. This condition is easily diagnosed by inspection, and pressure on the anterior portion of the ear, the tragus, compressing the canal, causes intense pain. Prophylactic eardrops of vinegar (15 drops) and alcohol (1 ounce) can decrease the rate of occurrence if used during the swimming season.

Testing for decreased hearing should be done. Most often, the reduction is a result of repeated bouts of otitis media years before, but it could be a concomitant of Alport's hereditary nephritis. Decreased hearing can also be the result of continued exposure to loud music, firing guns during hunting, tuning engines for drag racing, etc.

The eyeball grows with the rest of the body during adolescence, and myopia is a frequent result. Infections and allergic conjunctivitis are regularly encountered. Prophylactic administration of sodium cromolyn eyedrops during allergy season may be the answer for allergic conjunctivitis.

MOUTH

The oral cavity's major presenting problem in adolescence is dental caries, especially when water is not fluoridated. A great many adolescents are also in need of orthodontic intervention for their malaligned teeth. Sports injuries often fracture teeth, and prompt treatment by a dentist is necessary.

Although tonsillitis is more frequent in younger children, it still occurs during adolescence. Swelling, redness, flecks of whitish exudate on the tonsils, associated with mild tenderness and enlargement of the anterior cervical lymph nodes, are likely to be caused by the streptococcus. Cultures should be made, and, if positive, penicillin should be given as the drug of choice. At times, there is great pain in swallowing; the patient can barely open the mouth, and it is difficult to see the tonsillar areas. If the tonsil is greatly enlarged and protrudes toward the midline, it is likely that a peritonsillar abscess is present. The tonsils and pharynx are often red and swollen, sometimes with exudate, in mononucleosis; it is not rare for a superimposed streptococcal infection to be present in this disease.

NERVOUS SYSTEM

Two serious problems of the central nervous system can severely impair many areas of adolescent development and function. They are epilepsy and mild mental retardation. Seizure disorders often begin de novo during puberty, and preexisting epilepsy can worsen. Most often, seizure disorders do not cause subnormal intelligence. The goal of medical management is the achievement of as normal a life style as possible. Diagnosis of epilepsy relies most heavily on a detailed history, because the physical examination is usually normal. Approximately 20% of all seizure patients have normal electroencephalograms[12] so that one cannot rely on a negative electroencephalogram to rule out epilepsy. Phenytoin and phenobarbitol are the mainstays of therapy. Grand mal seizures are usually relatively easy to control, whereas psychomotor seizures can be more difficult to treat. Sometimes a balance must be struck so as to minimize both the number of seizures and the degree of side effects of medication. Unfortunately, the most serious problem that young people with epilepsy must overcome is society's attitude toward them. Obtaining a driver's license and getting a job can be harrowing tasks for these adolescents but often serve to increase compliance with treatment.

Mild mental retardation can be an insidious impediment to cognitive and psychosocial growth. An adolescent with this problem usually appears normal and functions adequately in most everyday experiences. We define mild retardation, for our purposes, as the intellectual inability to keep up with peers in school. A teenager who is mildly retarded can become quite frustrated and often develops a very poor self-image. Efforts must be made to identify these young people, to give them extra help, and to channel them into vocations in which their abilities can be best utilized and their deficiencies minimized. Experience is often necessary for an examiner to be aware of mild retardation.

CARDIOPULMONARY SYSTEM

Pulmonary or cardiac conditions can surely handicap adolescents. For example, a young girl with cystic fibrosis may not develop sexually at the same time as her peers. She cannot keep up in the physical activities so important in this group. She has difficulty in achieving independence because of her need for physical therapy, hospitalization, and financial support. Yet her cognitive functions may mature at a normal rate. She eventually comes to realize that her future is bleak. Early death is a real possibility. Much help will be needed by such an adolescent to achieve any goals within her capacity.

New rheumatic fever cases occur during adolescence, but more important to consider, perhaps, are those patients who had heart damage from rheumatic fever as children but who are functionally well until physical growth during adolescence causes the heart to be overburdened and to decompensate. Most congenital heart lesions have been diagnosed and treated by the time a child reaches his teenage years.

GASTROINTESTINAL SYSTEM

Gastrointestinal problems occur in adolescence; the most common disorders are temporary bouts of gastroenteritis. Appendicitis with typical lower right quadrant pain and a history of vomiting can be confused with gonorrhea in girls, although gonorrheal pain is usually bilateral and other symptoms are present. Sickle cell crisis should be excluded in the diagnosis of abdominal pain in black adolescents. Peptic ulcer disease increases in incidence during adolescence, as does inflammatory bowel disease. Crohn's disease (regional enteritis and granulomatous colitis) achieves peak incidence between 15 and 35 years of age. A thorough history is very important and often reveals that the disease was present long before obvious or present manifestations occurred. In young children and early adolescents, failure to grow—particularly failure to achieve sexual maturation—should suggest the possibility of Crohn's disease. Generalized or specific abdominal tenderness or the presence of one or more masses demands further investigation. Ulcerative colitis is usually more dramatic in onset with explosive diarrhea being more common than it is in Crohn's disease. However, an insidious onset does occur in this disease. Proctosigmoidoscopy and radiographic contrast studies are necessary to confirm the diagnosis of either disease.

ENDOCRINE SYSTEM

As might be expected, endocrinologic aberrations are not uncommon in adolescents. Disorders of the thyroid gland make up a significant proportion of these problems during adolescence, more commonly in females than in males. Though one must keep alert for systemic signs of hypo-or hyperthyroidism in one's patients, most often a problem is signaled by enlargement of the gland.

Graves' disease (thyrotoxicosis) accounts for the greater portion of hyperthyroidism in adolescents. It usually presents with enlargement of the gland and with some symptoms of hypermetabolism such as weight loss or weakness. Nervousness, anxiety, decreased school performance, and general irritability can usually be elicited on taking the history. Physical examination typically reveals a symmetrically enlarged thyroid gland with a bruit over the surface. Confirmatory laboratory tests include an elevated thyroxine (T_4), tri-iodothyronine (T_3), and thyroid index with suppressed thyroid-stimulating hormone. Treatment includes antithyroid drugs and/or subtotal thyroidectomy. Irradiation is rarely if ever indicated in adolescents.

Hypothyroidism is less common in adolescents, but one must be on guard for it. Any adolescent who displays growth retardation and/or unexplained lethargy should be investigated for hypothyroidism. Chronic lymphocytic thyroiditis (Hashimoto's struma) presents with nontender thyroid enlargement without a bruit. T_4 is low or normal, and antithyroid antibodies are usually elevated. Treatment utilizes thyroid replacement medication. Thyroid nodules demand investigation, including scintillation scanning. Thyroid carcinoma, however, is rare in adolescence.

Diabetes mellitus is probably the most important chronic disorder of adolescence. The peak incidence occurs between 9 and 12 years of age. The diabetes that occurs in adolescents is almost always of the insulin dependent variety known as juvenile-onset diabetes mellitus. Symptoms, e.g., weight loss, weakness, polyuria, and polydypsia, usually progress rapidly from their onset to clinical recognition of the disease. Diagnosis is confirmed by the finding of glycosuria and hyperglycemia. Glucose tolerance tests are rarely necessary for diagnosis. Ketonemia and ketonuria are common at presentation, but symptomatic ketoacidosis is unusual.

After initial stabilization with insulin, the adolescent usually experiences a "honeymoon" phase in which insulin requirements decrease significantly. This period may last for a few months, after which insulin requirements rise to or above "pre-honeymoon" amounts. Some adolescents can be managed with one insulin injection per day, given in the morning. This is usually a combination of an intermediate-acting and a short-acting insulin. Many adolescents, however, require an additional, though smaller, amount of insulin in the evening for optimal stabilization of carbohydrate metabolism. Dietary management consists of maintaining a well balanced, nutritionally sound diet with no excesses of carbohydrates.

In many instances, management of juvenile diabetes mellitus in adolescents presents no major problems. These adolescents incorporate the constraints imposed by the disease into their life styles with minimum difficulty. However, a fair number of teenagers have great problems with diabetes, and frequent bouts of ketoacidosis may occur which necessitate hospitalization. Often such an adolescent lives in a disturbed psychosocial milieu. Alternatively, diabetes occurred prior to puberty, and the stress of adolescence precipitates management difficulties of the diabetes. The point is that the combination of an unstable home, a developing psyche, and a chronic disease requiring daily management is often too much for the young person to handle. Attempts to manage the medical aspects of the patients's problem are doomed to failure if the psychosocial problems are not attacked as well. Fortunately, a number of these "brittle" diabetics achieve adequate control of their disease just by maturing, provided they can be kept somewhat stable during their stormy adolescence.

REPRODUCTIVE SYSTEM

The genitalia and all aspects of the reproductive system and sexuality are of prime importance during adolescence. Aside from the general increase in body size and changes in body shape, the development of secondary sex characteristics is the significant biologic event of adolescence. The problems, real and imagined, related to the sex organs and to sexuality occupy a proportionately large part of the trials of adolescence. In males there are concerns about size, shape, and function. Misconceptions about masturbation and sexually transmitted disease abound. Nocturnal emissions can be frightening to the uninitiated boy. Hernias and hydroceles may be present. Either condition is almost always unilateral. A hernia can usually be reduced, but a hydrocele cannot. Hydroceles also transilluminate and generally hernias do not. A varicocele is a collection of enlarged blood vessels along the spermatic cord, most often on the left side; it rarely demands any treatment. Phimosis occurs if the foreskin is so tight that it cannot be retracted over the glans, and in such an instance circumcision is indicated. Undescended testicles are usually diagnosed in childhood but occasionally are present in adolescent boys, and these should be referred for surgical treatment. Males may also be greatly concerned if only one testicle is present; often they have restricted their activities or they have received much misinformation, which should be corrected.

Females are often concerned with breast size and shape, with menstruation, and with sexuality. Breast masses do occur in adolescent girls. In our experience at the Adolescent Clinic at the University of Alabama in Birmingham, a mass has never been malignant in a series of more than 300. Almost all of the masses were fibroadenomas, which are firm but not hard and are movable. More than one mass was present in 25% of the patients. Nevertheless, fibroadenomas can cause discomfort and concern. If they persist unchanged or if they enlarge through two menstrual cycles, we recommend surgery for excision.

Menstrual problems fall into two main categories. The first encompasses irregularity or lack of menstruation; the second involves abnormal quantities or periods of bleeding. Primary and secondary amenorrhea must be differentiated. First, girls who have developed secondary sex characteristics have to be distinguished from those who have not.

Although the average age of onset of menstruation is 12 years 3 months, many girls have an earlier or later onset. One occasionally encounters a girl of 14 or 15 years of age who has never menstruated. If this is the case, a thorough history and physical examination should be done. If the girl is at a sex maturity rating of 3 or 4 and has no abnormal anatomical findings, she should be reassured that periods will probably start within a few months. If there are real emotional problems associated with being left behind by her peers, a trial of progesterone for five days can be done. If there is bleeding in the week following cessation of treatment, the girl is reassured that she can menstruate and that when her own hormone production is adequate, she will do so. If there is no bleeding, estrogen can be given for three weeks, and then discontinued; bleeding should then occur. Or, progesterone can be added immediately after the estrogen is discontinued. If bleeding does not occur, further endocrine examinations are warranted. However, if bleeding is present, the girl (and probably her mother) should be reassured that menses will occur.

The most common cause of secondary amenorrhea is pregnancy; the examiner should not rely on the history given by an adolescent girl, for many wish to deny the possibility of being pregnant. If the teenager is not pregnant, cycling with estrogen and progesterone can be done, but it should be remembered that long periods of amenorrhea are common when girls first begin to menstruate. Turner's syndrome (XO chromosome pattern) is rare but should be suspected if a girl is less than five feet tall and has retarded sexual development and no menses.

Dysfunctional uterine bleeding, i.e., excessive bleeding during or between menstrual periods, can be a distressing problem. Most commonly it is due to prolonged estrogen effect on the endometrium with prolonged breakdown of the lining. The possibility of an incomplete abortion must be considered. Tumors of the uterus are very rare at this age. Therapy, following a normal vaginal examination, involves administration of estrogen to stabilize the endometrial lining followed by withdrawal to induce normal menses. This therapy can be given intravenously or orally, depending on the severity of the bleeding. The hematocrit must be checked to see if anemia due to blood loss has occurred. If so, replacement therapy with iron is indicated.

Dysmenorrhea is another complaint of many adolescent girls. Menstrual pain usually does not begin until periods become ovulatory. This usually does not occur at menarche. Most girls have several anovulatory periods after menarche, so that cramps do not become a problem until several months later. If in a thorough physical examination other abnormalities (which are rare) are not revealed, treatment of this very real problem must be considered. Depending on the number of days when pain occurs and on the severity of the pain, various therapies may be considered. These include non-narcotic and narcotic analgesics, exercise, and hormonal intervention in the form of oral contraceptive pills, among others.

A male with failure of sexual development after 13½ years of age should usually be evaluated endocrinologically. In the great majority of cases short stature is also found and growth records reveal normal prepubertal height increases. Most commonly a history of similar late development in closely related males will be found. Bone age radiographs will reveal a lag. Usually, assurance that all is normal and that proper development will occur is all that is needed. If the boy is 14 or 15 years of age and endocrine investigation was normal, a six-month course of monthly testosterone injections will induce some sexual development and help to restore the young man's self-confidence. If height records reveal a flattening of the growth curve after several years of normal height increase, hypothyroidism and hypopituitarism should be considered as causes. Hypothyroidism, however, does not usually cause a delay in sexual maturation. If, upon examination, an adolescent male is found to have small, soft testicles, a buccal smear should be obtained to check for Klinefelter's syndrome (XXY).

A majority of adolescents over 15 years of age are at least occasionally sexually active.[13] Therefore one must always be conscious of the possibility of sexually transmitted disease (STD). The most prevalent of the serious sexually transmitted diseases is gonorrhea; more than a million cases are reported yearly. The actual number of cases is certainly somewhat larger. Females present most frequently with symptomatic cervicitis and/or salpingitis, whereas males usually present with a yellowish purulent urethritis. It must be noted that up to 80% of females infected with gonococcus and 40% of male contacts of females with gonorrhea are asymptomatic. Syphilis occurs much less frequently than gonorrhea, and the incidence has declined in the past two or three years, as has that of gonorrhea.

In males, the other significant sexually transmitted disease is nonspecific urethritis, which is caused by a chlamydial organism. It generally presents with dysuria and with very little discharge (which is usually mucoid), but it may progress to florid epidydimitis. An obvious case of gonorrhea, properly treated, but which does not seem to resolve, may actually have been a double infection in which the gonorrhea masked the chlamydial urethritis prior to treatment. Chlamydial genital infections have recently acquired a more ominous reputation as evidence accumulates that the organism can be transmitted to and can infect the newborn infant.

Females frequently experience symptomatic vaginal discharges, with or without urethral irritation, that are not caused by gonococcus. These are, most commonly, nonspecific vaginitis (caused by *Hemophilus vaginalis*), trichomonas vaginitis, and candidal vulvovaginitis. Diagnosis can usually be made by examination of vaginal swabs. Additionally, one must be aware of herpetic infections and various granulomatous infections.

VASCULAR SYSTEM

Hypertension is a condition being accorded much greater attention in adolescents than was formerly the case. It is being more commonly acknowledged that essential hypertension in adults has its onset, if not in childhood, then, in many instances, in adolescence. Heredity plays a definite etiologic role, as does environment, in the form of high salt diets and, most probably, stress. Hypertension in childhood, in the main, is secondary, and a diligent search must be pursued for the primary cause. In adolescents, however, the majority of the cases are of the idiopathic, i.e., essential, type. Problems occur when an attempt is made to define that blood pressure at which intervention should be initiated. Is the 95th percentile a valid cutoff point? Different criteria should probably be used for each sex at each level of sexual maturation. As yet, no definite standards are at hand. For our purposes we use criteria of three successive weekly readings in excess of 142/90 in males of SMR 4 and 5, and 138/88 in females of SMR 4 and 5, for defining hypertension. The importance of proper consistent recording techniques cannot be too heavily emphasized. In those adolescents found to be hypertensive, a thorough history and physical examination usually give one enough information to decide whether or not to pursue an investigation for a primary cause. In the great majority of our hypertensive patients, the history and physical examination are normal aside from the blood pressure. A minimal laboratory workup then ensues. This includes a hematocrit, a urine analysis (looking particularly for protein), an electrocardiogram (more sensitive in detecting cardiac hypertrophy than a chest Xray), and determination of serum electrolytes, blood urea nitrogen, serum creatinine, and serum uric acid. The last is used as a baseline in adolescents treated with thiazide diuretics which may elevate uric acid in the blood.

The dilemma of whether to treat or not to treat is considerable. A systolic pressure greater than 160 mm of mercury and a diastolic pressure greater than 110 mm are definite indications for drug therapy. But whether or not to treat a male or female with a level between 140/90 and 160/110 is not clear. This is especially true because we do not know which of these "borderline" adolescents will go on to have significant hypertension as adults and because the drugs used for treatment have side effects. We have tended to begin therapy when diastolic pressure remains in the high 90s.

Summary

The preceding pages show that adolescents can and do have significant organic problems in addition to cognitive and psychosocial ones. Too often even health workers view adolescents as having only behavior or drug abuse problems, venereal disease, or pregnancies outside of marriage. It is impossible in a chapter of this length to discuss in detail many of the important illnesses and handicaps affecting adolescents; standard texts must be consulted for further information.

It is readily admitted that a great deal of time would be required to take a detailed history as suggested and then perform a careful, complete physical examination. It should be obvious that under many circumstances all of this is not done at the time of a first visit. Essential information needed to diagnose and treat the medical condition is obtained at that time, and a return visit is scheduled during which the complete workup of the patient is done. Busy clinics and office practices rarely permit an hour or more for one patient but, depending upon the complaints and the situation, adjustments must often be made.

It is again stressed that the health provider should develop a tripartite concept in which the physical, cognitive, and psychosocial aspects of adolescence form a whole that affects growth and development and also the management and outcome of disease. Illness and handicaps can also affect each of these three important areas, and it is necessary to consider their effects. Adolescence can be an opportunity to correct past damages and to provide new opportunities for good health and also social and preventive measures that are extremely important. Most adolescents are appreciative without expressing appreciation. However, they can be forthright and candid, though often biased and misinformed. The adult who sincerely tries to understand them and respect them will find them a delightful group of persons with whom to work.

REFERENCES

1. Cosgrove, M., et al. "Male Genital Urinary Abnormality: Maternal Diethylstilbesterol." *J. Urol.* 117:220–221, 1977.
2. Bibbo, M., et al. "Follow-Up Study of Male:Female Offspring of Diethylstilbesterol Treated Mothers. Preliminary Report." *J. Reproductive Med.* 15:29, 1975.
3. Gill, W. B., et al. "Pathological Semen and Uncommon Abnormalities of Genital Tract in Human Male Subjects Exposed to DES in Utero." *J. Urol.* 117:477–480, 1977.
4. Tanner, J. M. *Growth at Adolescence,* 2nd ed. Oxford, England: Blackwell Scientific Publications, Ltd., 1962.
5. Frisch, R. E. "Weight at Menarche: Similarity for Well-Nourished and Undernourished Girls at Differing Ages, and Evidence for Historical Constancy." *Pediatr.* 50:445–450, 1972.
6. Barnes, H. V. "Physical Growth and Development During Puberty." *Med. Clin. N. Am.* 59:1305–1317, 1975.
7. Daniel, W. A., Jr. "Hematocrit: Maturity Relationship in Adolescence." *Pediatr.* 52:388–394, 1973.
8. Garn, S. M., Smith, M. J., and Clark, D. C. "Race Differences in Hemoglobin Levels." *Ecol. Food Nutr.* 3:299–301, 1974.
9. Vaughan, V. C., and McKay, R. J. *Nelson Textbook of Pediatrics,* 10th ed. Philadelphia: W. B. Saunders Co., 1975.
10. Daniel, W. A., Jr. *Adolescents in Health and Disease.* St. Louis: C. V. Mosby Co., 1977.
11. Gallagher, J. R., Heald, F. P., and Garrell, D. W. *Medical Care of the Adolescent.* New York: Appleton-Century-Crofts, 1976.
12. Daniel, W. A., Jr. *Adolescents in Health and Disease.* St. Louis: C. V. Mosby Co., 1977, p. 301.
13. *Eleven Million Teenagers.* New York: the Alan Guttmacher Institute, Planned Parenthood Federation of America, 1976.

BIBLIOGRAPHY

Daniel, W. A., Jr. *Adolescents in Health and Disease.* St. Louis: C. V. Mosby Co., 1977.
Daniel, W. A., Jr., and Bennett, D. L. "The Use of Anabolic-Androgenic Steroids in Childhood and Adolescence." In Kochakian, C. D., *Handbook of Experimental Pharmacology.* New York: Springer-Verlag, Inc., 1976, pp. 441–482.
Daniel, W. A., Jr. "Hermatocrit: Maturity Relationship in Adolescence." *Pediatr.* 52:388–394, 1973.
Davis, S. *Rights of Juveniles.* New York: Clark Boordman Co., Ltd., 1974.

Emans, S. J., and Goldstein, D. *Pediatric and Adolescent Gynecology*. Boston: Little, Brown & Co., 1977.

Farber, M. L. *Theory of Suicide*. New York: Funk and Wagnalls Co., 1968.

Jacob, J. *Adolescent Suicide*. New York: Wiley-Interscience, 1971.

Konopka, G. *Young Girls: A Portrait of Adolescence*. Englewood Cliffs, N. J.: Prentice Hall, Inc., 1976.

Lipsitz, J. *Growing Up Forgotten—A Review of Research and Programs Concerning Early Adolescence*. Lexington, Mass.: D. C. Heath & Co., 1977.

Loggie, J. M., ed. "Hypertension in Childhood and Adolescence." *Pediatr. Clin. N. Am.* 25:1978.

Moriarity, A., and Toussing, P. *Adolescent Coping*. New York: Grune & Stratton, 1976.

Muus, Rolf. *Theories of Adolescence*. New York: Random House, Inc., 1975.

Rice, F. P. *The Adolescent: Development, Relationship, and Culture*. Boston: Allyn & Bacon, Inc., 1975.

Tanner, J. M. *Growth at Adolescence*. Oxford: Blackwell Scientific Publications, Ltd., 1973.

7

The Adolescent in the Hospital

MARILYN SAVEDRA, R.N., D.N.S.

"Today I'm leaving this god-awful place. I'm walking out on my feet, not in a gurney or a wheelchair but just my own two feet. Well I'm outside now and feeling great. You wouldn't believe how good it feels to have the wind blow against my face. It's so nice, it leaves me speechless. The sun feels hot, and the breeze is nice and cool. It's a beautiful day for a person to get out of the hospital. It was a long haul and a terrible experience. I hope it never happens to me or anyone else again." These are the words of an adolescent writing of his hospital experience resulting from a fractured femur. He typifies the many adolescents hospitalized unexpectedly following traumatic accidents. Although he had an uneventful recovery from a medical standpoint, the several weeks of hospitalization were anything but uneventful for this teenager, as his hospital diary reveals.

Other adolescents may also experience hospitalization unexpectedly, but for shorter periods and without the traumatic, life-threatening suddenness frequently associated with accidents. These patients may actively seek care when symptoms of an acute illness such as appendicitis are present. Though treatment and hospitalization may be no less threatening, it is purposefully sought by the adolescent and/or his family.

Still another group of adolescents, those suffering from chronic and/or life-threatening diseases, may enter the hospital hurriedly, but they enter a setting where the people, the routines, and the facilities are more than familiar. For example, the adolescent with asthma or cystic fibrosis may have been in and out of a given hospital for the major portion of his life.

A much smaller segment by far of the adolescent patient population enter the hospital for elective tests or surgery. Although the hospitalization may not be without stress, it is nevertheless a planned, expected event. The anticipated outcome, as, for example, in the case of corrective cosmetic surgery, is usually eagerly sought by the young patient.

The adolescent may find himself in any one of a number of locations when he is admitted to a hospital. With increasing frequency he may find himself in a unit especially designed and organized to care for adolescents. The ages of patients in such a unit may range from a lower limit of ten years to an upper limit of 21 years.[1,2] At the other extreme, the patient may find himself in a unit with adult patients of all ages who may or may not be understanding or tolerant of adolescents and their behavior. The majority of patients will most likely find themselves in a pediatric unit designed to care for patients from birth through adolescence, the top age figure varying from institution to institution. Thus the adolescent may find himself in a room with patients his own age or considerably younger. With the decline in inpatient pediatric patients as a result of greater emphasis on disease prevention and health maintenance, adolescent patients who were once admitted to adult units because of lack of space in the pediatric wards are now being assigned to these wards; this increases the numbers of teenage patients found in general pediatric units. Adolescents may also come to the hospital to seek care on an outpatient basis; adolescent health clinics are being established at an increasing rate for this particular age group.[3] Though this chapter focuses on the inpatient and the implications for nursing care, much of the material presented is applicable to the adolescent in the clinic situation as well.

There is increasing awareness on the part of nurses and other health professionals that the adolescent patient has unique needs and can be effectively treated neither as a child nor as an adult.[4,5] Assessment and interventions must be made in the context of adolescent development and the teenage patient's perception of his illness.

Illness and the Adolescent

Illness with resulting hospitalization is not part of the experience of the average adolescent. Any illness—no matter how minor or seemingly insignificant to the adult—presents a major concern to the adolescent patient. For some, a given problem may be a new and threatening event such as acne, venereal disease, or scoliosis. For others, the present disease—as in the case of diabetes or nephrosis—may have had its beginning in childhood and may be carried over into the adolescent period. Although adolescents with long-term or chronic conditions may be more familiar than other young people with the disease process and its effect on their bodies, the condition is no less threatening and disturbing to them when they are facing, at the same time, a number of new developmental tasks.

Understanding of the impact of illness on the adolescent can be increased by consideration of the major developmental concerns and tasks of this stage, as described in Chapter 1. Just as important as an understanding of these tasks, however, is an awareness that all of the tasks do not have equal priority throughout the adolescent period. The early adolescent, for example, is focusing on three tasks as defined by Havighurst:[6] achieving new and more mature relations with agemates, achieving a masculine or feminine social role, and accepting and using his or her body more effectively. The attention of the middle or late adolescent is focused on achieving emotional independence from parents and selecting and preparing for an occupation or career that will insure economic independence. Cultural and socioeconomic status are other important variables that influence the timing of focus on a given developmental task. Two major developmental concerns which emerge from the tasks and have major implications for health professionals are concern about body function and body image. Awareness of cognitive development is also necessary for the health care professional who deals with adolescents.

DEVELOPMENTAL CONCERNS

All teenagers are concerned about the proper functioning of their bodies, and illness of any nature heightens this concern. Many young teenagers are experiencing new and unfamiliar sensations as part of normal physiological changes. This unfamiliarity with their changing bodies often makes it difficult for them to distinguish between illness and normal sensations. Hofmann and associates[5] speak of the hyperresponsiveness of adolescents to pain and other abnormal sensations; their reactions may seem quite out of proportion to the presenting biological condition. The seemingly exaggerated response to these perceived sensations is indeed age-appropriate. What is inappropriate is an expectation on the part of the health professional that the adolescent will behave either as a child or as an adult. Treatments that affect body functioning are also viewed with a high degree of anxiety by the adolescent if he is not given an adequate explanation of them while they are going on.

In addition to his heightening concern about what is happening to his body, the adolescent has an equally great concern about its appearance. Even a seemingly trivial or minor blemish can be shattering to an adolescent. Anything that makes one seem less than perfect and/or different from one's peers makes the task of becoming comfortable with oneself more difficult. To the adolescent, and particularly the girl, attractiveness is viewed as a vital asset in achieving desired relationships with the opposite sex. The result of this increased concern about body functioning and perfection of appearance is a normal hypochondriasis.[5] It is understandable that the adolescent with genuine physiological changes and alterations of appearance such as obesity, skeletal deformity, clubbed fingers, and disfiguring scars will experience added stress as he or she struggles both to accept his or her body and use it effectively and to achieve satisfactory social relations with peers of the opposite sex.

COGNITIVE FACTORS

At this stage in his cognitive development the adolescent becomes capable of abstract thinking. According to the developmental schema of Piaget he achieves the stage of formal operations. Flavell,[7] in his summary of Piaget's work, identifies the major characteristics of thinking at this stage as being concerned with the real versus the possible, propositional in nature, and geared to combinational analysis or the exhaustive inventorying of variables. Thus the adolescent can appreciate physiological changes resulting from illness and often seeks answers to his questions based on scientific evidence. His level of cognitive ability enables the adolescent to think beyond the present to the future and to participate actively in a plan of care during and following hospitalization. At the same time the adolescent has a rich fantasy life which may cause him to see an illness in a way that is vastly different from reality. He may view a serious condition such as osteosarcoma as relatively minor, or on the other hand may consider a weight gain of a pound or two as a major threat to his future.

Responses to Hospitalization for Illness

The developmental stage, although it is one of the most valuable predictors of adolescent response to hospitalization and also provides a basis for understanding adolescent behavior, cannot in itself supply adequate information to guide a plan of care. For adolescents, as is true of all ages, hospitalization is perceived as stressful and as containing elements of a life-threatening experience.

FACTORS AFFECTING THE RESPONSE

Numerous factors have an influence on how any adolescent will respond to illness and hospitalization; they should be considered in the initial and ongoing assessments. While no one factor can be identified as being more significant than another, all of the following should be noted.

The expected or unexpected nature of the illness and resulting hospitalization has numerous implications. If the hospitalization was unexpected, there is a high likelihood that preparation for the experience was minimal or nonexistent. Wolfer and Visintainer[8] found that children, aged 3 to 14, who received psychological preparation and continued supportive care when they had minor surgery were less upset during hospitalization and following discharge than children who did not receive information about events, experiences, expectations, and responses along with previews of procedures through play techniques. Pediatric nursing textbooks also stress the value of preplanning and knowledge of what is to take place in relation to coping effectively with the situation.[9,10,11] Schowalter and Lord's[1] study of 100 adolescents indicates that 87% of the subjects agreed that some preparation is desirable. However, 61% indicated that the waiting period should be no longer than one week.[1] Unexpected events of any kind are frequently disruptive of plans and long-anticipated activities. An adolescent, for example, who is hospitalized with an injury during the final month of high school when a prom is anticipated, may find the experience far more devastating than the adolescent who is admitted for a planned tonsillectomy during the school break.

Linked with the expected or unexpected character of the hospitalization are the nature of the illness and the anticipated duration of the hospitalization. Is the problem acute, chronic, or terminal, and what is the expected outcome? Is a relatively brief hospitalization expected, as in the case of an appendectomy, or will the hospitalization be prolonged, as in the case of idiopathic scoliosis, causing extended absence from school and estrangement from peers? Blake[12] speaks of the impatience of youth in waiting for health to improve.

Numerous combinations of factors can often occur. Although hospitalization for scoliosis may be extended, the eventual prognosis is good. On the other hand, an adolescent's brief hospitalization for diabetes that is out of control carries with it the knowledge that he is faced with an imperfect body for the rest of his life. Because of his great concern for attractiveness and normality, the visibility of the illness or of the effects of treatment will affect the adolescent's response. Severe acne, while not life-threatening, may cause excruciating distress. An abdominal incision which appears small and insignificant to the adult may appear altogether different to the 14-year-old girl who anticipates wearing a bikini swimsuit during the approaching summer. Another major factor influencing response is the factor of restrictions that must be imposed because of the illness. Restrictions may be physical, as in the case of the patient in traction or in a cast, or may be related to diet or other activities of daily living. Pain, whether resulting from the disease process itself or from the imposed treatment, must be considered when assessing an adolescent's responses. As was mentioned in the preceding section, a teenager often responds to pain in a manner felt to be most inappropriate by the adult. There are other factors—more difficult to identify than those already mentioned but nevertheless significant—that influence the teenager's response to the hospital experience; they are his self-concept and degree of emotional stability.

ADOLESCENT COMMENTS ON HOSPITALIZATION

Research on hospitalized adolescents has been minimal to date. One study, though unsophisticated in design, revealed some interesting data. Chambers and associates,[13] in an attempt to find out how adolescents would feel about hospitalization, asked adolescents on the streets of Leicester, England, what would be their immediate reaction to hospitalization. Some typical responses were: "Bloody awful!" "Oh hell, what a waste of precious time!" "Very frustrating and claustrophobic," "Scared stiff at the prospect of lying in bed having horrible things stuck in me," "Don't fancy it because I'm going to a party on Friday." Schowalter and Lord,[1] wishing to determine adolescents' reactions to hospitalization in an adolescent unit, interviewed 100 randomly selected adolescents, ranging in age from 10 to 17 years, and their parents. Among other things, the findings showed that though parents tended to be more pessimistic about their children's conditions, they also tended to underestimate their children's concerns. The adolescents' focus of concern was on daily discomforts, as opposed to the parents' long-range concerns. Parents underestimated the fears experienced by the patients in relation to medical procedures and separation.

EXPECTED BEHAVIOR IN RESPONSE TO HOSPITALIZATION

Of greatest concern to the nurse and other health professionals who care for adolescents, whether in an adolescent unit or in a setting with other children and adults, is the behavior elicited by the response to illness and hospitalization. Hammar[14] characterizes this response as variable and unpredictable and considers the adolescent less likely to be the "ideal patient." Whatever the adolescent's response, it is imperative to assess what is happening, for according to Hofmann and associates[5] the matter is critical and assessment is essential if constructive behavior is to be reinforced and maladaptive behavior is to be deterred.

The majority of adolescents who enter the hospital are anxious. As described by Conway,[15] this anxiety may be external and relate to the new and strange environment with its unknown and often painful procedures and its isolation from family and friends, or it may be internal and arise from perceived threats to body concept and identity. The adolescent attempts to manage his anxiety by a variety of coping strategies, which he has customarily used in the past when stress or crisis have arisen. The number and sequence of coping strategies varies with the individual and may or may not prove successful for the immediate situation. The ideal response is insightful acceptance—the adolescent realistically accepts the condition and views the illness without any sense of personal devaluation. This constructive response is rare in any individual and extremely unlikely in an adolescent who is grappling with developmental tasks related to self-identity.

When a serious illness with a possible life-threatening outcome occurs, the most common device used by adolescents, and often by their families, is denial that the illness exists. Or if, as in the case of the early adolescent, the diagnosis is accepted, the outcomes and anticipated alterations in activities may not be acknowledged. This strategy of denial may have positive implications or may be potentially destructive. If the adolescent is cooperative and complies with the plan of care, initial denial may be useful. If, on the other hand, he refuses to carry out treatments, take prescribed medications, and keep follow-up appointments, the results of denying the illness may have dire consequences. For instance, an adolescent—who formerly accepted a condition and complied with the needed care—may suddenly have a reversal in behavior, as in the case of a teenager with a bleeding disorder who chooses to engage in contact sports. Denial in adolescents is usually temporary, for most feel that they can deal with the condition and consequently begin to use other strategies.[2]

The acutely ill adolescent who may also have experienced a surgical procedure almost universally returns to a more childlike mode of behavior. He is accepting or demanding of attention from nurses. He dislikes being alone and calls for services which he often appears capable of performing himself. He desires the presence of his parents. He may be whiney and irritable. All of the behaviors associated with the mechanism of regression are not only to be expected but are appropriate and healthy in the acutely ill, postsurgical, or immobilized adolescent. They enable the adolescent to set aside the burden of dealing with tasks he is physically and emotionally unable to handle at the time and return to the more dependent state of early childhood. The ability to regress, as in the case of a severely burned adolescent or an adolescent suffering multiple injuries, may offer the most realistic way of dealing with the situation. An adolescent may even find temporary enjoyment in the oversolicitousness and increased attention of his parents. Responding to their child's regression may be helpful to parents who are also coping with the stress of the situation. Regression as a coping strategy does become unhealthy when it carries over into the convalescent period. As the patient feels better and no longer is experiencing severe pain, his behavior should again reflect the previous drive to achieve normal developmental tasks.

To nurses and doctors, some of the most distressing behaviors exhibited by adolescents include manipulation strategies, verbal abuse, physical attacks, sexual suggestiveness, and refusal to cooperate with the plan of care. Case studies appear frequently in the nursing literature which graphically portray the young person who copes with his situation by acting out.[16,17,18,19,20] Unlike the strategies already discussed, these behaviors are not healthy. They indicate both a real fear engendered by the situation and the desire to escape. They may indicate an attempt by the adolescent to secure reassurance about his self-worth.[5] These behaviors are not those most frequently seen. In their five-year experience on an adolescent ward, Schowalter and Anyan[21] found that sexually aggressive behavior was not a usual acting-out behavior and that patients who are ill behave in a way that is more characteristic of the latency period. Acting-out behaviors are often indicative of a more serious behavior problem that has antedated the hospitalization. Hospital staff members, unfortunately, frequently respond to patients who are acting out in an equally ineffective manner. Rational appeals, verbal threats, and retaliative measures do little to alleviate a stressful situation. Though it may not be possible in a brief hospitalization to alter this type of behavior, seeking to understand the underlying cause and developing a nursing plan to carry out when the behavior is exhibited can be helpful.

Less outwardly distressing than manipulative and acting-out behavior, but at times equally frustrating, is that of the adolescent patient who withdraws and walls himself off. This type of behavior, like regressive behavior, is normally present on a temporary basis during the acute phase of illness. Withdrawal may be severe—as in the case of a teenager who does not talk, turns away when people enter his room, lies quietly immobile and refuses to watch television or listen to the radio—or it may be expressed by temporary refusal to see peers during a time when the visible manifestations of the disease are disfiguring. When used to conserve energies during the critical stage of illness, withdrawal may be a healthy strategy. As in the case of regression, it becomes maladaptive when it continues into the recovery phase. When the circumstances appear to warrant a degree of withdrawal it is appropriate to accept the behavior while at the same time helping the adolescent to move toward resuming involvement with friends and usual activities.

At times, adolescents who feel guilty or responsible for the situation they are in, as in the case of injury from a motor vehicle accident, blame the nursing staff for being uncaring and inconsiderate of their needs. Parents also are berated for being inattentive to the teenager. Frequently the outbursts can be perceived by the nurse as a personal attack and are not seen as a device to ease the anxiety and guilt of the adolescent patient.

Another strategy commonly used by adolescents and made possible by their stage of cognitive development is to focus on the factual aspects of the illness and its treatment and suppress the emotional aspects. The result is a patient who is interested in gaining information about his condition and responsive to the teaching initiated by the nurse and other members of the health team. This behavior is generally approved and results in responsiveness from the nurse. Although this strategy may be a positive way of coping, it has some inherent difficulties. Even when given accurate information, the adolescent may nevertheless fantasize and consequently end up with a distorted view of the condition. If the illness is of a severe nature, such as leukemia, it may not be possible to continue to suppress the emotional aspects. When an adolescent freely discusses his diagnosis, staff members may infer that he is coping well and overlook the anxiety underlying this strategy.

One of the most frequently observed behaviors in the hospitalized adolescent is his constant complaining about food. Schowalter and Lord[22] found during patient meetings that even such items as milk, gelatin, and other relatively unalterable items were denounced as being poorly served and poor tasting. This verbal behavior is actually a helpful means of defusing the anxiety that may arise when a young patient is awaiting the results of tests, anticipating surgery, or tolerating temporary immobility. Other similar behaviors are preoccupation with the condition of a roommate, concern about school work, and engrossment in books or games brought from home. All of these activities distract the adolescent from his major concern, over which he has no control. This strategy of displacement is most effective when the situation causing the anxiety is of relatively short duration, such as the usual illness and/or hospitalization.

Developmental Tasks Altered by Illness and Hospitalization

The energy used in coping with illness and the hospital experience may take away the energy needed to master the developmental tasks of adolescence.[14] Since a nursing care goal for patients of any age is to enable the individual to achieve his developmental tasks, it is important to consider how hospitalization may enhance or impede the process.

The early adolescent's attention is focused primarily on his changing body and on using it effectively. Hofmann[23] states that "the impact of illness on early adolescence poses its greatest threat in the real or fantasized insult to physical integrity." The early adolescent is concerned with anything that affects the appearance of his body or its function. Though illness might seem to have an essentially negative impact on his hope of achieving this task, being hospitalized may place the young teenager in contact with professional people who can teach him about his body and its functioning and with peers who are also coping with the same developmental tasks while under stress. If he is physically disfigured he should be exposed to those who show acceptance of him as he is and who can also help him to achieve acceptance of himself. If the hospitalization is for repair of a defect that will enable the adolescent to be more like his normal peers, the experience should also have a positive influence on the task of achieving comfort with his body.

Another task of early adolescence that may be hindered by hospitalization is the achieving of new and more mature relations with peers.[4] Hospitalization, with its possible immobilizing aspects—i.e., traction, intravenous therapy, and enforced bed rest—separates the adolescent from his usual friends. If prolonged, it can have a marked effect on the accomplishment of this task unless measures are taken to keep the adolescent patient in contact with his agemates. Often hospital visiting policies exclude the young adolescent's peers. The early adolescent is just beginning to achieve emotional independence from his parents and other adults; the dependency imposed by hospitalization will not pose quite as great a threat to him as it will to the midadolescent.

The task of achieving emotional independence from parents and other adults is a major focus of the midadolescent. At a time when emancipation conflicts are at their peak, illness or injury that is severe enough to require hospitalization can pose a serious threat to the achievement of this independence. Enforced bed rest, with possibly greater immobility due to traction or a cast, places the midadolescent in a state of extreme dependency. He is incapable of dealing with even his most basic needs for nourishment, hygiene, and elimination. He is frequently isolated from persons who could help him attain mastery of the developmental tasks of this stage. His sense of loss of control, when superimposed upon a condition that alters his appearance or body functioning, can result in the same body image concerns that were a preoccupation of the early adolescent. This can have a major effect on his need to attract members of the opposite sex and to achieve a gender-appropriate sexual role. The adolescent may fear that illness and hospitalization may result in the loss of a relationship with a newly acquired girl or boy friend. This thought may be devastating. Some midadolescents may have begun the task of preparing for a life career. Others may have secured jobs which afford them at least a degree of financial independence. A prolonged hospitalization therefore may pose problems in keeping up with studies and may threaten the job.

On the positive side, if an adolescent is in a unit specifically designed for this age group he will have opportunities for associating with others of his own age and for receiving needed support from peers of both sexes. The hospital experience may also open up new possibilities for a future career, or at least maintain his schoolwork responsibilities at an appropriate level so that he does not fall behind his classmates.

The late adolescent, for the most part, has gained independence from his parents—if not economically, at least emotionally. He is now focusing more on a special partner than on the opposite sex in general. Marriage and future children may be seriously considered at this time. If a job or career has not been previously selected it may now become a major focus. The adolescent also develops an awareness and concern for his social and civic responsibilities.[4] Illness and hospitalization at this time may pose the greatest threat, because job, career, marriage, and life style goals may have to be altered. The teenager with cystic fibrosis or epilepsy may seriously wonder if he should marry and what the job possibilities are for him. The diabetic girl may be concerned with the effect of her disease on childbearing. In some cases, a job may have been selected but may no longer be feasible because of permanent disabilities resulting from an accident. Even when the illness is not of long duration and no long-term results are expected, the adolescent may be concerned about possible implications.

Implications for Nursing Care

Although implications for nursing care have been alluded to and the reader may have begun to come to his own conclusions regarding the type of care that would be most effective for hospitalized adolescents, the final section of this chapter will speak to this point.

Nursing care must be based on the needs of the individual adolescent. Though it is logical to assume that many of the adolescent's needs and concerns will be related to his developmental stage, it is essential to consider the individual differences that correspond to variations in timetables for anticipated physical and psychological changes. During the assessment process considerable time must be given for evaluating all of the factors which may affect the adolescent's response to illness and hospitalization, including the expected or unexpected nature of the experience, the degree of preparation, the timing in relation to important events, the nature of the illness and its anticipated prognosis, the expected duration, the visibility of the illness, the degree of restrictions imposed, the pain engendered by the illness and its treatment, the degree of separation from family and peers, and the adolescent's self-concept and degree of emotional stability. Information is also needed about the individual adolescent's typical coping strategies that have been helpful to him in past experiences with stress.

THE SETTING

Based on a knowledge and understanding of what adolescents are like, consideration should be given to providing a setting that can most effectively meet their physical, psychological, and social needs and foster the accomplishment of developmental tasks.

It is generally agreed that a ward exclusively for adolescents is the ideal situation. Studies have shown that adolescents and their families overwhelmingly approve of the arrangement.[1,24] In the Schowalter and Lord report, those who were not in favor of the adolescent ward were 13 years old or younger. The chief complaint, which is understandable in terms of developmental level, was that the unit was not restricted to their own sex.

Numerous articles,[4,25,26,27] as well as a section in *Changing Hospital Environments for Children,*[28] discuss the desirable characteristics of a hospital setting for adolescents. It is essential that adolescent rooms, whether in a separate unit or in a pediatric unit, should provide privacy. The writer recalls vividly the acute distress engendered in adolescent patients by the initial lack of curtains or screens in a newly opened unit. Rooms that are bright and cheerful, with age-appropriate decoration, are helpful in maintaining morale. Bulletin boards or walls that provide space for posters and items selected by the adolescents themselves are greatly appreciated. Adequate light for reading is essential. Adolescents should be encouraged to wear their own clothes, or, when this is not appropriate, should be provided with something other than the usual pediatric pajamas decorated with bunnies or the like. Because of their great concern for their bodies, adolescents need adequate facilities clearly marked for private bathing. Eating is a major activity of most adolescents and sneaking food is a characteristic way of life. A kitchenette with a refrigerator filled with milk, juices, ice cream, sandwiches, and fruit is a most welcome part of the unit for teenagers. Because of the need to communicate with friends and families, telephones should be readily available for any hospitalized adolescent. A recreational area for adolescents is also a must. The usual playroom found in pediatric wards does not meet the needs of this group and will rarely lure an adolescent to use the available activities. Most needed by this age group is a room with a television, record player, radio, table games, puzzles, magazines, and possibly a Ping-Pong or pool table. Space and facilities for more physical activities are important.

Although rules or policies are needed on any unit, for adolescents they should be few, appropriate to the needs of the age group, and enforceable. As discussed by Fuszard,[27] rules, rather than being a negative factor, are beneficial in that they reduce anxiety by pointing out what is expected of the patient and his or her peers. Peck[29] suggests that rules for an adolescent service should be based upon appropriate hospital behavior—i.e., no sleeping together, no fighting, no rough joking, and no pinching of the nurses. Policies need to be established regarding visitors, boundaries, and timing of activities. Liberal visiting hours that allow contact with peers are desirable, since they answer the need of the adolescent to socialize. It may be necessary to set limits on number and on the use of the recreational facilities by visitors. Adolescents need to move about and, when their condition warrants, to be able to go to the coffee shop, other wards, and, if possible, to outside areas. Adolescents may prefer to stay up late and sleep late. Flexibility about hours and routine activities, such as bathing, often makes for a happier and more cooperative patient who can cope with the many procedures and treatments that do not allow for flexibility. It does have to be communicated that the needs of an acutely ill roommate may necessitate limitations on noise and visitors for a given time.

More important, however, than the setting, the rules, and the policies of the ward are the people who staff the unit and the approach they use in caring for adolescents. Ideally, those who work with adolescents will not only have an understanding of this age group, but will choose to work with them because they are interested in them and enjoy them. Because, as was mentioned earlier, adolescents are neither children nor adults, they must be treated as the unique group that they are. Recognition of the need to establish independence from family and adults should play a major role in the approach used when working with teens. They need to be allowed as much freedom of choice as possible and from the onset should be involved in planning their care. Choice should be possible in such things as selecting their menus, setting a schedule of care, and what they wear. Adolescents, though still very much in need of support from family, also need time to communicate with the staff when parents are not present. It is generally not appropriate for parents of an adolescent to room in. If the hospital is some distance from home, parents may need help in finding suitable accommodations. Nurses frequently serve as needed role models as the adolescent seeks to establish an identity that is independent of his parents. If dependency behaviors appear to be extending beyond an appropriate period it may be necessary for the nurse to supportively set limits and thus encourage the adolescent in his task of independence.[30]

Recognition of the great concern about body functioning and appearance is another factor influencing an approach to care. As is stated by Gallagher,[31] the adolescent has a need to know the difference between ''not being average and being abnormal.'' Explanations must be given to the adolescent about what is happening to his body. In most cases he can be assured that what appears abnormal is not a permanent condition. A 17-year-old boy in traction as the result of a motor vehicle accident was asked if he would be willing for a nursing student to do a chest examination on him. He readily agreed and later expressed how reassuring it was to know that at least one part of his body was functioning normally. Throughout his rather extended hospitalization he had expressed numerous concerns about the various parts of his body.

Of vital importance—with respect not only to concerns about body functioning and possible death but also to concerns about school, finances, relationships with peers, and future career and family plans—is the adolescent's need to have someone to listen to him, someone who will hear not only the words he is saying but the fears and anxieties hidden beneath the words. Tiedt[30] suggests that the nurse in the process of listening to the adolescent must pay as much attention to him as to his symptoms. Patients' group meetings, as exemplified in the adolescent unit of Yale-New Haven Hospital, may give an added opportunity for adolescents to share their feelings.[32] Teens are often concerned about the matter of confidentiality. They need assurance that any information they give that might be destructive to them will be shared only with appropriate individuals.

Although little has been said about the family of the hospitalized adolescent, they too have concerns and anxieties related to the illness and cannot be ignored. As in the case of any other pediatric patient, the adolescent is supported when the needs of the family regarding the situation are identified and addressed. Duran[33] outlines three objectives of family-centered care that are related to the adolescent: (1) supporting the adolescent in his task of achieving independence, (2) identifying a parent's relationship with his adolescent child and assisting the parent in active participation in the adolescent's goal, and (3) providing an atmosphere that will help the parent in accomplishing his task.

PROBLEMS

In settings where adolescents are hospitalized, the major problems usually arise because of staff members who are inexperienced with this age group and lack knowledge of the adolescent's needs and concerns. While some nurses may feel comfortable in dealing with the adolescent when he is acutely ill, they become far less tolerant when, as his condition improves, he resumes some of his normal noisy, unruly behavior. Rigg and Fisher[24] identify two other situations that can present difficulties. One is the boredom that results from lack of activities. This is particularly true in units not geared to the teenager. The other problem is that of the adolescent who was troubled before hospitalization; in such a case, the present situation only accentuates what was already a problem.

Summary

Illness with hospitalization is not the usual experience for the adolescent. Coming at a time when the youth is dealing with major developmental tasks regarding independence, sexual identity, peer relations, and future job and career goals, it adds an extra stress to an already critical period. Though hospitalization may impede the accomplishment of the developmental tasks, it may also aid in their accomplishment. Whether hospitalization is ultimately a positive or negative experience for the adolescent depends to a large degree on the understanding, interest, and sensitive care of the nurse and other members of the health team.

REFERENCES

1. Schowalter, E., and Lord, D. "Admission to an Adolescent Ward." *Pediatrics* 44:1009–1011, 1969.
2. Daniel, A. *Adolescents in Health and Disease.* St. Louis: C. V. Mosby Company, 1977, pp. 11, 108.
3. Wolfish, M. G. "A Clinic for the Ambulatory Adolescent: Essentials, Scope, and Patterns of Operation." *Clin. Pediat.* 12:13–17, 1973.
4. Jackson, D. W. "The Adolescent and the Hospital." *Pediat. Clin. N. Am.* 20(4):901–910, 1973.
5. Hofmann, A. D., Becker, P. D., and Gabriel, H. P. *The Hospitalized Adolescent.* New York: Free Press, 1976, pp. 19, 20, 25, 38, 58.
6. Havighurst, R. J. *Developmental Tasks and Education.* New York: David McKay Co., Inc., 1948, pp. 33–71.
7. Flavell, J. H. *The Developmental Psychology of Jean Piaget.* New York: Van Nostrand Reinhold Co., 1963, pp. 204–211.
8. Wolfer, J. A., and Visintainer, M. "Pediatric Surgical Patients' and Parents' Stress Responses and Adjustment." *Nurs. Research* 24(4):244–255, 1975.
9. Klinzing, D. R., and Klinzing, D. G. *The Hospitalized Child: Communication Techniques for Health Personnel.* Englewood Cliffs, New Jersey: Prentice-Hall, Inc., 1977, p. 63.
10. Waechter, E. H., and Blake, F. G. *Nursing Care of Children.* Philadelphia: J. B. Lippincott Co., 1976, p. 11.
11. Marlow, D. R. *Textbook of Pediatric Nursing.* Philadelphia: W. B. Saunders Co., 1977, p. 856.
12. Blake, F. "Immobilized Youth—A Rationale for Supportive Nursing Interventions." *Am. J. Nurs.* 69:2364–2369, 1969.
13. Chambers, P., Dutson, C., Burke, A., and Gunby, G. "The Adolescent Patient." *Nurs. Times* 64:1240–1242, 1968.
14. Hammar, S. L., and Eddy, J. *Nursing Care of the Adolescent.* New York: Springer Pub. Co., 1966, p. 40.
15. Conway, B. "The Effect of Hospitalization on Adolescents." *Adolescence* 6(21):77–92, 1971.
16. Meyer, H. L. "Predictable Problems of Hospitalized Adolescents." *Am. J. Nurs.* 69(3):525–528, 1969.
17. Wiley, L. (ed.) "Manipulative Adolescent." *Nurs. '73* 3(7):36–41, 1973.
18. Dolan, M. "Shelly was Angry." *Nurs. '74* 4(6):86–88, 1974.
19. Earhart, M. "Beverly—Dealing with a Difficult Adolescent Patient." *J. Pract. Nurs.* 24:24–25, June 1974.
20. Guthrie, D. "Debbie Got Attention . . . The Hard Way." *Nurs. '75* 5(11):52–4, 1975.
21. Schowalter, J. E., and Anyan, W. R. "Experience on an Adolescent Inpatient Division." *Am. J. Dis. Children* 125:212–215, 1973.
22. Schowalter, J. E., and Lord, R. D. "On Writings of Adolescents in a General Hospital Ward." *Psychoanal. Study of Child* 27:181–200, 1973.
23. Hofmann, A. D. "The Impact of Illness in Adolescence and Coping Behavior." *Acta Paediat. Scandinavia,* supplement #256, 1975, p. 30.
24. Rigg, C., and Fisher, R. C. "Is a Separate Adolescent Ward Worthwhile?" *Am. J. Dis. Children* 122:489–493, 1971.

25. Bach, W. G. "Teen-Age Patients." *Hospitals* 44:51–53, 1970.
26. "Characteristics of an Inpatient Unit for Adolescents." *Clin. Pediat.* 12:17–21, 1973.
27. Fuszard, Sr. M. "Rationale and Planning for an Adolescent Unit." *Supervisor Nurse* 3(9):37, 1972.
28. Lindheim, R., Glaser, H. H., and Coffin, C. *Changing Hospital Environments for Children.* Cambridge, Mass.: Harvard University Press, 1972, pp. 77–98.
29. Peck, R. L. "Teaching Hospitals: The Adolescent Service Comes of Age." *Hosp. Phys.* 8(3):34–37, 1972.
30. Tiedt, E. "The Adolescent in the Hospital: An Identity-Resolution Approach." *Nurs. Forum* 11(2):121–140, 1972.
31. Gallagher, J. R. "General Principles in Clinical Care of Adolescent Patients." *Pediat. Clin. N. Am.* 7:185–195, 1960.
32. Schowalter, J., and Lord, R. D. "The Hospitalized Adolescent." *Children* 18(4):127–132, 1971.
33. Duran, M. T. "Family Centered Care and the Adolescent's Quest for Self-Identity." *Nurs. Clin. N. Am.* 7(1):65–73, 1972.

BIBLIOGRAPHY

Louis, M., and Lonejay, F. "Adolescent Attitudes in a General Pediatric Hospital." *Am. J. Dis. Children* 129:1046–1049, Sept. 1975.
Meldick, M. E. "Health Problems During the Adolescent Years." In Kintzel, K., ed. *Advanced Concepts in Clinical Nursing.* Philadelphia: J. B. Lippincott Co., 1977.
Oremland, E. K., and Oremland, J. D. *The Effects of Hospitalization on Children.* Springfield, Ill.: Charles C Thomas, Pubs. 1973, Chapter 5: The Adolescent in the Hospital.
Schowalter, J. E. "Psychological Reactions to Physical Illness and Hospitalization in Adolescence. *J. Am. Acad. Child Psychiat.* 16(3):500–517, Summer 1977.

8

The Adolescent with a Handicapping, Chronic, or Life-Threatening Illness

Eugenia H. Waechter, R.N., Ph.D., F.A.A.N.

Chronic illness has always been regarded as a personal tragedy. For an adolescent, chronic illness or a handicap may represent the loss of all hopes and plans for the future. For teenagers who have been living with an illness or handicap since childhood, the period of adolescence is particularly stormy, since they face additional problems in achieving developmental tasks and are asked to cope with awesome responsibilities in preparation for an uncertain future. For individuals who acquire a handicapping condition or illness during adolescence, the sudden catastrophic threats to present and future life styles may be overwhelming and may induce panic.

Increasing numbers of children with severe, chronic, disabling conditions are now reaching adolescence and adulthood. Although the prevalence of disabling and chronic conditions in the young population of this country is difficult to estimate because of ambiguities and overlap in diagnoses and inaccuracies in case finding, it has been estimated that there are almost eight million individuals, from birth to 19 years of age, who have physical handicaps.[1] When adolescents who have chronic illnesses are added to this number, along with family members who are also deeply affected by the condition, the problem becomes formidable indeed.

Many difficulties in early development, deficiencies in experience, and developmental gaps may prevent an adolescent from ever reaching maturity in some areas. Development may also be impeded both by personal and environmental factors that influence response and by the very nature of the condition. However, social disabilities, which are far more serious than physical limitations, can be ameliorated or prevented entirely.

Professional personnel and society alike are beginning to explore the causal relationships between physical limitations on the one hand and psychosocial development and adjustment on the other. In most cases this relationship is reciprocal. Physical illness or limitation vastly complicates the difficulties associated with mastering normal developmental tasks. Similarly, the stresses of adolescence often exacerbate the chronic illness or handicap.

A knowledge of normal adolescent development can be a valuable instrument for nurses who are helping adolescents with disabilities, and their families, through this perhaps most difficult of all developmental periods. To intervene most effectively, they must consider that what is important is not so much the disability or disease itself, but the manner in which it affects adolescents and those close to them. Their twofold responsibility is to help adolescents cope with their problems and to become advocates for families within the health care system.

Factors Influencing Response

It is generally expected that different types of chronic illness will have somewhat different effects on the development and behavior of an adolescent. There is some support for this belief in the results of a number of recent research studies. For example, Linde[2] found that young people with heart disease often expressed denial more than did adolescents with other chronic diseases; they also displayed greater noncompliance and overparticipation in activity. Similar behavior has been noted in individuals with hemophilia[3] and those with fibrocystic disease.[4] Such adolescents have also been seen to encounter more difficulties with identity; since the disease is marginal and not overtly apparent to others, it therefore less readily evokes sympathy and support from the environment.[5,6]

Other intrinsic and extrinsic factors, however, also influence the adjustment of an individual to physical disability. Since the ultimate goals of rehabilitation depend upon psychological adaptations, the interaction of such factors with the additional difficulties posed by physical limitations must be understood in order for professional personnel to be of maximal support to the chronically ill adolescent. It may be useful to discuss these factors at this time.

STAGE OF DEVELOPMENT

In order to understand the process by which the adolescent masters the task of moving from childhood to the point where he assumes adult roles, it is helpful to divide adolescence into three stages. Early adolescence can be considered the period of puberty, middle adolescence the period of identification, and late adolescence the period of coping.[7]

In early adolescence, physical growth and sexual changes occur at a rapid pace. The first developmental task, acceptance of the physical self, is difficult even for the normal teenager, who as yet has vague and undefined feelings about his body. Young adolescents are very much aware of their bodies, often wonder if they are normal, and frequently feel out of control as they experience the unexpected changes that accompany altering relationships of body parts to each other. Chronic illness or physical imperfection occurring at this developmental stage when a body image is being formed will dominate the teenager's life, whereas loss of function, disfigurement, or mutilation often causes panic. Therefore, when a severe handicap is incurred during early adolescence, great efforts will be required to establish a realistic body image. These efforts are the more difficult, causing uncertainty and increased anxiety, if the chronic illness is not stable or if it involves deterioration or remissions alternating with exacerbations of the illness.

Young adolescents are also faced with the dilemma of seeking independence from their parents while also relying on them for necessary physical and emotional support. Such conflict results in contradictory behavior toward parents and other authority figures. Handicapping illness at this stage of development catapults the teenager into a sense of helplessness and dependence from which he may see no future relief. A sense of hopelessness about ever achieving mastery of the environment may result, since the young individual feels insufficient resources within the self to cope with an uncertain future. With a lowered self concept, communication between the teenager and his or her parents may further deteriorate, since it has been found that the lower the self concept, the more negative is perceived communication.[8]

During middle adolescence, preoccupation with body changes and the seeking of independence from parental domination decreases, permitting fuller interaction with peers and greater efforts toward the establishment of an individual identity and value system. Such peer relationships are made extremely difficult for the chronically ill adolescent because of rejection by friends who are as yet uncertain about their own physical adequacy and who feel threatened by the limitations of others. Such low peer acceptance produces great emotional distress unless vigorous efforts are made to support former peer relationships and/or encourage the formation of new ties with other chronically ill adolescents.

During late adolescence, parents and society increase their demands on the teenager to achieve self-sufficiency and to assume responsibility for independent living, career choice, and consolidation of identity. A chronic illness or handicap at this developmental stage threatens all of the goals of adult living, necessitating major alterations of plans for the immediate present; all dreams for the foreseeable future may disappear.

CONGENITAL VERSUS ACQUIRED HANDICAPS

Recent early childhood development research has heightened our awareness of the obstacles that the handicapped child must circumvent and of the possible consequences of congenital disabilities on long-term development and functioning. We now know that the psychological damage which accompanies a congenital physical handicap can be more extensive than the physical handicap itself.

Emphasis has long been placed on the influence of early experience on later development, but we are now becoming aware of the various elements that affect the realization of potential. Recent research[9,10] on the critical nature of maternal-infant bonding in the first hours and days after birth gives rise to speculation about the possible consequences when opportunities for such bonding are not provided. Massive investigative efforts have also been directed to the infant's needs for sensory stimulation[11] and adequate nutrition[12] as factors in the realization of future intellectual potential. Research has also been directed toward the consequences of parental discipline,[13] the effects of cultural values on parental attitudes, and the effects of parental attitudes and security on the child's levels of self-esteem, intellectual growth, and behavior.[14]

The child born with a congenital handicap can be considered vulnerable and psychologically at risk, as can all members of his family. Such children may look vulnerable and behave vulnerably from birth, but the impact of deprivation and trauma in this earliest period may lead to further increases in vulnerability in the years to come. There can now be no doubt that genetic, constitutional, and environmental factors interact, deciding the ultimate vulnerability of the person. Constitutional factors, such as sensory or communicative limitations or restricted mobility, may in themselves impede the child's potential at adolescence. When these limitations are compounded by deficiencies in environmental support, the resulting psychological and physical damage may be profound.

Parents who have been less than optimally supported in their grieving and in coping with their feelings of guilt and shame about the birth of a child with a chronic disease or disability may become incapable of fulfilling their parental roles toward their child. Parental fear or inability to form an attachment may force the child into an unproductive relationship in which he fails to develop his capacities for strong relationships with others.

Lack of parental mutuality leaves the handicapped child vulnerable to early experiences which convey to him that the world is chaotic, painful, and capricious. Later parental attitudes of overprotection may prolong the natural maternal-child symbiosis and lead to immature patterns of functioning in the child.

Lack of support in learning behavioral controls also tends to increase the child's insecurity and can later lead him to attempt to control any situation in which limits are either lacking or unclear. The child's consequent lack of ability to delay gratification eventually results in weak conscience development and in failure to develop resources for coping with future deprivation, tensions, and developmental crises. During adolescence, such inadequate preparation for coping with increased stress may lead to partial or complete breakdown of behavior.

It is also known that intellectual development depends to a great extent on the opportunities the child has had to receive optimal levels of stimulation, to explore the environment, and to solve problems as age increases. In any situation where there is deprivation of sensory and tactile experience, optimal cognitive development may be at risk. During adolescence, while normal peers are hypothesizing about possible futures, the handicapped adolescent may continue to operate very much in the present, may revert to immature patterns of cause-and-effect reasoning, and may persist in seeing treatment procedures as hostile and punishing.

Development of autonomy and self-control of body processes are often jeopardized when physical limitations interact with residues of parental conflicts. The young person's sense of body integrity may have been defective from early child-hood, and unsuccessful attempts at mastery may produce apathy and the unconscious conviction that it is easier to remain dependent on others. Such continued dependence on adults is often compounded by lack of socialization with peers outside the home. Lack of adequate limitations on behavior may make the child unacceptable to peers, with lasting detrimental results; the teenager who continues to resort to socially unacceptable methods of expression of hostility and aggression will encounter rejection. Because of increased surges of energy in adolescence, combined with greater frustrations, the acting-out behavior of the handicapped teenager may be difficult for others to tolerate or control.

Parents may have difficulty in resolving their resentment and feelings of guilt related to the child's disability and may therefore be unable to provide the supportive environment the child requires to master age-appropriate developmental tasks. When this is the case, certain patterns of behavior in later childhood and adolescence are predictable. Mattsson[15] describes the following psychological profiles encountered in clinical practice:

1. The child is fearful; inactive; markedly dependent on his family, especially his mother; and lacks outside activities. The child is passive-dependent; the mother overprotective.

2. The child is overly independent, often daring; engages in prohibited and risk-taking activities. The child uses strong denial of realistic dangers; the mother is oversolicitous and guilt-ridden.

3. Less commonly the child is shy, lonely, and resentful, directing hostility toward normal people. His family usually emphasizes his defect and tends to hide and isolate him. The child develops a self-image of the defective outsider.

Some conditions, such as cystic fibrosis and renal disease, may become more serious and threatening with the sudden changes of puberty and the disruption of the steady growth rate. This greater threat, combined with lower energy levels and the necessity of confronting new developmental tasks, may induce a sense of hopeless-ness and despair. It is at such a time that an adolescent may contemplate or actually commit suicide either directly or indirectly by refusing to follow the prescribed treatment regimen.[16] Many a health professional has encountered the adolescent diabetic who, though under reasonably good control during childhood, consumes nothing but cola drinks for four days and comes into the hospital in a coma.

On the other hand, chronic diseases or handicaps which occur during adolescence present a more variable picture, depending on the nature of the condition, on whether the condition is sudden or gradual in onset, and on the adolescent's previous experience. Many adolescents who have had a secure childhood bring great strength and a repertoire of coping strategies to bear in dealing with crises. However, adolescents who have had to contend with chronic illness since birth, as previously described, do not possess such coping skills.

The nature of the handicap is of great importance. For example, the child with congenital deafness may go through childhood without the benefit of language, and this deprivation influences thought processes and communication patterns, perhaps for a lifetime. The adolescent who becomes deaf through illness or accident can draw on rich prior physical and emotional experience, so that secondary psychosocial damage is minimized.

On the other hand, certain levels of adaptation are possible when an individual has lived with a handicap over time. For example, a child born without an extremity may function quite well by the time he reaches adolescence, whereas the adolescent who loses an arm or leg through accident must go through intense grieving and cope with a sudden massive assault on body image.

It is also true that when a disability is acquired gradually during adolescence the individual is given the time to adapt to change by degrees. For example, because of the time involved, the adolescent who acquires paraplegia from a slow-growing tumor of the spinal cord may be able to accept limitations and mobilize resources more easily than the adolescent who suddenly becomes paraplegic from an accident. In the latter case, abrupt loss of sensation is accompanied by rapid destruction of the previously formed body image.[17]

In acute disease or trauma, however, the disability usually becomes stabilized in a circumscribed period of time. The boundaries of limitation become known fairly soon and are usually quite specific. Despite greater initial psychological shock, the adolescent can be helped to learn his limitations and to build on residual capacities.

In the case of an adolescent who has a progressively debilitating disease or one with remissions and exacerbations, such as arthritis, the degree of disability from one period of time to another may be unknown or unpredictable, which causes great uncertainty and anxiety.

SEX

The sex of the chronically ill or handicapped adolescent may be of significance aside from the fact that some diseases occur more often in one sex than in the other; for example, hemophilia occurs very rarely in females. Responses to a handicap may vary according to differential societal pressures for engaging in physical sports, for vocational training, for communication skills, or for attractive appearance. The female adolescent with a defect of the face or head may suffer particular anguish.

INTELLECTUAL ABILITY

Most normal adolescents who have had the prerequisite physical and emotional experience enter puberty at the level of what Piaget has termed "formal operations."[18] At this stage, the individual is no longer bound to the manipulation of real objects but is able to hypothesize possibilities conceived before any manipulation and to consider possible future events. He is able to use logic and to cooperate with others for future gain.

Many adolescents, however, have not reached this level of thinking and are unable to perform age-appropriate scholastic tasks. When intellectual ability lags significantly behind physical and sexual development, it is very difficult for the young person to comprehend body changes, to think abstractly, to see cause-and-effect relationships in illness or accident, to plan realistically for a vague future, or to cooperate fully with treatment goals.

Inability to project thought into the future toward the goals of rehabilitation or the prevention of later recurrences may prevent compliance with prescribed treatment. For example, this inability, coupled with the teenager's great concern about being different, can result in the discarding of medication by adolescents with cystic fibrosis or other diseases whenever they are with age-mates. When the adolescent is oriented to the present, procedures which must be continued over a long period of time mean little. The teenager's expectations for the future may also be inaccurate if explanations are not given honestly and clearly or are stated in abstract terms. When rapid improvement through treatment is expected and does not occur, the adolescent may repudiate any further efforts at cooperation, become angry and hostile, or become convinced that ultimate improvement is hopeless.

It is also true that levels of ability influence the educational and vocational goals that are possible with chronic illness or sudden handicap. Parents of children with chronic illness may have aspirations for them which they are incapable of achieving. Pushed beyond their ability, these young people acquire a failure identity. Through a sense of hopelessness, they may drop out as an alternative to their constant feelings of inadequacy. The next step is social failure. Many such adolescents may turn to drug abuse through peer pressure. Through anger at their parents, others may become daring in testing limits in order to prove that they are better than others in some way. Accidents—some of which are not wholly accidental—may be frequent. The ultimate accident is suicide.[19]

Adolescents who have acquired a handicap through sudden illness or accident may have to revise drastically their long-term plans and dreams of the future. Such sudden loss is also accompanied by deep grieving, both for the adolescent and for his parents. Along with the loss of future aspirations for vocation or profession, the adolescent may also question and doubt his social and sexual identity and his abilities in many other areas of living.

REACTION OF OTHERS

Current as well as earlier developmental problems discussed previously may affect the adolescent's response to chronic illness or handicap. Parental support may be inadequate because of previous or current conflicts, problems, or preoccupations. Friends may be indifferent or rejecting, or may hold unrealistic social expectations. Relatives or professional personnel may encourage inappropriate dependency. Societal mores and expectations may determine the depth of the identity crisis and the level of success which the adolescent can accept for the future.

Parents of children with developmental disabilities or congenital handicaps must live with constant pain and experience grief anew as their children fail to measure up to others at each developmental milestone. Simon Olshansky has termed this psychological response "chronic sorrow."[20] Residual guilt, shame, anger, and depression may resurface at each milestone despite general resolution of the intense feelings engendered by the child's birth.

The period of adolescence is particularly difficult for parents of a chronically ill or handicapped individual because they must now cope with new or increased responsibilities. Adolescence also rekindles past emotions as the young person begins to question who he is and what he is about to become. At a time when parents of normal adolescents look forward to the eventual self-sufficiency of their child, parents of chronically ill children must anticipate continued responsibility until their own or their child's death.

Parents who have established a relationship of overprotection with their child may feel threatened as he enters adolescence and attempts to achieve greater independence. The parents' needs to see themselves as "good parents" may be frustrated as the adolescent attempts to extricate himself from a symbiotic relationship. The adolescent's attempts to transfer affection to others may elicit anger and wounded pride, adding to normal parent-adolescent conflicts.

Families are also confronted with new decisions and major problems when their ill or handicapped child enters adolescence. Normal children have had many opportunities throughout childhood for testing and considering possible vocational choices. The handicapped or ill young person may have had few of the experiences which normally color and influence career selection, such as interaction with peers, play, and encounters with other adults. He may therefore deny limitations or continue in unrealistic fantasies.

Parents of children who become disabled or chronically ill in adolescence must also meet new demands for care and for emotional and financial support which may significantly alter their own life style. In addition, they must cope with their own shock, guilt, and resentment and the pitying responses of their relatives and friends. Denial and disbelief may lead them to seek many medical opinions before they are able to accept this sudden threat to their dreams of the future for themselves and for their child.

Initially, most parents wish to provide the best care possible for their ill or injured adolescent. Displays of false cheerfulness, however, are frequently resented by the adolescent and disturbances in communication are inevitable. Parents may then feel that their efforts are not appreciated and may retreat into their own frustrations and resentment.

As time passes and parents envision permanent caring and financial responsibilities and major disruption of all future plans, some may become hostile or rejecting, particularly if former relationships have not been smooth. If they are not emotionally strong, or if they have additional problems or responsibilities or limited intellectual abilities, they may feel incapable of meeting such great demands. In such instances, their expectations for their adolescent's recovery or improvement may be unrealistic, which only increases the young person's frustrations and hostility. On the other hand, they may be unable to support and encourage their adolescent's efforts toward self-sufficiency.

Other parents, who have emotional strength, a strong marital relationship, and previous constructive relationships with their child, are able to meet necessary changes for the entire family adequately. Meaningful communication with each other and with their adolescent may continue or become reestablished, and cooperative and realistic plans can be initiated for the future.

However, when parents do not have strong marital ties or emotional strength, the stress may become so great that family disruption is inevitable. This possibility is greatly increased if professional, environmental, and societal support is lacking or inadequate. Blame for the condition may be attributed to one or the other parent; the father usually leaves the home, and the mother may dedicate herself to the care of the adolescent.

The responses of siblings may also be crucial in determining family adjustment. The necessity for increased attention to the ill or injured adolescent, the disruption of patterns of family life, and the financial hardships are eventually—and understandably—resented by the other children in the family. If siblings are also entering, or in, adolescence, they see their future as also threatened, along with the possibility that they will have to assume heavy responsibilities when their parents are no longer able to do so.

COMMUNITY RESOURCES

Each state and community provides some resources for individuals with chronic or disabling conditions. However, these vary in quantity and quality in terms of financial support available and facilities and services provided. Special schools, rehabilitation facilities, and vocational training and counseling services may be available only in metropolitan centers. For those families living in rural areas or small communities, access to such services may be limited and may entail frequent travel and parental absences from home—causing further family disruption. In some instances, families may have to relocate, which further separates the adolescent from a known environment and previous peer support.

Additional Development Problems of the Chronically Ill or Handicapped Adolescent

BODY IMAGE

Although temporary illness during the adolescent period threatens all developmental tasks, chronic illness or handicap is a much more massive threat in that there is no foreseeable end to struggles for independence, for self-actualization, for personal and sexual identity, and for formulation of realistic future plans and goals.

Without a firm and realistic sense of body image, the adolescent will have great difficulty in achieving personal identity. Threats to body integrity at a time when the body already seems out of control may induce a sense of helplessness and, later, of hopelessness. Achievement of idealized body image may seem impossible. This is often accompanied by the feeling that since the adolescent cannot change his physical self, he is also helpless to alter the circumstances of his life. If the illness or handicap occurs after a body image has been formed, the adolescent is called upon to deal with acute anxiety and to revise drastically his previous sense of self.

Frequently, treatment for chronic illness compounds the adolescent's problems with body image. Corticosteroids and immunosuppressive drugs may stunt growth, produce obesity, and promote acne and prominent striae. For the adolescent who fervently wishes to be like his or her peers, this can be devastating.

DEPENDENCY

When normal adolescents are beginning to loosen ties with their parents and do things on their own, chronically ill or handicapped adolescents may be forced into increased dependency. Struggles against physical dependency may be intense, particularly when parents unconsciously or consciously encourage such dependence by posing restrictions as a method of retaining their adolescent. The adolescent who is constantly reminded of his limitations may either rebel against them or become fearful of any personal ventures into dependence. Conversely, the adolescent may use his illness in his struggle for independence. An attack of illness may be used to end a quarrel with parents, to gain power over them, or to gain privileges he sees his peers enjoying.

The adolescent's need to see himself as independent and self-reliant may also result in denial of the illness, refusal to cooperate in a treatment regimen, or indifference to rehabilitation goals. Conversely, the adolescent who has been fearful of independence may use the illness to maintain the comforting childhood dependency relationship with his parents. The additional attention received because of the illness may be so enjoyable that the responsibilities which achieving maturity entails may be indefinitely avoided.

IDENTITY

The task of forming an identity is often compounded for the chronically ill adolescent because, in his bleak condition of enforced isolation, he is estranged from his peers. If the condition has been of long standing, peer relationships may never have been optimal or growth-producing. If the illness or accident is of recent origin, accessibility to former friends may be limited and separation from them can be most disorienting. In addition, normal adolescents who are uncertain of their own identity and physical adequacy may feel threatened by the physical imperfections of others and may avoid their less fortunate friends. In all instances, the paucity of peer relationships retards the development of identity, which is partially built on the mirror image reflection of others.

SOCIAL MATURITY

The development of social maturity also depends on previous and current peer relationships and on ties to family and other adults. Without friends to reflect the worth of ideas and personal values, to clarify emotions, and to assist in the development of understanding and empathy for others, the adolescent may continue in the egocentrism of childhood. Essentially self-centered, he may never learn to know himself completely or to reach out to others in true communication. Without such communication and validation of personal worth, the adolescent may never aquire confidence or the ability for self-assertion.

SEXUAL ADEQUACY

An important aspect of both body image and identity is the adolescent's sense of sexual adequacy and acceptability. Many chronic illnesses, such as diabetes or fibrocystic disease, directly affect sexual functioning. Other conditions, for example, ulcerative colitis or chronic kidney disease, entail many examinations which require exposure, exploration of body orifices, and invasion of the adolescent's greatly needed privacy. Sexual development may also be delayed either by the illness itself or by its treatment. Any of the above can prove humiliating. When this is compounded by alterations in appearance caused by corticosteroids or other drugs, the combination may be devastating to an adolescent's sense of himself as a sexually adequate human being. Frequently, critical remarks about his masculinity are heaped upon the adolescent boy who cannot compete athletically. Adolescent girls, for whom physical appearance is an index of sexual attractiveness, may respond by sexual promiscuity in order to prove their femininity.[21]

For many chronically ill adolescents, the outlets for sexual and aggressive feelings available to healthy teenagers may not be available. Participation in athletics and contact sports may be prohibited or severely limited; this may lead to acting-out or disruptive behavior, verbal aggressiveness, or other antisocial behavior. However, such challenging of authority is far preferable to the alternative response of depression. When the adolescent suppresses his feelings or becomes frightened of his own aggression and hostility, he may lapse into withdrawal and depression and become incapable of relating to others.

DELINEATION OF FUTURE GOALS

The delineation of future goals may seem impossibly difficult for the chronically ill adolescent who feels sad and hopeless and who is still struggling with current problems and developmental tasks. Because of frequent absences from school, scholastic attainment may have lagged. Previous underachievement may have resulted in the expectation of failure in any endeavor of importance. Such expectation of failure may also be tinged with reality because of societal prejudice against the chronically ill or handicapped individual. Usdane[22] reports that "although for more than 53 years the State-Federal program of vocational rehabilitation has responded to the needs of the disabled individual over the age of 16, there has been little assistance available for the handicapped child or young adolescent to prepare him vocationally."

The goals of intimacy with another, including parenthood, and that of fully participating in society as an accepted, contributing member may also seem impossible of achievement for the chronically ill adolescent who has low self-esteem and many doubts regarding future self-sufficiency. The realities of physical limitations may indeed prohibit full participation in many activities. Such adolescents require much counseling and assistance in recognizing and capitalizing on their talents, their potential, their strengths, and the successes in living which they have achieved.

DEFENSE MECHANISMS

A number of defensive maneuvers used by chronically ill and handicapped adolescents are also counterproductive; they can impede adjustment to the condition and threaten further developmental progress. Some problems caused by *denial* have already been mentioned. Such a defense can become destructive if the teenager refuses to seek medical care, learn about the condition, or follow a treatment regimen. *Projection* of blame for the illness or handicap onto his parents or others results in strained relationships and communication difficulties and often in refusal to accept responsibility for self care. *Introjection*, or the personal assumption of blame and guilt, frequently ends in deepening depression and loss of contact with the environment. *Suppression of feeling* requires the expenditure of enormous amounts of energy which then becomes unavailable for constructive resolution of problems. *Acting-out behavior*, though more healthy, often earns the adolescent retaliatory hostility and delays or prevents the development of trust relationships. *Regression*, though normal and to be expected, may result in overdependency if continued indefinitely. All of these defensive maneuvers, as well as others, are inimical to progress if they persist over an extended period of time or if one mechanism is used consistently to meet all concurrent and future threats.

Support for the Adolescent and His Family

All adolescents need attention and understanding. This is particularly true of the chronically ill or handicapped adolescent who is in both developmental and physical crisis. The nurse who is aware of her own attitudes toward disabled individuals, who is knowledgeable about the developmental process, and who has a sincere interest in adolescents can become the friend, support, and advocate of the disabled young person, who is passing through the most difficult period that he or she may ever be called upon to face.

This chapter cannot deal with all the various and important nursing interventions which are of such great value during this period. However, certain basic principles may be summarized as follows:

1. Chronically ill or handicapped adolescents require a basic respect for themselves as worthwhile individuals who have great strengths and who can trust in their own abilities to come to an eventual resolution of the major problems that impede healthy adjustment.

2. They require support for self-esteem through the provision of an environment which maintains their contact with others, encourages open communication, and enables the individual to experience success through his own efforts.
3. They require nurses who are understanding of challenges to their authority, who do not feel threatened by agressive or acting-out behavior, and who do not retaliate with hostility but rather assist the adolescent to discover why it was necessary to behave in a socially disapproved manner.
4. They require advocates who will demand appropriate resources for them from the health care system, who will enable them to participate in decisions which affect them, who will help them to learn about their illness, and who will protect their rights until they are able to act as advocates for themselves.
5. They require nurses who, because they understand their developmental needs, will enable them to maintain or establish ties with friends, retain previous modes of dress and interests, and protect their privacy, and who will encourage them to become increasingly self-sufficient and to live openly with their handicap.
6. They require nurses who can set limits on their behavior until they are able to develop internal control. Such intervention prevents the ego-destructiveness of loss of control through temper outbursts or overt demonstrations of apprehension and fear.
7. They also require nurses who consider it important to listen to their fears, anxieties, hopes, plans, and ambivalent feelings within a trusting relationship.

Parents and siblings also require assistance and support when a family member is ill or disabled. In addition to the need for knowledge about adolescent development and the manner in which a chronic condition impinges on developmental tasks, they need to learn about the condition itself, the treatment that is required, procedures that must be continued, and methods of encouraging their adolescent to participate in his own care, so that he may develop self-sufficiency and progress in health and psychosocial development.

Parents also need assistance in understanding their adolescent's responses to his condition—and the responses of other children within the family—and a nurse who will understand and listen to their own fears and anxieties about the condition and their present relationship with all of their children. Often the nurse can be the agent who reestablishes meaningful communication within the family and assists in the reintegration of important relationships.

The Adolescent with Life-Threatening Chronic Illness

Many people living in the United States today have had little contact with death. Our society has been characterized as one which denies death and avoids it in ways which are sometimes unreasonable, illogical, or bordering on fantasy wish fulfillment. Although there is now more open discussion of death and more concern about the philosophical, ethical, and moral issues surrounding life and death, anxieties and fears about death still seem to have increased in the past decade.

Attitudes toward death were different several generations ago when the death of a young person was not a rare occurrence. Parents accepted the possibility that not all of their children would survive into adulthood. They also had greater experience with death, since many older family members were cared for and died in the home, surrounded by those they loved. Because of closer acquaintance, death was not considered an uncomfortable topic of conversation, and adults, in acknowledging death as a natural part of existence, formed personal philosophies of living and dying.

Although the death of the elderly, disabled, or infirm in our society today is often considered a ''blessing,'' the death of children or adolescents is seen as the ultimate tragedy. Inasmuch as they have just begun to live, and because of our youth-oriented society, the young are highly valued in themselves as well as for their future potential. Adolescents on the brink of living fully are seen as having everything to live for. Yet, adult society also views adolescents with ambivalence. Whereas the death of a young college student is greatly mourned, far less compassion may be shown for adolescents who have fatal accidents while speeding in automobiles or who become fatally ill while addicted to drugs, alcohol, or a way of life that is opposed to society's standards. These adolescents are often written off as ''no great loss'' and receive little sympathy from society or even from their parents and relatives.

Professional caretakers, as products of their society, may have difficulties in caring for adolescents, particularly those who are facing imminent death. Yet ill and dying adolescents are perhaps more in need of understanding and of knowledgeable, empathetic, and concerned care than are individuals in any other developmental phase of life. In order to give such care, health professionals of every discipline must examine their own attitudes toward life and death, have a sincere interest in and respect for all adolescents as individuals of worth and dignity, and become knowledgeable about the ways in which adolescents view death, the possible responses to incurable illness, and techniques of communicating with them when they are anxious and afraid.

THE ADOLESCENT'S CONCEPT OF DEATH

A mature concept of death is built slowly throughout childhood, both as a result of experiences with death and as a function of expanding intellectual awareness that encompasses aspects of time perspective, logic, and reasoning ability. In Western society, adults often ''protect'' children from what they feel are the harsh facts of life and death, and this practice can lead to a sense of unreality and distortion of the concept of death. Such misconceptions are further reinforced through the influence of television programs, since an actor may appear to die in a given play and yet reappear alive and happy on subsequent days.

Studies of child development by Inhelder and Piaget in Switzerland,[18] Nagy in Hungary,[23] Gesell and Ilg in America,[24] and Anthony in England[25] all agree that up to the age of about three years, children have little or no mental picture of death. To them separation and death are synonomous. They have not yet learned to ask the question "Why?" which signals the awareness of function. They are at first puzzled by death; death is inexplicable and is a mysterious phenomenon, since in their experience anything that happens is wished so, or controlled, by themselves or by their parents.

Children's first experiences with death (usually of an insect, bird or animal) lead them to equate death with separation, sleep, or going into a grave, coffin, earth, or water. Children under the age of five also have a sense of reversibility or lack of finality in death, since individuals who "go away" do return and characters on television appear and disappear inexplicably.

During the early school years, children are aware of the reality of death but may conceptualize it as gradual or temporary. Because of early experiences with the death of animals, they often view death as the end result of violence or agression. They may also personify death as someone (a "death man" or a skeleton) who comes to carry people away,[23] and they elaborate the concept of death with many religious and cultural meanings. In fact, many six-, seven-, and eight-year-olds may be intensely interested in the rituals surrounding death and spend considerable time in enacting burial scenes. Children of this age are often much more preoccupied with death than many adults are willing to admit. Though one reason for this activity is to gain intellectual mastery over a mystery, such preoccupation is also partly due to a growing suspicion that they also are mortal.

From the age of nine until adolescence, children usually accept death realistically and are aware that death is the common lot of humanity; many are interested in what happens after death. However, many also are secretly in great fear and terror of nonexistence. They often invent rituals to lessen their anxiety, behave recklessly and take chances to prove themselves invulnerable, or cover their fear by jokes and tough attitudes. They may also deride death by mutilating or killing insects and small animals. Such cruelty may serve the purpose of giving them a sense of control over death at a time when they are feeling very helpless in averting death for themselves or their loved ones.

There is still much room for research regarding the concept of death during adolescence. Most developmentalists and health professionals assume that by early adolescence most individuals have reached a level of cognitive growth at which the finality and inevitability of death are comprehensible, though they may not yet be accepted emotionally. It is also assumed that the adolescent's aptitude for hypothetical-deductive reasoning allows him to dream about the future, to anticipate and to concern himself with philosophical issues of life, death, and reality.

This is true for many adolescents, particularly for those in the middle and late stages of the developmental period. However, it is not true for all. Many individuals have not and may never reach the level of formal thought described by Piaget.[18] Others may have had previous experiences with death which have led to a distortion of the concept. For some, death may still be seen either as a redeemer or as an avenger that punishes for sins committed.[26] For many adolescents, who already have a tendency to feel guilty as they attempt to separate from parents, death may be seen as a confirmation of essential badness. This is reinforced by the inevitable breaking of many family and cultural rules as they test their independence.

In a small research study in Canada, Olsiak[27] asked 14- to 19-year-old healthy adolescents about their concepts of death. She found that young adolescents often had vague, strange, frightening, and mysterious concepts of death, whereas older adolescents tend to have more definite conceptions of an afterlife. Philosophical convictions grew stronger with age, as did definite concern for others, should they learn of their own fatal illness.

The adolescent who is under personal sentence of death is even more deeply convinced that his dying is a dreadful retribution for his offenses. Many adolescents do indeed die as a result of breaking the rules of society in regard to alcohol, drugs, and speeding automobiles. Many accidental traumas are a result of testing and exploration. To some it seems that a punishment as severe as death can only be due to essential badness.

In addition to guilt and depression, however, the adolescent with a life-threatening condition or illness is also bitter, angry, and bewildered. He may know that he has broken many rules, but he is deeply shocked at the magnitude of the punishment, which also implies rejection by parents, by society, and by God.[28] Because he is resentful toward those people whom he still depends on and cares for deeply, his quiet depression and helplessness deepen. Many dying teenagers feel that no one can understand them, and they face death lonely and alone.

RESPONSES OF THE ADOLESCENT TO LIFE-THREATENING ILLNESS

Such a sense of isolation is also a result of separation from the peer group, which has become all-important as the ties to parents and family loosen. This is particularly difficult for those adolescents who have disrupted family bonds abruptly or drastically. Teenagers who have felt deprived or rejected by parents during childhood and those who have been very close to parents and siblings may, of necessity, become extremely dependent on peers for direction, for support, and for the comfort of companionship. These teenagers are extremely vulnerable when faced with life-threatening illness, for the group may be of little help.

Younger adolescents are struggling to establish their own independence, self-sufficiency, and plans for the future. The serious illness and possible death of a friend is threatening to them, in that it points up their own vulnerability and frailty. At a time when strength, beauty, and body image are of utmost concern, they are uncomfortable with illness, mutilation, or disfigurement. In order to cope with feelings they may not have had to face before, they must withdraw from former close relationships.

Dying adolescents also contribute to the loosening of such ties. In defending themselves against the threat of abandonment by friends, they often deny their need for them by emphasizing their own self-sufficiency and independence. Fearing rejection by friends, they may repulse friendly overtures. Feeling very different, they set themselves apart to prevent exclusion and to avoid pity they do not want.

Alienation from former friends intensifies conflicts with parents, conflicts that may previously have been partially solved. If the teenager turns to his parents in his loneliness and need for understanding, he may feel that he is surrendering and returning to a former, outgrown, childlike state. As he becomes increasingly dependent on them, he resents his overdependence. Longing to be cared for and protected, he may violently reject his parents and the caring and concern they offer. Admitting such feelings to himself is infinitely threatening to his sense of control over himself. Wanting attention desperately, but proud, he may cut himself off from all warmth. When marital discord and financial strain affect his parents, the adolescent is further burdened with the knowledge that he is the cause of the strain. Often communication between the teenager and his parents deteriorates to stoical role playing—the teenager misinterprets his parents' protectiveness as sympathy and the parents feel rejected and helpless.

Young teenagers are also very aware of their bodies. They are extremely sensitive to the feelings they are experiencing and most perceptive of the world around them. They feel and live intensely, experience deeply, and live completely. They perceive acutely the beauty of a sunset, the beat of music, the sensation of walking barefoot through the grass.

The young adolescent wants to live. Acutely aware of his body, he senses its deterioration, whether or not his diagnosis and prognosis have been shared with him. At a time when the whole world is opening up, he is led to the mountain like Moses and shown the promised land and adulthood—but he learns that it is not for him.[29]

Understandably, the young adolescent is bitter and resentful and asks, "Why me?" "To whom can I assign blame?" Deeply living life, he can appreciate losing everything in dying. He has just come to realize what life can hold when the visions and dreams are snatched away. Not knowing where to direct his anger and bitterness, he often struggles on alone.

Although he may previously have loudly disclaimed agreement with the established social system and his parents' standards and religious principles, contemplation of his own prognosis may force him to consider some aspects of religion. He asks himself, "Is there a life after death? If so, will the sins I have committed in anger and rebellion against God and parents prevent me from getting there?" Unsure and ambivalent, he attempts to find answers to profound questions and meaning for his sufferings. If discouraged from asking such questions, his emotional isolation deepens.

Teenagers in midadolescence have developed more self-confidence, self-control, and pride in themselves as individuals. They take great interest in their appearance and are more comfortable with a consolidating body image. Self-esteem is high as they see themselves as individuals in their own right for the first time and contemplate a future which may now hold more concrete plans for college, career, or the work world.

Death can only mean defeat for the adolescent on the threshold of mastery. The 16-year-old youth is well aware that death will take away all of his physical and mental powers, will strip him of his competency and of his future. The 16-year-old young woman often, in addition, faces the destruction of her physical attractiveness through deterioration, deformity, or disfigurement. It is not surprising that young people who are undergoing such major alterations of body image and destruction of hopes have self-doubts and low self-esteem, or that they withdraw from contacts with the opposite sex and reject the advances of others. This is a cruel reality, and the adolescent will reasonably react with anger, bitterness, and hopeless rage at the futility of life—rage at the waste; rage at his powerlessness to change his fate.[28] Because the adolescent at this age has tasted mastery and self-achievement, the deprivation is the greater.

Those adolescents, however, who have become more secure in their own individuality may not need to reject their parents as violently as does the young teenager. With greater self-confidence, they no longer need to defend themselves as strenuously against love and comfort lest they become children again. Even though they feel bitterness and rage, the need is less intense to direct such feelings toward parents, particularly when communication lines have been maintained and concerns can be discussed openly. When such communication lines are closed, however, and the young person is not allowed to disclose feelings, bitter episodes of fighting between the adolescent and parents may occur until the adolescent finally becomes severely depressed and withdrawn. Neither side knows how to break the silence, which may last to the end.

When communication is open, the adolescent's rage may periodically erupt against his family, but usually the older teenager will attempt to control and direct these feelings elsewhere. Explosions are usually triggered by changes in treatment procedures, lack of proper explanations, or threats to the adolescent's sense of independence—for example, not allowing him to have a voice in decisions that concern him. When the adolescent is the last to know about a new therapy which is being considered, he rightly explodes and considers it unfair, for, after all, it is his body "they're doing it to." Though angry and hurt, he may continue to smile at hospital personnel for fear of being further excluded from decision-making processes in the future.

When the older adolescent, on the threshold of maturity, is faced with death, his worries and concerns also encompass lost relationships. These relationships may be infinitely dear and important, since they may involve present or future marital partners and hopes for the security of family life. Peer relationships now are also more mutually rewarding and constant. Ties with parents and siblings have been re-formed on a new basis of understanding. The older adolescent grieves for the loss of all of these close, rich, and meaningful emotional bonds. This mourning is all the more intense because the dying late adolescent cannot reinvest emotionally as can those he will leave behind.

The late adolescent has just arrived at the door of adulthood. Concrete plans must now be relinquished. If the young man or woman is married, he or she may make efforts to have a child, even though it is medically ill-advised, so that something of themselves will live after them. This investment in the future is assurance that their fading existence will not be completely erased.

Reigh and Feinberg[26] have delineated three distinct phases which adolescents go through as they progress toward death. The first phase is characterized by anxiety, depression, and a gradual withdrawal from the environment. The second phase is one of motor activity, which represents a return to earlier developmental patterns when tension and anxiety were relieved through motor discharge. The third phase is a regression to an even earlier developmental period when touch and closeness brought relief from anxiety.

In coping with the intense threat of premature death, adolescents use much denial, which often permits them to live with their illness. As time progresses, both the adolescent and his family may begin to grieve in anticipation of death.[30] This "grief work" often allows the adolescent to accept, at last, the inevitability of his own death. As death approaches, the world of the adolescent narrows to his bed and to a few loved members of his family. Even the young adolescent is able to accept the caring of warm and loving relatives. He can allow himself to be babied, as death grows nearer, as long as he is not treated disrespectfully.

FAMILY RESPONSES TO LIFE-THREATENING ILLNESS

When an adolescent becomes seriously ill, it is natural for parents to ask "Why?" "Did this happen because of something I have done?" "If I had noticed the symptoms earlier; if I had brought him to the hospital or doctor earlier, would he have gotten so sick?"

Such feelings of guilt are almost universal. Despite the fact that most parents know intellectually that illness is not divine retribution for sin, guilt is still *felt* on a deeper emotional level. The question is still there. "How could God let this happen? Has He stopped listening to us? Has He deserted us?"

Guilt is the feeling experienced most intensely by parents—along with disbelief or shock. The parents are concerned that they may have been neglectful in not watching their son or daughter closely enough, and their self-chastisement extends to every level of the relationship. They worry that they have not loved enough, have not gotten to know their child well enough, have not given enough attention. Each parent has different feelings about how he or she has failed, and the desolation of each is very real. This is particularly true during the time of adolescence, when family quarrels, misunderstandings, and miscommunication may be a way of life.

Such guilt must be affirmed as normal. It does no good to tell parents, "You shouldn't feel guilty". In fact, this only leads them to suppress their real feelings, to feel that they are abnormal—or even losing their minds. It is much better to say, "I can see why you would say that. Most parents feel that way." Then parents must be helped to see that they now have a choice: to be overwhelmed and engulfed by their natural feelings of guilt, or to admit them, accept them, let them subside gradually, and go on with attending to their son or daughter *now*. They can share *now* and appreciate him or her and bring the family closer together.

Just as guilt is a normal part of grief, so is anger. Parents are understandably angry at this total disruption of their lives, because of the threat to the future and to all of the plans they had for their adolescent who is now on the threshold of justifying them as parents. Most of all, however, they are angry because of the sense of helplessness they feel. They usually do not know what caused the illness, what to expect now and in the future, what they may be called upon to bear, and what their responsibilities might be. Because of this sense of helplessness to alter events, they are also very afraid.

Because of these feelings of guilt, anger, and fear, and because they do not know where to direct such feelings, they frequently direct hostility toward the staff as an alternative to directing it inward or toward God. Though it is often difficult for the staff, such hostility is actually an indication that the parents have moved beyond the phase of denial in the grieving process.

Other parents may avoid the threat of death for a considerable period of time in order to protect themselves from overwhelming anxiety. They may be unable to function if these avoidence mechanisms are taken away early in the course of the disease.[30] Denial can be considered adaptive behavior when nothing can be done to alter the threat. It has also been noted that such behavior is usally abandoned as the illness and deterioration progress.

On the other hand, if denial is perpetuated through the illness, communication with the adolescent—who is always aware of what is happening—may break down. Further isolation of both adolescent and parents is the inevitable result. Anticipatory grief is also impeded, and, as a result, the terminal phase of the illness is a greater shock, because they have not had time to prepare and much may have been left unsaid and undone.

Not all parents are able to support their dying adolescent. For some, the relationship with their son or daughter was so stormy prior to the illness that they are unable to reestablish a meaningful relationship at a time when the adolescent is also feeling guilty and irritable, and perhaps projecting blame towards them. Other parents need to intellectualize; they may spend much time in learning all of the medical details of the illness yet may avoid seriously discussing the illness with their adolescent child. Some parents find the stress and guilt so painful that they are unable to visit their adolescent when he is hospitalized or to function effectively when they do visit without concerted staff support.

During the time when the adolescent is acutely ill and hospitalized, families live "one day at a time." The former smooth operation of the family is disrupted and life revolves around the ill teenager. When the illness is chronic, the disruption is also a long-term problem. In many instances, the pattern of family life will be changed from the initial period of diagnosis until some time after the adolescent's death, when a reorganization of family roles takes place. In some cases, the family may be completely and permanently disrupted through divorce or separation of the parents.

Long-term illness is usually also accompanied by remissions and exacerbations. Because of this, the family must adjust and readjust constantly in an effort to retain equilibrium. Further, as the disease progresses, and as the family grows and changes, the home situation may also be constantly changing. The needs of family members and the interactions between them change, as siblings mature and develop and as parental needs vary. Therefore, the family must always learn to cope anew.

Parents of adolescents with life-threatening illness tend to be less sociable and more withdrawn than other parents. This is partly because the community of "normal" families does not understand the changes which must occur in a family that is supporting a seriously ill member. It is also partly because of the fact that "differentness" and the words "cancer" and "leukemia" still carry stigmas in our society. Chronic illness may also cause families to adopt a pattern of illness behavior as an integral part of their lives. For example, families with an adolescent who has cystic fibrosis are confronted with seemingly unending responsibilities related to treatment regimens and diet restrictions. They can never forget for a moment that their adolescent has a serious illness and that the state of his health is their constant responsibility.

Financial troubles are a chronic problem for many families with high medical expenses. Income may be reduced and expenses are generally greatly increased. Frequently, additional employment is needed, and this further reduces the time that parents can spend together. The inaccessibility or unavailability of community resources enhances the vulnerability of the family to other problems.

Many families are not informed about resources which are available to help financially and in other supportive ways. Other families are fearful and therefore unable to use the resources; or they may be unsophisticated about finding their way through our often fragmented maze of medical and supportive services.

Siblings also have many problems when an adolescent member of the family becomes seriously ill. Young children are often thrust very much into the background of the medical crisis. They are often left with various members of the extended family and may suffer greatly when deprived of parental care. When young children are at home, living conditions may have deteriorated severely, especially because of the inevitable disruption of routines necessary to their security. As their insecurity increases, their demands for attention increase. However, where previously parents responded to demands, they may now see them as unreasonable. In addition, siblings may take responsibility for the illness and feel generally guilty, ''bad,'' and unlovable.

Older children also have many problems. Although they are intellectually better able to understand the situation and no longer ascribe guilt to themselves through magical thinking, they still react on a deep emotional level. They still resent deeply the decreased attention to their needs and the disruption in their lives. Many are asked to take on new responsibilities in the household. Though they may appear to pitch in willingly or even enthusiastically, in reality they may deeply resent their new responsibilities. Because of their cheerful outward manner, parents may become comfortable and not look deeply into the true feelings below the surface.

Many children are also afraid that their siblings' disease may strike them at any moment. Not wishing to ask the fearful question, they may withdraw from friends and involvement with others, wishing only to be left alone.

Because of decreased personal attention from their parents, older children also often feel less loved and therefore less lovable. Lack of finances and increased responsibilities prevent them from enjoying many things that their peers have and do and limit interaction with them. Often older girls resent the premature role of mother and choose never to accept it again. Others eventually become hostile to their parents and never again have the same warm and loving relationship with them.

Some recent studies[31] indicate that neglect of siblings results in hostile and aggressive responses to the affected child or adolescent. They also document the fact that siblings have a higher incidence of school problems, emotional problems, obesity, and school failure.

It has also been noted that when a child or adolescent in the family dies, siblings may again accept blame, which can result in a sense of hopelessness, anxiety, and pervasive feelings of personal ''badness'' and unlovableness. They may also fear that other members of their family may die and they may therefore experience other separations with deep distrust and anxiety—perhaps for a lifetime.

FURTHER ASPECTS OF NURSING SUPPORT AND INTERVENTION

The care of fatally ill adolescents has frequently been referred to as one of the most difficult tasks faced by nurses. Students of nursing are frequently close in age to the dying adolescent and can therefore identify with him or her intensely. This close association makes it difficult for them to handle the situation from a professional standpoint rather than from a personal point of view. They fear that they will be unable to talk to the adolescent or listen to his or her fears and concerns without revealing their own personal responses. Some may never have had an experience with death or may not have formed a personal philosophy of life and death. For these reasons they also need support when dealing with a dying adolescent and his family.

Nurses who work with adolescents who are facing death need to understand that outbursts of hostility and rage are usually not meant for them personally, but are a result of the situation in which the teenager finds him- or herself. Teenagers cannot be expected to handle their emotions as adults do. On the other hand, nurses can convey the expectation that with help and support the adolescent will be able to handle feelings more appropriately. Providing activities into which he or she can channel furious rage will help to work out some of the bitterness, support self-esteem and a sense of self-control, and prevent disruption of the treatment regimen. Parents can also be helped to understand the reasons behind their adolescent's anger and bitterness. If they can continue to show by their actions that they still support and love him or her, despite behavior, the adolescent may be better able to accept comfort without losing face. Attention from relatives expressed in cards, letters, and visits also helps the adolescent to appreciate that he or she is not really alone, despite the feelings of desolation that are always present. Though unable to express gratitude for such attention, the loneliness and bitterness may become less acute.

Though the teenager may have become isolated from former friendships, much can be done to promote friendships with other adolescents who have similar interests and problems. Together, they may be able to share their fears and frustrations, discuss their relationships with family, and consider their thoughts or philosophies about life and death.

Nurses can also promote adolescents' sense of independence and control over their situation as far as possible. They can be advocates for them to ensure that they have a voice in decisions and play a role in their own care. Answering all questions honestly, avoiding condescending treatment or attitudes, and keeping restrictions to a necessary minimum will protect the personal dignity of adolescents.

Dying adolescents, above all, need nurses who will listen to them when they are able to share concerns, fears, and frustrations. They will usually indicate by their questions the kind of information they wish. If the teenager initially needs to deny absolutely, he should not be obliged to face unpleasant and unbearable realities that he cannot yet tolerate.[28] When he is strong enough to face reality more directly, he will usually indicate by his questions that he now wants to discuss his situation more fully. At no time do adolescents appreciate false cheerfulness, to which they are very sensitive. Hope, however, can realistically be offered for shorter-term goals as the disease progresses. Most of all, dying adolescents appreciate adults who can sit with them and be comfortable in an atmosphere of silence.

In the terminal phase, adolescents usually select one or two adults to share their thoughts and feelings. Knowing that they cannot get well, they are often ready for death to come and are resigned to the inevitable. Some younger adolescents may resist to the end, lonely and proud, but this is relatively rare. In many cases, as death nears, adolescents show amazing strength, comforting their parents who are in pain and providing meaning to this tragedy by teaching parents and nurses the value and ideals of living.

REFERENCES

1. President's Committee on Mental Retardation. *Mental Retardation: Century of Decision,* Washington, D.C.: U.S. Government Printing Office, 1976.
2. Linde, L. M., Rasof, B., Dunn, O. J., and Robb, E. "Attitudinal Factors in Congenital Heart Disease." *Pediatrics* 38:92–101, 1966.
3. Wolfish, M. G., and McClean, J. A. "Chronic Illness in Adolescents," *Pediat. Clin. N. Am.* 21:1043–1049, 1974.
4. Gayton, W. F., and Friedman, S. B. "Psychosocial Aspects of Cystic Fibrosis." *Am. J. Dis. Children,* 126:856–859, 1975.
5. Bruhn, J. G., Haupton, J. W., and Chandler, B. C. "Clinical Marginality and Psychological Adjustment in Hemophilia." *J. Psychosomat. Res.,* 15:207–213, 1971.
6. Garson, A., Jr., Williams, R. B., and Reckless, J. "Long Term Follow-up of Patients with Tetralogy of Fallot, Physical Health and Psychopathology." *J. Pediat.,* 85:429–433, 1974.
7. Miller, D. *Adolescence: Psychology, Psychopathology and Psychotherapy* New York: Aronson, Jason, Inc., 1974.
8. Flora, R. "The Effect of Self Concept Upon Adolescents' Communication with Parents," *J. School Health* 44(2):104–108, 1974.
9. Ainsworth, M. D. "The Development of Infant-Mother Attachment." In Caldwell, B., and Riciuti, H., eds. *Review of Child Development Research,* vol. 3. Chicago: University of Chicago Press, 1973.
10. Klaus, M., and Kennell, J. *Maternal-Infant Bonding.* St. Louis: C. V. Mosby Co., 1976.
11. Hebb, D. O. "The Effects of Early Experience on Problem Solving at Maturity." *The Competent Infant, Research and Commentary.* In Stone, L. J., and Murphy, L., eds. New York: Basic Books, Inc., 1973.
12. Cravioto, J. "Nutritional Deficiencies and Mental Performance in Childhood." In Glass, D., ed. *Environmental Influences.* New York: Rockefeller University Press, Russell Sage Foundation, 1968.
13. Madsen, C. K., and Madsen, C. H. *Parents/Children/Discipline.* Boston: Allyn & Bacon, Inc., 1972.
14. Weininger, O. Rotenberg, G., and Henry, A. "Body Image of Handicapped Children," *J. Personality Assessment,* 36:248, 1972.
15. Mattsson, A. "Long Term Physical Illness in Childhood: A Challenge to Psychosocial Adaptation," *Pediatrics,* 50:801–811, 1972.
16. Schowalter, J., Ferholt, J., and Mann, N. "The Adolescent Patient's Decision to Die," *Pediatrics* 51:97–103, 1973.
17. Daniel, W. R. Jr. *Adolescents in Health and Disease.* St. Louis: C. V. Mosby, Co., 1977.
18. Inhelder, B., and Piaget, J. *The Growth of Logical Thinking From Childhood to Adolescence.* New York: Basic Books, 1958.
19. Janeway, C. "The Adolescent Patient." *Northwest Med. J.,* Feb. 1974.

20. Olshansky, S. "Chronic Sorrow: A Response to Having a Mentally Defective Child." *Soc. Casework* 43:191–194, 1962.
21. Leichtman, S., and Friedman, S. "Social and Psychological Development of Adolescents and the Relationship to Chronic Illness." *Med. Clin. N. Am.,* 59:6, 1975.
22. Usdane, W. M. "Vocational Planning for the Handicapped Adolescent." In Downey, J. A., and Low, N. L., eds. *The Child with Disabling Illness.* Philadelphia: W. B. Saunders Co., 1974.
23. Nagy, M. H. "The Child's Theories Concerning Death," *J. Genetic Psychol.* 3:73, 1948.
24. Gesell, A., and Ilg, F. *The Child from Five to Ten.* New York: Harper & Row, Pubs., Inc., 1946.
25. Anthony, S. *The Discovery of Death in Childhood and After.* New York: Basic Books, Inc., 1972.
26. Reigh, R. and Feinberg, H. "The Fatally Ill Adolescent." In Feinstein, S., and Giovacchini, P., eds. *Adolescent Psychiatry,* vol. 3. New York: Basic Books, Inc., 1974.
27. Olsiak, M. "Adolescence and Impending Death." *Canad. J. Pub. Health,* 67:65, Jan/Feb. 1976.
28. Easson, W. *The Dying Child.* Springfield, Ill.: Charles C Thomas, Pubs., 1970.
29. Aune, R. "Adolescence and Death." Unpublished manuscript, 1974.
30. Lowenberg, J. S. "The Coping Behaviors of Fatally Ill Adolescents and Their Parents." *Nurs. Forum,* 9(3):269–287, 1970.
31. Madison, D., and Raphael, B. "Social and Psychological Consequences of Chronic Disease in Childhood," *Med. J.* 2:1265, 1971.

BIBLIOGRAPHY

Brown, A., and Bjelic, J. "Coping Strategies of Two Adolescents with Malignancy." *Mat.-Child Nurs. J.* 6(2):77–85, 1977.
Duran, M. "Family Centered Care and the Adolescent's Quest for Self Identity." *Nurs. Clin. N. Am.,* 7(1), 1972.
Gyulay, J. *The Dying Child.* New York: McGraw-Hill Book Co., 1978.
Herrmann, N. *Go Out in Joy.* New York: Simon and Schuster, Inc., 1977.
Jelneck, L. J. "The Special Needs of the Adolescent with Chronic Illness." *MCN. Am. J. Mat. Child Nurs.* 2(1):57–61, 1977.
Kikuchi, J. "A Leukemic Adolescent's Verbalizations about Dying." *Mat.-Child Nurs. J.* 1(3):259–264, 1972.
———, "An Adolescent Boy's Adjustment to Leukemia." *Mat.-Child Nurs. J.* 6(1):37–49, 1977.
Lacasse, C. "A Dying Adolescent." *AJN.* 75:433, 1975.
Lopez, R., ed. *Adolescent Medicine,* vol. 1. New York: Spectrum Pubns., Inc., 1976.
Mitchel, M. *The Child's Attitude to Death.* New York: Schocken Books, Inc., 1967.
Saintz, M. L. *The Nurse and the Developmentally Disabled Adolescent.* Baltimore: University Park Press, 1977.
Schneidman, E. *Death and the College Student.* New York: Behavioral Pubns., Inc., 1972.
Steele, S., ed. *Nursing Care of the Child with Long Term Illness.* 2nd. ed. New York: Appleton, Century, Crofts. P-H, 1977.
Stevens, C. *Special Needs of Long Term Patients.* Philadelphia: J. B. Lippincott Co., 1974.

9

Drug Use Among Adolescents

FREDERICK H. MEYERS, M.D.

Let it be said explicitly at the outset that the term ''drugs'' includes ''our'' drugs as well as ''their'' drugs: the highly dangerous, if legally countenanced, ones, such as alcohol and cigarettes, as well as the ones that have come into use more recently and are more emotion-laden. Then a comparison of drug use among adolescents in their culture and among adults in their culture shows more similarities than differences, and the importance of attitudes in the dominant culture successfully inculcated into our youth must be constantly mentioned.

There are, however, good reasons for examining drug use separately during the individual's period of identity formation. For a young person, the consequences of abuse of drugs for a relatively brief period during a time of rapidly progressing social, academic, or vocational development or opportunities can be more intense than the effects of drug abuse in an adult who has either achieved stability or abandoned efforts in these areas. Furthermore, the age at which experimentation and first use are most common is the period when efforts to prevent or contain drug use should be most productive.

Why Do People Take Drugs?

The answer to this question is generally made needlessly complex. Answering it now can facilitate the understanding of the more complete discussion that follows. *Pleasurable Relief of Anxiety:* There are several reasons why adolescents or others might use a drug once or a few times. If, however, a drug is used regularly, it must provide some physiologic or behavioral reward that is pleasurable.

By far the most common mechanism by which drugs give pleasure is the dissolution of anxiety by disinhibiting agents such as alcohol or marihuana. Sometimes the sensory reward is so great—e.g., the orgasm-equivalent from intravenous heroin or speed (amphetamines) or the mild stimulation of nicotine—that drug use becomes a compulsive act and anxiety is suppressed by repetition of the act. Anxiety, both situational and neurotic, is pervasive, and the rewards of drug use are correspondingly commonly experienced. This simple explanation is actually the consensus, but it is expressed so variously that the agreement may be obscured: pleasure seeking, euphoria, oblivion seeking, stress relieving, relief from memory, social lubrication, and the like.

Testing and Exploration: Drugs are a new and, in the case of some drugs, a dangerous or challenging experience and will be part of the expected exploration and testing during the adolescent process.

Peer Group Pressure: Peer group pressure or social acceptance is often given as a factor or explanation for increasing adolescent drug use. Certainly it is an important permissive factor in experimentation, acting through mere availability as well as through social acceptance. As an explanation for continued drinking or other drug use, it is a peculiarly circular argument: Drug use among adolescents is very common because many adolescents use drugs.

Imitation: Such data as are available (which relate to cigarettes and alcohol) suggest that family habits and generally manifest societal attitudes are probably more important factors than peer pressure in determining whether adolescents use drugs. We will return to the responsibility of the adult in the discussion of prevention.

Marker for Change: The use of a drug such as LSD may be followed by changes in life style or in other behavior that are unrelated to any possible pharmacologic effect. Such ritual use of drugs is discussed in the section which follows.

Patterns of Drug Use and Abuse

There is, of course, no "drug problem" but multiple problems involving many drugs and several patterns of use carrying different dangers and degrees of danger. Therefore, one further preliminary but essential matter is to provide definitions that will allow us to describe the multiple drug problems—definitions that will replace ambiguous terms such as addiction and dependence.

Experimental: Obviously, the use of each drug by each person involved must have its first use, and this experimental use continues until the individual either rejects the drug or passes on to another pattern of use. Such a statement sounds like a nominal gesture toward pedantic completeness but is actually crucial to most of the thinking about prevention.

Abstinence: It is important to consider that any single drug (with the exception of alcohol and tobacco) is totally rejected by most people and that, even for alcohol and tobacco, abstinence is not an impossible goal. Nevertheless, when the uses of all of the psychoactive drugs—therapeutic and illicit—listed below are summed, only a small minority of people approach abstinence.

Social Use: The majority of people adopt one or more drugs to use socially—i.e., using them temperately in the company of others to facilitate relaxation and sociability. The consensus would designate this pattern social *use* rather than *abuse*. However, to introduce the crucial idea of this chapter, social use is extremely dangerous because it tests every person for his vulnerability to progress to a more dangerous pattern. The reason why our culture contains so many alcoholics is that we methodically test each member of each emerging generation and identify and destroy the vulnerable personalities. We are able to tell a group of young people that it is a statistical inevitability that a certain percentage will use alcohol to such an extent that they will lose family, vocation, and health as a result. Unfortunately, we are not able to identify the vulnerable individuals before the fact, and, logically, the only safe course is to avoid social use, however unrealistic a goal that may be or appear to be.

Episodic Abuse: Another danger of social use is that it may from time to time become immoderate. Excessive amounts of a drug may be used periodically. If the drug is alcohol or some other sedative, the user may in his disinhibited state damage himself and others. The abuse is, however, still elective rather than compulsive.

Compulsive Abuse: In a number of individuals who have experimented with one drug or another, its use becomes a compulsion, i.e., an act based on emotion rather than volition, recognizably irrational even to the user, but senselessly repeated to avoid the anxiety that appears if he does not repeat his compulsive act.

The hazard of developing such a compulsive pattern of use depends in part upon the personality of the individual. However, considering the portion of the population that at some time adopts a compulsion—e.g., cigarette smoking, coffee drinking, nail picking, or masturbation—the vulnerability must be so widely distributed as to escape being called abnormal.

The probability of a given act's becoming a compulsion also depends upon the sensory or pharmacologic reward that reinforces the behavior. Thus, injected opiates and injected amphetamine carry a great hazard because of the "rush," or feeling of orgasm, that occurs at the time of injection. The mild CNS (central nervous system) stimulating properties of nicotine make cigarettes a common vehicle of compulsion; statistically, 85% of adolescents who smoke more than one cigarette become regular smokers and cannot substitute nicotine-free cigarettes. Relief of anxiety by sedatives must also be an important reward, or reinforcing factor. The percentage of drinkers of alcohol who become compulsive alcoholics is smaller than the percentage of heroin users or cigarette smokers who become that dependent, but the widespread use of alcohol ensures that a huge number of chronic alcoholics will develop. The compulsive drug user ("addict") has difficulty giving up his habit even when given maximal assistance.

Ritual Abuse: Drugs may be used with a philosophic basis or preconception. For example, LSD may be used with the expectation of achieving a religious or psychotherapeutic experience. In such a situation the pharmacologic effects of the drug are less important than the significance attributed to the drug by the proselytizer. The ritual pattern of use is not a part of the above-mentioned sequence—i.e., it does not develop from social use or progress to compulsive abuse. Ritual drugs are not selected to provide some hedonistic reward, and, if the user is protected by other group members during the drug effect, the dangers are minimal. One is not committed by such a judgment to agreement with the philosophic basis for the use of the drug or to sympathy with any associated life style.

Statistics on drug use for adolescents are inaccurately reported and thus misleading. Also, when incidences of use are reported by clumping all ages, the higher incidences of drug use that occur with increased age are obscured. Available percentages for drug use by adolescents in 1972[1] indicate that: among 12- to

19-year-olds, 33.4% used alcohol and 22.8% used tobacco; among 12- to 17-year-olds, 23% used marihuana, 6.4% used glue and other inhalants, 4.8% used LSD and other hallucinogens, 1.5% used cocaine, and 0.6% used heroin.

Drug Factors

At this point, the pharmacologic effects of abused drugs will be reviewed. Many agents are misused; however, drugs can be put into classes, and the variety of agents is not as great as it first appears.

SEDATIVE-HYPNOTICS

There is a huge number of agents that have as a direct pharmacologic effect the ability to relieve anxiety. Drugs of this class—e.g., alcohol, marihuana, sleeping pills, and other "downers"—are the most widely used and misused of drugs because of the ubiquity of anxiety in human behavior.

The following list identifies many of the antianxiety agents. They can be placed in two large groups: (1) those that have a rapid onset but short duration of action either because of their inherent physicochemical properties or because of their usual route of administration, and (2) those whose effects develop more slowly but persist for a longer time.

1. Short-acting, rapid onset substances:
   Alcohol
   Marihuana (*smoked*) ("grass," "weed," "joint," and many terms based on geographic origin ["Colombian," "Thai sticks"] or strain ["sin semilla"])
   Hashish (*smoked*)
   Prescription hypnotics: pentobarbital (Nembutal, "yellows"), secobarbital (Seconal, "reds"), methaqualone (Quaalude, "Ludes"), diazepam (Valium), meprobamate (Miltown), amobarbital (Amytal and in Tuinal).
   Nitrous oxide, ether, etc.
   Airplane glue, gasoline, other hydrocarbons
   Freon-type propellants
2. Long-acting substances:
   Marihuana, hashish (*ingested*) ("hash" in tea, brownies)
   Phencyclidine (PCP, phenyl-cyclohexyl-piperidine, "Angel Dust," "Peace Pill")
   Prescription sedatives: phenobarbital, chlordiazepoxide (Librium)

What is the basis for grouping all of these drugs together and thereby implying that information that you have about one can be extrapolated to the others? All of the drugs listed have common properties that are best established by describing the effects of giving increasing doses to a human. The resulting sequence of effects will already be familiar to you from (depending upon experience) the stages of anesthesia, an objective view of the effects of alcohol in yourself and others, recollection of the action of nitrous oxide in the office of your dentist, or, possibly, observation of someone who has attempted suicide with an overdose of sleeping pills.

Progressing from small to lethal doses, the following effects may be seen. Relief of anxiety or sedation is described by the recreational user and often prescribed by the physician. Synonyms for this experience were mentioned above.

Excitement appears with larger doses and under conditions of continued stimulation. All of the drugs listed, taken at bedtime by a subject who does not try to continue to function, will encourage sleep or, if the dose is large enough, guarantee it. If, however, stimulation continues, that is, if the drug is taken in a social setting that requires continued functioning, the subject may respond to ordinary stimuli with inappropriate and exaggerated responses. Whether he is happy or belligerent depends not upon the drug but upon the setting and the personality of the subject. This is the high of "grass" or the "stimulation" of alcohol.

However, excitement is not the same as stimulation, and the observed effects of large doses and data from neurophysiologic and behavioral studies establish that the state is one of disinhibition. The inhibitory effect of higher centers and the inhibitory effect of recently acquired behavior are depressed with the release from inhibition of phylogenetically older behavior.

Behavioral disinhibition is accompanied by impaired psychomotor performance and impaired judgment. The sedatives thus cause antisocial behavior by a direct pharmacologic effect. The distorted behavior may result only in an "unintended" insult or it may lead to an unwanted pregnancy or to felonious acts. In half of the annual 50,000 fatalities due to automobile accidents in the United States, alcohol is a factor. In half of the homicides, statistics show that either the aggressor or the victim had been drinking. Amnesia for the period may be present.

A dreamy, fantasizing state may be induced under proper conditions with each of the sedatives but has been best described for nitrous oxide because of its use in anesthesia. Unfortunately, the state has been misperceived by some observers and has led to the classification of marihuana as a "mild hallucinogen." However, the reaction produced by marihuana is comparable to that seen after the use of other sedatives, not after the use of LSD.

With large doses, the more or less normal sleep that may be induced is superseded by anesthesia: sleep from which the subject cannot be awakened and the loss of protective reflexes that normally keep the airway open. In the extreme stage, respiration is stopped.

With chronic or continued administration, additional effects appear which are useful in classifying and understanding these drugs. For example, an anticonvulsant effect has been demonstrated for most of the drugs categorized as sedatives. Marihuana has such an effect—one of the properties that justifies our placing it in the sedative category and that also allows us to anticipate the claims of therapeutic usefulness that are now being made for marihuana. It is a rapidly acting sedative (if smoked), but no shortage of such agents is apparent and possible therapeutic effects have no bearing on its recreational use.

Tolerance of two types develops to the effects of sedatives. Both are very limited in degree. Behavioral tolerance develops as the subject learns and anticipates the effects and adapts his behavior to a small extent to his impaired ability. Many, if not most, "bad trips" are anxiety reactions in a naive user reacting to a new experience.

Metabolic tolerance develops as the rate of metabolism of the drug by the body increases with continued use. The degree of tolerance to sedatives is always small—that is, to maintain a constant effect the administered dose need be increased only slightly (10–50%). In contrast to the sedatives, metabolic tolerance to the narcotics is so great that many doses that would be lethal to the nonuser are tolerated by a regular user with a large habit.

A withdrawal state, reflecting the development of physical dependence, has been demonstrated for all of the sedatives listed except for a few of the volatile agents. After the sedative has been administered regularly and in adequate dosage for a few days, continued administration of the drug is necessary to maintain normal physical health. Or, stated differently, abrupt discontinuation will lead to the appearance of physical abnormalities or a withdrawal state.

After the use of small amounts of a sedative, for example, the usual doses of a sleeping tablet or capsule for a week or two, withdrawal may be limited to a disturbed sleep pattern or some daytime tremulousness and anxiety. After the use of large dosages, the withdrawal hyperexcitability may progress to excitement, convulsions, and a toxic psychosis.

Cannabis as a Special Case. Marihuana and hashish, forms of cannabis or hemp, are sedatives like alcohol but appear distinctive because they are usually smoked rather than ingested. The active ingredient, THC, actually has a long life in the body, and, if taken by mouth, looks like a "long-acting alcohol." However, when it is smoked, the small amounts rapidly absorbed are carried quickly to the brain, because blood flow to that organ is great. Within a few minutes an effect is noted. The effect is then rapidly terminated not by chemical alteration of the THC but by redistribution of it to other fatty areas of the body with lesser blood flow.

All of the properties used as criteria for membership in the sedative group have been demonstrated for cannabis or its active ingredient THC. This conclusion is abhorrent both to the users of cannabis and to opponents of its use. Cannabis does not have the organic toxicity so characteristic of alcohol abuse and its use generally involves small doses. So long as large amounts of concentrated hashish are not available, it appears that cannabis can be faintly praised as not as bad as distilled alcoholic drinks. Unfortunately, young people are more and more given to combining it with alcohol, confirming the pharmacologic teaching that the effects of all the sedatives are additive.

NARCOTICS

The term "narcotic" should be applied only to opiates such as morphine that are extracted from opium and to synthetic and semisynthetic equivalents. These include codeine, Talwin, Demerol, Percodan, morphine, Dilaudid, heroin, and methadone.

Given by any route other than intravenous (oral, subcutaneous, or sniffing), the opiates are comparatively slowly absorbed and the effects are those associated with the therapeutic use of the drugs. Not only is the perception of pain altered, but the subject is isolated or insulated from other stimuli, however anxiety engendering they may be. Such a state is pleasant for some people and may lead to misuse of the drug. However, the resulting problem is comparatively benign and easier to treat than the problem resulting from the intravenous use of a narcotic—usually heroin, because of its availability.

When heroin is injected, the immediate ''rush'' at the moment of injection is more important to the user than the late effects described above. The rush is an intense sensual experience often described as a total body orgasm, although it centers in the epigastric region. The explosive relief of anxiety that this sexual equivalent provides makes most heroin use very likely to progress to compulsive use.

Heroin use is invariably destructive to the individual even though it is not inherently dangerous to the user, nor does it cause antisocial activity, as the disinhibiting agents do. The heroin user is either depressed by his drug or shows no effect, if he is ''maintaining'' on a habit of unvarying size. He is driven to antisocial acts not by the drug effect but by a compulsive need to guarantee the availability of the next fix. The dangers and the objections of society must be based on the associated criminal activity resulting from the illegality and expense of heroin—i.e., the societal reaction rather than the drug effects.

The argument that the narcotics are not inherently and inevitably destructive can no longer be opposed, now that society has established its willingness to provide heroin users with large daily doses of methadone, another synthetic narcotic. On daily doses of methadone large enough to last for 24 hours, the heroin user is so tolerant to narcotics that he cannot ''get off'' on affordable amounts of heroin.

The theory of the treatment also holds that methadone will quell the desire for heroin that the compulsive user or addict feels. However, the drug is given by mouth and is not quite equivalent to heroin. Deprived of the experience of intravenous injection, the patient remains anxious; drug use among patients on methadone maintenance remains high and involves heroin, alcohol, Valium, and the like. Methadone maintenance as treatment is probably judged unsatisfactory by most therapists and patients.

Tolerance to and physical dependence on the opiates are less important than might be predicted because heroin (owing to its expense) is supplied in diluted form. Fear of withdrawal is, however, a factor in maintaining the habit and is the first barrier to treatment. However, withdrawal is repeatedly imposed on the average user, either by detention or therapy, without curing him. Heroin users, like alcoholics, often revert to their compulsion even after prolonged periods of abstinence (as during incarceration), when physical withdrawal sickness cannot be present.

MAJOR STIMULANTS

Cocaine and the amphetamines are stimulants of the CNS (central nervous system) and also have peripheral sympathomimetic (epinephrine-like) effects on blood pressure, pulse rate, pupil size, and other functions. They are identified as major or sympathomimetic stimulants. Within the amphetamine group are included amphetamine itself (dextroamphetamine, Dexedrine, ''Bennies''), methamphetamine ("speed," Desoxyn), Ritalin, Preludin, and a host of slightly less potent diet pills with many trade names.

In small doses, the amphetamines cause a pleasurable stimulation or euphoria. With larger doses, and especially with chronic use, the subject experiences wakefulness, deferred fatigue, anxiety, tremulousness, excitement, and, ultimately, distorted perception and a toxic psychosis.

Amphetamine, methamphetamine, and other diet pills are prescribed in huge amounts as anorectic agents. They soon lose their effectiveness for this purpose, but patients and others are persistent in their efforts to maintain a continuing supply of the medication. They are obviously being used as euphoriants rather than as anorectics. Amphetamine abuse after oral administration is not usually a difficult therapeutic problem, but an occasional case of compulsive oral misuse has followed therapeutic administration. The cause of greatest concern, however, is that, when injected intravenously, methamphetamine ("speed," "crystal") causes an immediate pleasurable experience that imposes a hazard of compulsive abuse comparable to that of heroin.

An epidemic of intravenous methamphetamine abuse occurred in the young people's ghettos (e.g., the Haight-Ashbury neighborhood of San Francisco) during 1967–1969. Not only was the effectiveness of the drug-dominated individual destroyed, but much violent behavior was generated by the drug effect and by the new, poorly disciplined illegal marketplace. The users found heroin an effective drug for terminating the speed "run," and through this experience progressed to heroin use—and probably initiated the epidemic of heroin use that began in 1969–1970. Abuse of intravenous amphetamines is still seen today, but comparatively few people are now involved.

Cocaine is generally equivalent in its effects to amphetamine except for a much shorter duration of action. It is usually inhaled or sniffed and is rapidly absorbed across the pharyngeal mucosa. The effects are thus intermediate between those of intravenous and of oral "speed." The use of cocaine as a party or spree drug has increased markedly over the past few years. Its expense limits its extensive use to groups or individuals with a high cash flow. Unfortunately, such groups include pop idols and rock groups with status among adolescents. If cocaine use is not consequently increased, general drug use is.

Tolerance to the sympathetic stimulants does not develop, although a subject may adapt to the effect with repeated experience. Withdrawal is also not a problem except that a user may be exhausted after a period of use.

MINOR STIMULANTS

There are three stimulants which are less potent than the amphetamines but which are widely used.

1. *Nicotine:* Nicotine is the factor in cigarettes that leads to their compulsive use. Any formulation of the biology or psychology of cigarette use must begin with the observation that nicotine-free cigarettes cannot satisfy the compulsive

smoker. Indeed, controlled experiments together with the results of providing low-nicotine cigarettes to an entire population show that a reduction in nicotine simply leads to the smoking of more cigarettes down to a smaller butt. To be driven for a lifetime by a compulsive need as aesthetically and sensually unrewarding as smoking appears inherently undesirable. And, of course, the massive effect of cigarette smoking on the incidence of cancer and of cardiovascular and respiratory disease is established beyond question.

The example of cigarette smoking is useful to the therapist in that it provides an example of compulsive drug use familiar to most people and can be used to explain compulsions even to those who cannot recognize or acknowledge compulsions in their own behavior. The compulsive use of cigarettes is, like heroin use, an act senselessly repeated despite the certainty of damage — not so much out of a desire to smoke as because the confirmed smoker cannot tolerate the resulting intense, if transient, anxiety that follows quitting. The use of nicotine does not result in physical dependence and withdrawal. The apparent withdrawal is not organic in origin but is entirely the result of terminating a compulsion.

2. *Caffeine:* The caffeine in coffee or tea qualifies as an ''addicting'' drug in that use can become compulsive and physical dependence can be objectively demonstrated in subjects drinking seven or more cups per day.

3. *Propoxyphene:* Propoxyphene in its various forms (Darvon, Darvon-N, Darvon compound, Darvocette, and other mixtures and generics) is the drug for which the most prescriptions are written each year in the United States, although the dollar volume of prescriptions for Valium, another commonly abused prescription drug, is greater. Yet propoxyphene is virtually inactive for its nominal purpose of relieving pain. The CNS stimulant properties of the opiates are apparent to some patients who take codeine, and this stimulant effect, which is selectively increased in propoxyphene, is the explanation for its popularity.

HALLUCINOGENS

Drugs from several pharmacologic classes are able to disorganize neural function and produce a toxic psychosis or acute brain syndrome. The toxic state is characterized by alterations in perception that culminate in what have usually been called hallucinations, although, in all but the most severe states, the external stimulus being misinterpreted is usually apparent. These agents have been called hallucinogenic, psychotomimetic, or psychedelic drugs. Their use and importance are small today but their earlier extensive use is important in that it was the prototype of the many mystic, narcissistic therapies and life styles affected today by whites of ages well beyond adolescence.

The type compound of this class is lysergic acid diethylamide (LSD, ''acid''), a synthetically modified alkaloid from ergot. It is unusual in its potency — a dose of 50 micrograms produces subjectively apparent changes in behavior — and in its ability to cause the desired changes in perception with a minimum of sympathomimetic effects. The total duration of its effect is approximately eight hours. Tolerance develops after a single dose, and the effects cannot be duplicated within two to three days. The effects of taking acid can be separated into the more or less objective changes in behavior that occur and the meaning of these changes to the individual. *Altered Perception:* Initial effects or the effects of small doses may be limited to variable degrees of euphoria or anxiety and feelings of depersonalization. Subsequently, there is progressive alteration of perception of tactile, visual, and auditory stimuli. Colors and sounds develop unexpected qualities or objects change appearance. Delusions occur, i.e., objects or sounds actually present are falsely perceived. Finally, in a rare person after a large dose, hallucinations may occur, i.e., voices or objects are perceived in the absence of any stimuli. At this time, paranoid ideation and panic are common.

When acid or other hallucinogens are knowingly ingested, the subject recognizes that his symptoms are drug-induced—i.e., the ability to test reality is retained to a greater or lesser degree, and the drugs do not mimic a true schizophrenic experience. *Meaning to the Individual:* In the absence of preconditioning or philosophic preparation, the LSD experience is anxiety-laden, and only an occasional person will use the drug repeatedly for amusement or for the minor euphoria induced. If an individual accepts instruction from an enthusiast or proselytizer, the experience may develop one of two meanings: a mystical one or a psychotherapeutic one. Both groups believe that the altered perception extends to abstract ideas as well as to stimuli from physical sources.

The devout "hippie" uses LSD to achieve mystical understanding. The nature of this psychedelic or "consciousness-expanding" effect of LSD is no more susceptible to description than other mystical or religious experiences. Indeed, the analogy to religious conversion first suggested for other drugs by William James is impressive; the requirements are: an individual with a need to change, an experience that serves to mark the change, and, afterward, the continued support of a like-minded group.

Another group may use LSD as a substitute or accelerating technic in a process visualized as being close to psychotherapy.

Today, other processes have almost entirely replaced acid and the drug is generally used only experimentally.

Other sympathomimetic stimulants are sometimes used in place of LSD. Some of these are rarely available (peyote, mescaline, various tryptamine derivatives in mushrooms or as DMT). Several amphetamines, chemically modified to increase their CNS effects, are more commonly used, e.g. STP and MDA. STP and acid are frequently misrepresented by purveyors as one of the natural or organic hallucinogens such as mescaline.

Individual (Psychological) Factors

Drug effects are consistent, and, in a given culture, we can assume that the social factors establishing availability or sanctions change only slowly. In a given group, then, with those factors consistent, all members should be using the same drug to the same extent. This is obviously not the case; individual, psychological, or psychiatric factors must account for the different preferences in drugs and the different patterns or degrees of use.

It is tempting to conclude at this point that drugs are abused because they meet a psychological need imposed by some individual abnormality and to accept the attractive conclusion that drug use is symptomatic of some personality, social, or even organic problem, and that treatment must approach these underlying problems. There must be more than a kernel of truth to the idea or there would be no explanation for the fact that some members of a group may use a given drug to the point of death and others use the same drug temperately or not at all.

Consider, however, three important comments. First, the nature of the defects cannot be defined and vulnerability cannot be predicted. Even those few and generally unaccepted studies that claim to identify a ''user'' or ''addict'' personality (studying groups of selected patients without controls), claim only a statistical definition. Second, the defects, whatever they are, are so commonly distributed as to be outside the concept of abnormal. Abuse, at least episodically, of alcohol, cigarettes, ''grass,'' Valium, Darvon, or diet pills is modal behavior in the United States today. Even the liability of compulsion formation appears again to be the norm if one considers not only heroin, alcohol, and cigarettes but also compulsive nail picking, masturbation, overeating, and others. Finally, there is no evidence that drug problems are accessible to psychotherapy that is directed at personality change.

Group (Sociologic) Factors

The sociologist must certainly be credited with providing the bulk of the early literature in the area of drug abuse. However, much of the data are of value as sociology rather than as preparation for the therapist.

If a classification of drug-using subcultures considers not only the drug but age, ethnicity, sex, geographic location, source of income, meaning of use, and other factors, the resulting list is very long, and the amount of crude sociological data is large. These data are invariably interesting, but they describe behavior after drug use is established, and their importance to the origin and treatment of drug problems is easily overemphasized. Only a limited familiarity with the ritual and jargon of a particular group is necessary for the therapist, and this familiarity is rapidly acquired as needed. Undue emphasis on the practices of the group from which the client must be removed is often a show of virtuosity that can be as counterproductive as the ''show and tell'' style of drug education.

Nevertheless, sociological factors are of tremendous import in understanding, defining, and treating drug abuse. The group factors that interact with the properties of drugs and the individual personality can be simplified into two categories: the attitude of the dominant group in the culture and the often conflicting attitudes of members of the several subgroups in our society.

The attitudes of the dominant group are reflected in the laws. In our society, the laws are generally permissive with respect to alcohol and tobacco, which are actually quite harmful, but impose severe penalties for the mere possession of certain other drugs.

Much of the "drug problem" in the United States is actually a conflict between the mores of the dominant culture and the conflicting ideas of one or more subcultures. The youthful subculture, for example, has adopted marihuana as its social drug—comparable to alcohol. The essential similarity of these two drugs is discussed above, yet the sale of one is treated as a serious crime, whereas the use of the other is not only tolerated but openly advertised and promoted.

Does it matter that we are discussing adolescent drug use rather than the overall problem? Is there some age below which drug use is so ill-advised that provision of the drug should be defined as a crime, as it is now? Before making a judgment in this area of active conflict, a look at the recent changes in the youthful subculture is warranted.

THE NEW HIPPIE CULTURE

The adolescent personality (or process) has a degree of constancy from time to time and place to place. However, whether an adolescent tests himself by spearing a lion, "dropping acid," or mugging a neighbor depends on cultural factors.

What cultural change underlies the recent increase in total drug use, the increase in the number of drugs tested, and the decrease in the age at which experimentation and use begin? In my opinion, from the mid-sixties on, the dominant culture has been increasingly unable to transfer its values to the emerging generation. Not only have an important fraction of young people adopted the values of the new or alternate subculture, but that new, youthful, or "hippie," subculture has had a strong influence on the nominally dominant culture. The term "hippie" is applied to the large and influential counterculture to distinguish it from other small or moribund subcultures that arose just before the flowering of the hip subculture in 1967.

The hip counterculture is different and did not derive from the new left, radical activist, or adversary culture. Now that the controversial war in Vietnam is past, the nonpolitical or passive attitude of young people is apparent. That the radicals are now few and disorganized is a fact only slightly obscured by academic and literary melancholia.

Nor is the new drug-using subculture related to civil rights activism by blacks or whites. The counterculture is tolerant but segregated; blacks cannot drop out of a culture that they have not fully entered.

The barely recognized counterculture of today—barely recognized because it is so nearly dominant—is best introduced by reminding ourselves of the characteristics of the exploring, white, middle-class young people who built up youthful ghettos in the summer of 1967 and then returned to school and home to spread the new word.

The hip scene, which is now accepted without the furor of ten years ago, had the following characteristics (or brought the following message): Middle-class goals are no longer accepted. A new philosophic basis is sought, and no form of mysticism or superstition is too nonsensical for consideration. Individual freedom is paramount and the concept is applied not only to sex, dress, hair style, and vocational choice but especially to drugs.

The summer of love had barely ended in the Haight-Ashbury and similar ghettos in other cities, in 1967, when a then colleague, Fred Davis, published a remarkably prescient paper entitled, "Why All of Us May Be Hippies Someday."[2] He recognized that the emerging generation was rehearsing possible adjustments to problems of identity, work, and leisure that were looming in our affluent, cybernated, industrial society.

These adjustments have indeed taken place. Not only has drug use spread, but other aspects of the counterculture are widely influential and even in some matters accepted by a near majority. Since the problems to which the youthful counterculture is adapting are still present, the changes will continue and will include changes in the pattern and extent of drug use. The problems, not incidentally, that Davis identified were three:

1. The search for an appropriate attitude to be adopted toward a high-production, compulsively consuming but highly automated industrial system.
2. A need to find a way to play in the face of the passive spectatorship that has developed with the industrial revolution and professionalism in music and sports.
3. Finally, the unwillingness, based on absence of perceived need, to defer pleasure (including drugs) against future promise.

If our successors conclude that they will be provided with minimal economic security independent of individual effort, and if they conclude that it will be possible to provide only a fraction of them with interesting jobs and careers, the changes in life style and attitudes of the past few years will progress and control of drug use will be impossible.

Treatment

A discussion of individual treatment and of individual and societal response to adolescent drug use cannot be less complex and less ambiguous than the preceding discussion of factors that modulate drug use.

The matter is further complicated by the paucity of carefully collected and documented (quantified) experience with the adolescent user group and by the lack of controlled studies comparing approaches or comparing treatment with no treatment.

People, especially adolescents, do mature and grow out of bad habits and compulsions; therefore, in this age group with its rapidly changing behavior, the fact that a patient changes during treatment does not prove that the treatment was in any way efficacious! A pharmacologist, committed to the importance of quantitative evaluation of treatment efficacy by careful clinical trials, is embarrassed to present mere experience. Thus, the following generalizations about five groups of patients cannot be justified, but the experience of one circle suggests that they can be used productively as hypotheses to be tested in each client.

1. Individuals Who Acknowledge No Problem. There are large numbers of adolescent and other drug users who do not see themselves as threatened in any way by their drug use—and see themselves still less as ill or deviant. Included in this group are some who are perceived by others as requiring change. They will be referred from or to school, family, probation, parole, or "treatment programs" in large numbers. Such coercive referrals are generally unproductive, and treatment must wait until the person is hurt badly enough to seek help on his own. Ideally, all such referrals should be accepted, at least briefly, in order to identify those who finally acknowledge a problem because of the most recent difficulty.

It is especially important in working with this group to emphasize treatment evaluation. Like older clients subjected to involuntary treatment, this age group will also apply the "talk and you walk" method of enthusiastic participation in therapy for the duration of the appointment. A vain therapist who does not objectively evaluate change and who does not independently verify at least some information can waste most of his time.

2. Problems Unrelated to Drug Abuse. To the limited extent that drug use is symptomatic of some personality, situational, or social ill, the underlying problem should, obviously, be approached. Very commonly, however, drug use is a comparatively unimportant part of a total pattern of behavior, but it is a plausible, visible, and objective point of contention, The distinction between this situation and a problem of primary drug abuse must be made, or else the planning, and especially the evaluation, of treatment will be confused.

3. Acute Drug Reactions. The common drug reaction is simply intoxication from a depressant or stimulant drug in the wrong setting. Unfortunately for teachers, parents, and others, it is exactly the time when counsel cannot be comprehended and none should be attempted. Other drug reactions, such as withdrawal or a well-developed toxic psychosis, should be treated initially as medical problems.

4. Compulsive Heroin Use. Heroin abuse is an infrequent problem among adolescents, the prevalence remaining low even after the criminal skills and physical attributes needed to support a habit have developed. However, under our present system of laws, it is a terribly destructive practice, and treatment should be more actively offered. Since one of the prime goals of treatment is to keep the users out of one kind of ghetto or another and since effective treatment requires that the patient isolate himself from all other heroin users, the adolescent should be kept away from any "program," including methadone maintenance. If his socialization progresses in the company of a hundred junkies, all is lost.

Withdrawal—whether primarily organically based or due to the anxiety that attends the interruption of any compulsion—is an initial barrier to treatment and requires initial drug support.

5. Primary Drug Problems. There remain, then, a small group of young people who appear of their own volition and express a need to use less of a drug or, usually, drugs. Their situational bases for anxiety and their general development are within the expected range; that is, their home and family are not grossly pathologic and it is not possible to relegate the patient to any accepted diagnostic pigeonhole.

The following generalizations about treatment, it should be recalled, have already been denigrated as mere uncontrolled experience. These patients receive little benefit from conventional psychotherapy provided by a therapist trained in the traditional manner to be passive and uninvolved. Conventional therapy more often than not can provide an intellectualizing screen behind which the patient can hide from subsequent therapists.

Treatment should be highly directive and much help in environmental control should be provided. How the patient handles specific people on the phone, at the front door, and on the street is of great importance during the time when he is forgetting what his drug does.

Except for the instruction in avoiding anxiety-generating contacts with drug-using cues, treatment should not be drug centered. Assume that your treatment is worth the effort because it hastens maturation.

It is not always and not necessarily productive to involve the family. The patient may have to isolate himself emotionally and perhaps even physically from a drunken father, a drug-using brother, or a mother who is not so much interested as embarrassed.

Prevention or "Drug Education"

The common demand on the health professional is for treatment—treatment that is only irregularly successful and so consuming of therapist time and energy that it can be provided for only a fraction of those who solicit it, not to mention those judged by others to be in need. Health professionals should, therefore, consider that it may be more productive to involve themselves in prevention of drug abuse than to delegate the responsibility entirely to educators, law enforcement personnel, and individual citizens.

However, any efforts require great forethought, because the conclusion that "drug education" to date has been totally ineffective is a statistical imperative established by the increased prevalence of drug use.

The epidemiologic studies involving surveys, arrest figures, and emergency room experience are all subject to criticism but provide some approximations. Added to objective sales records for licit recreational and prescription drugs, they are consistent with the intuitive conclusions of those close to young people that alcohol, "grass," pills, cigarettes, and some more exotic agents have, during the past ten years, come into much wider use and at younger ages than ever before. The impression that the situation is relatively stable now as compared with a few years ago is factitious and reflects the acceptance by the older population of drugs and drug-related behavior that would have been defined in 1965 as problems—e.g., the regular use of marihuana, alcohol, and pills by high school students. Indeed, the change has been in process long enough that one may find that the "new" drugs may come from the supply of the parent and the approving attitudes from teachers.

At this point I must state my assumption that you are willing to be judgmental and that you find the present situation harmful. Such a conclusion is implicit in every offer to provide treatment, but, in the area of drug use, "judgmental" is used disapprovingly and leads, to repeat myself, to confusion between a nonpunitive and a permissive attitude, between decriminalizing and proselytizing.

The above suggests that whatever we have been doing in the area of prevention can be safely discontinued and also suggests the changes in approach that must be made. At the present time, drug education is directed at the youthful population felt to be at risk. No one who has experience with our children will be surprised by the statement that the didactic material of prevention has no impact compared with the effect of our observable behavior. This discussion to this point has been aimed at presenting something close to the consensus. With prior warning, it concludes with an idea that is probably discordant with the consensus.

The absolutely crucial idea is that efforts to abate drug use should be directed at the total population which imposes attitudes on the emerging generation. The general, adult population must project an attitude of disapproval toward the use of all drugs and must act concordantly. The educator's concept of responsible drug use must be abandoned and all drug use must be surrounded by an aura of guilt or disapproval. The goal of drug education would be to reduce *all* drug use—a goal easily evaluated from the sales of legal drugs.

This idea is as acceptable as prohibition. Advertisers and their allies in the media and entertainment business proselytize for an increasing number of nominally social drugs which will disable an increasing portion of our population through the sequence outlined above. We are not faced, as is often said, with an epidemic of drug abuse. There is no epidemic or increase in the incidence above the expected. However, there is a new cultural pattern for which the present level of drug use is the expected—and is seen as alarming by a small group and one of decreasing size.

REFERENCES

1. Millar, H. E. C. *Approaches to Adolescent Health Care in the 1970s*. Rockville, Md.: U.S. Dept. Health, Education, and Welfare. PHS, DHEW Pub. No. (HSA) 76–5014, 1975, p. 11.
2. Davis, F. "Why All of Us May Be Hippies Someday." *Transaction* 5(2):2–8, 1967.

BIBLIOGRAPHY

Brecher, E. M., and the editors of Consumer Reports. *Licit and Illicit Drugs*. Boston: Little, Brown & Co., 1972.

Klagsbrun, K., and Davis, D. I. "Substance Abuse and Family Interaction." *Fam. Process* 16(2):141–164, 1977.

Meyers, F., Jawetz, E., and Goldfien, A. *Review of Medical Pharmacology*, 6th ed. Los Altos: Lange Medical Pubns.,1978.

Whiteside, T. "Annals of Advertising: Cutting Down." *New Yorker*, November 18, 1974.

Wiker, A. "Dynamics of Drug Dependence." *Arch. Gen. Psychiatry* 28:611, 1973.

10

The Enigma of
Adolescent Suicide

Sister Penny Prophit, D.N.Sc.

Is there a word more whispered than suicide? We speak in masked messages and euphemisms of the unmentionable—and yet suicide is part of the experiential knowledge of thousands of young people who commit self-inflicted death and of the hundreds of thousands who attempt suicide each year.

Startling Statistics

Since 1950, the suicide rate for adolescents has increased by approximately 300%. Internationally, the problem of suicide is growing, but no rate is escalating faster than that of adolescent suicide. Suicide is the second leading cause of death for the 12 to 24 age group in the United States; automobile accidents rank in first place.[1] However, one-car/one-person accidents, when viewed in the context of recent psychological events, might often be considered probable suicides. The addition of these cases to existing figures would make self-inflicted death the leading cause of adolescent mortality. What a chilling realization! Whatever happened to that generation "coming at you, going strong," who told us, "if you're living, you belong?"

In terms of these alarming statistics, sociologists attribute the dramatic rise in adolescent suicide (some call it the "hidden epidemic") to the breakdown of institutions—home, family, and church in particular—that used to provide stability; psychiatrists think it may be due to the premature growing up forced upon youth; moralists blame it on promiscuity; liberals blame it on puritan rigidity; conservatives blame it on "being too easy with the kids." *NOBODY REALLY KNOWS*. And, understandably, those who study suicide and its causes and who are involved in active prevention, intervention, and postvention work are extremely concerned. Presumably, young persons would have the least reason for ending their lives. Growing up can be challenging, but surely not so difficult that one would put a gun

226

to one's head (the exit of choice for males, but increasingly that of females also), or take an overdose of pills, or hang oneself. There is agreement on one major point among behavioral scientists, theologians, clinicians, and concerned persons: suicide is one of the nation's leading mental health problems and is *the* major mental health problem for the adolescent.

Adolescence in Our Day

It is suggested that we are moving from an age of anxiety to an age of depression: witness the emergence of mood clinics for the isolated, alienated, and lonely "Eleanor Rigbys" of our day. To the casual observer, it might seem that the average adolescent is anything but isolated and lonely. Together, teenagers congregate in spontaneous groups, dress in peer-governed styles, unite in special causes, and, viewed from a distance, perhaps, seem a close, cohesive group. However, closer scrutiny of adolescents reveals a sense of isolation and rootlessness that the so-called adolescent subculture rarely satisfies. In their peer groups, adolescents find little of the interpersonal security, consistency, and intimacy for which they so long. Moreover, they are haunted by the briefness of adolescence and the fact that whatever small comfort they have found in special groups will soon slip from their grasp. Few can put it into words, but it gnaws at them. They feel it.

The helping professions are only now recognizing that adolescence is a time in which truly unique and special events happen, and that we can no longer apply the categorizations and norms of adult healthy behavior as criteria for adolescent healthy behavior. Attempts at the demystification of adolescence have begun; we have embarked upon new and exciting research. Mark the development of adolescent clinics and health care units embodying the philosophy that adolescents are different and need a specialized environment for their unique developmental concerns.

Even a general discussion of normal adolescence may prove a gargantuan task! Inconsistency, uncertainty, and disharmony with adults seem to be frequent states of being for adolescents. In fact, adolescents seem to be in a very fluid and loose period of development which often puzzles them as much as it puzzles adults. Children realize that certain behaviors bring parental approval or disapproval. They have a good idea about which activities will bring love and which will bring wrath. As adults, we learn the behaviors expected of individuals in various life situations and we have learned how adults are expected to act in our society. But since the adolescent is no longer a child, childlike behavior on his part calls forth a plea to act his age; on the other hand, when he attempts to relate in a more sophisticated fashion, adults remind the young person that he is still a child. No wonder there is confusion! One adolescent defined his stage of development in the words: "an adolescent is someone who doesn't have his act together." This seems an astute observation: his childhood indentity is being altered, but he has not "got it together" enough to be considered an adult. Another adolescent put it this way: "I just can't take hold. . . . I just can't seem to take hold of some kind of life." Adolescence *is* the generation gap between childhood and adulthood and there are truly myriad reasons why adolescence seems to be such a disturbing period. In reference to this notion,

Josselyn[2] noted in a joint commission study on the mental health of children that there seems to be no symptom of the disturbed adolescent that does not in some way or another fit into a category of normal adolescence. Some—in frustration—might be tempted to consider adolescence a psychiatric diagnosis rather than a developmental period!

An adolescent develops his identity by bouncing ideas, values, and feelings against a solid family structure or a clearly defined person, identifying ways in which he is similar and ways in which he is different. If this is true, then the flux and lack of defined structure in our society today would seem to make this task doubly difficult. The outer flux and confusion of society are mirrored in the inner flux and confusion of the adolescent. Family structures are under question and political, economic, and social structures are under severe scrutiny. Developing an identity today is therefore a much more formidable task than it was in years gone by.

Adolescence is a time of moratorium and transition. It is a period which in itself provides a unique call. It offers the polar risks of freedom and commitment and heralds conflicts concerning dependency and a natural striving for independence. Fears of loss of control over self or environment often result in rigid and sometimes compulsive behavior. Fears of homosexuality or sexual inadequacy arise from the developmental task which requires the adolescent to establish an adult sexual identity, again greatly intensified by our changing society which provides more sexual options. Hormonal changes seem not only to precipitate many obvious physical changes, but also to stimulate and intensify an adolescent's emotional life. All of these emotions and feelings simmer together, building up the pressures which are part of every adolescent's inner life. What a challenge to be a normal adolescent!

Adolescents speak to us in many ways of their loneliness and pain. Have you noticed the adolescent folk-rock music lately? Are poets and minstrels still prophets? Do you listen to the music of the young? The melodies are haunting and beautiful, with poignant lyrics for the listener, one who hears. Do they speak for adolescents today? The messages of their fears, aloneness, and even self-destructive thoughts are strikingly present.

Adolescent suicide evokes many powerful and complex emotions within all whose lives have been touched by this tragedy. The inevitable question is posed: "Why?" The very fact of adolescent suicide raises existential questions that are largely unanswerable.

Theoretical Attempts to Explain Adolescent Suicide

There are few theories concerning adolesent suicide; there is no one comprehensive theory that adequately explains, describes, and predicts the tragic event. In fact, relatively little research has been conducted in this area since it is almost impossible to study suicide prospectively and experimentally; the clinician and researcher must rely on retrospective data. The general theories that provide frameworks for the analysis of adolescent suicide dynamics reflect the following three dimensions: (1) developmental, (2) sociological, and (3) psychological.

THE DEVELOPMENTAL DIMENSION

Developmentally, adolescence is characterized as a time of storm and stress, due in no small way to the physiological changes that are occurring both internally and externally. The adolescent is preoccupied with his physical appearance and experiences great distress if his body is in some way different from the peer group norm. Adolescents mature at different rates, with the result that many feel out of step with the group. Even within the adolescent's own body, development occurs in an asynchronous manner, in that various organs and subsystems grow at different rates, causing the teenager to look and feel awkward. One adolescent expressed a vivid perception: "It's not that I'm awkward; it's just that these days my head seems so far away from my feet!"

The adolescent also experiences awkwardness in relation to other persons. He moves from childhood into adulthood with ambivalence and uncertainty. Childlike qualities may be dominant at one moment, only to be replaced by more mature modes of behavior in the next. It is an understatement to say that adolescence can be a trying time for the family; since both parents and child must learn and relearn one another and adjust to new role relationships, it is indeed demanding.

The adolescent is very dependent upon his peers; their role is important in the process of self-definition. He is constantly striving to be as much like his peer group as he can, while at the same time he recognizes that he must be singularly different in some special way to gain his unique identity. Responding to the polar needs of competition and cooperation becomes his paramount and stressful concern. Psychologically, identity is the primary challenge of adolescence, and this often results in highly critical analytical behavior, for the teenager is forever measuring himself against others. It is a time in which a fragile raw self may bleed easily; tragically, the bleeding may occur literally as well as symbolically.

In sum, the teen years are a period of considerable normative stress when coping mechanisms are being stretched to their utmost in the search for psychological identity, independence, and a meaningful social role. If the new life experiences are coupled with other stresses and if balancing and supportive factors are lacking, a situation of suicidal risk might be an outcome.

THE SOCIOLOGICAL DIMENSION

Other theorists suggest that suicide is better explained by viewing society as a whole; individual motivation is perceived as less important than the ways in which that particular society supports or ultimately may produce suicidal persons. The social philosopher Durkheim[3] analyzed various kinds of suicides that grew out of different social conditions. He grouped suicides into three major types and used special terms to describe each. Egoistic suicide, according to Durkheim, comes about when a person feels alienated from society and has few binding ties; the suicidal person is a lonely, friendless individual, perhaps an adolescent runaway. Altruistic suicide represents the polar opposite in that it occurs among persons so dedicated to a cause or to the values of society that they put duty far ahead of their own needs. An example might be the adolescent who destroys himself as an anti-war protest. Anomic suicide, the third category in Durkheim's system, occurs when a person experiences sudden and great changes in his position in society—as in present-day situations of hypermobility and the modular society. We live in a society that Durkheim would have classified as anomic—involving rapid social change, increased mobility, family breakdown, and economic distress—one which, according to the sociological model, would suggest or predict the high suicide rates presently prevailing.

THE PSYCHOLOGICAL DIMENSION

Social theories explain a great deal about the stresses and tensions that may lead to young suicides, but they do not and cannot explain why some adolescents take the drastic step of killing themselves while others manage to cope with the same pressing social conditions and live. Psychological theory offers insight along these lines. In contrast to the societal perspective, Freud[4] sought intrapsychic answers to the question of suicide. Although he never published a book on the subject, his ideas permeate many of his most important works; one of those ideas has become a cornerstone of suicide theory. Freud's view of suicide as a form of aggression turned inward against oneself, or retroflexed rage, proposes that people who kill themselves are actually killing the image of a hated parent or significant other within them. Freud assumed that in a love relationship one person attaches energy to another, and when the loved person is lost, the angry feelings toward the lost loved one are turned inward. If the anger is great enough, the ego acts to destroy that identification and, in doing so, actually destroys itself. In this situation, one might say that suicide is murder in the 180th degree.

Some of the behavioral scientists[5] suggest that the roots of suicide are established in infancy, when basic trust is the developmental issue. It is theorized that if the mother-infant bond either is never established or is interrupted by death, abandonment, or even severe depression on the part of the mother, a seed is planted for later suicide.

This theory also relates to the perplexing clinical situation of the adolescent "starving sparrows"—the predominantly female youngsters who experience the self-destructive behavior known as the anorexia nervosa syndrome. Other clinical phenomena related to self-destructive eating patterns (such as the purging-gorging syndrome), identity formation, and parental influence await further clarification.

Alternative Answers

The isolation of the normal adolescent, the polarities and strains that he experiences, and his needs for security and consistency are factors that have been underscored in a casebook of psychological autopsies which examines instances of committed suicide by adolescents.[6] In the reconstruction of the events preceding death, in almost all of the examples cited, the profound sense of aloneness and isolation of the adolescent had become paramount. Stress was placed by the authors[6] on the fact that suicide was not the result of a few isolated events, but rather the end of a process of extremely frustrating situations which pushed the adolescent toward an irreversible decision to terminate his own life. The authors make the case that only an adolescent who has in his own deliberations reached the end of hope takes his own life, and that it is a deliberated decision.

One of the many issues that surround the enigma of suicide is whether suicide is simply an impulsive gesture of the ''hysteric'' for attention or whether it is the outcome of a series of disconfirming events which could threaten the vital balance of any of us to the extent that self-destruction might be viewed as the only way out of an intolerable situation. Shneidman[7] and Teicher,[8] both suicidologists, are convinced that suicide in adolescence is not an impulsive act but one that is actually almost determined by significant life events occurring at critical periods.

According to Teicher and Jacobs,[9] there is a characteristic presuicidal biography of the adolescent who eventually arrives at the conclusion that self-destruction is the only solution to his life problem. Teicher and his associate studied the life situations of adolescents who attempted suicide to discern whether a common pattern could be found in them. Fifty teenagers who had attempted suicide were matched with a comparison group for age, race, sex, and family income. The entire group was asked to chronicle life events, using a life history chart, from birth until the actual suicide attempt for the adolescent suicide group, and up to their present life situation for the nonsuicidal adolescents. Analysis of the data revealed that the suicide attempters had experienced a sequence of events that led to progressive unhappiness and pessimism. The suicidal adolescents had become increasingly isolated from the few important people in their lives, whereas the comparison group had not. The biography involved an identifiable three-stage progression to an intense feeling of isolation in the period preceding the suicide attempt:

1. A *long-standing preadolescent history of problems* of various kinds (broken homes, rejection by parents, early losses).
2. A *period of escalation* which was coincidental with adolescence, often associated with the appearance of new problems; these essentially involved a series of failures in the resolution of the normal tasks of adolescence, such as the struggle for autonomy, failure to achieve adequate identity, school failure with attendant lack of self-esteem, and also, perhaps, the inadequate working out of sexual conflicts.
3. A *final stage* which was described as a chain reaction involving any meaningful person relationships or associations; events were often mistaken as the reason for the suicide but in reality only represented the precipitating cause. Frequently mentioned examples were fights with the family, inadequate romance and breakups, school truancy and dropping out, pregnancy, running away, and delinquent behavior.

The adolescent has special ways of expressing depression. Situations such as those listed in the third stage may well be the classical, cardinal symptoms of depression in adolescence. Teenagers who attempt suicide consistently have histories of trying first to communicate their distress by these nonsuicidal means. Suicidal adolescents appear to have in common long-standing histories of ''downs'' which include one of, or complexes of, the following events:

1. Parent who attempted suicide, or relative or close friend.
2. One or both natural parents absent from the home.
3. Unwanted step-parent.
4. Both parents working.
5. Perception by the adolescent of family conflict as extreme.
6. Alcoholism of a parent.
7. Living with person other than natural parent.
8. Mobility.
9. Loss: death, hospitalization, frequent school change, etc.

Further supports for Teicher's findings are demonstrated by the work of Moss,[10] who in a review of 50 case histories of seriously suicidal patients, observed that the loss of a significant person in the life of the individual had occurred during childhood in 60% of the cases. Similarly, in a review of 137 cases of suicidal persons, Lester and Beck[11] found a significant relationship between the loss of both parents before the age of ten years and suicide (or suicidal attempts). Rohn and associates[5] studied 65 young persons who attempted suicide and found that social isolation was a major factor; 50% of the teenagers described themselves as loners. These authors discovered a high rate of family disruption—59% of the young persons came from one-parent families. In this same group studied, 75% had poor school records, 19% had failed one or more grades, and 35% were dropouts or chronic truants. Jacobs[12] studied various life situations which seemed to be associated with adolescent suicide. He found that frequency of residential moves and school changes, amount and severity of discipline, and living with step-parents distinguished the attempters from the normal adolescents.

Adolescent Suicide as a Family Problem

Adolescent suicide most frequently takes place in the context of family problems and often is directed toward bringing about a resolution of these problems. Often, of course, the attempt has an opposite effect and further alienates the adolescent, if he survives the suicidal gesture. Suicide among young people is so horrifying and unthinkable to adults that many of us are compelled to be complacent about the troubles of the adolescent. Shakespeare's Romeo and Juliet are to most of us romantic and innocuous literary tragic figures. Yet, many adolescents cling to one another in similar love and desperation. A modern Juliet is likely to be a frightened and pregnant young woman; the contemporary Romeo might be an adolescent who feels rejected, alone, and lonely. Both feel isolated and forsaken. Again, the consistent theme of loneliness and alienation prevails.

When, in a survey of adolescents who had attempted suicide, the young people were asked to whom they would turn if in trouble, almost 75% responded that there was no one who really cared or who would understand them.[8] In a similar study,

Teicher and Jacobs[9] reported that 46% of the group studied had indicated their intention to commit suicide to other people and that fewer than half that amount had shared the information with their parents. This is particularly significant since 88% of the adolescent suicides occur at home, very often with the parents in the next room. In every instance, the lack of communication between parent and adolescent was identified as a significant factor in the period preceding the suicide.

The Void of Relationships

Two essential concepts that recur throughout the singularly meager literature on adolescent suicide continue to be tragically pertinent. First, there is a void of meaningful, consistent, and caring relationships in the life situations of a suicidal adolescent. Second, the conspiracy of silence that surrounds this usually secretive and private period of growth and development is coupled with the deep silence that shrouds the suicidal situation.

In the fascinating prologue to his book on the human search for meaning, Frankl[13] describes his efforts to help clients find meaning in their lives. He asked them, ''What has prevented you from committing suicide?'' This author conducted a survey of 330 university students using Frankl's approach. A questionnaire was developed around similar questions, such as ''What factors would prevent you from committing suicide?'' The significant factor identified by the group of male and female adolescent respondents was the presence of at least one meaningful relationship with a person. The major element identified which they perceived would promote suicidal thoughts and possible action was a sense of being alone and lonely, heightened by being with people (as in a dormitory) but alone. The universal theme of aloneness seemed once again to be prominent in these adolescents.

Shneidman[7] edited a book of essays written by Harvard students which reflected the themes of suicide and death. One chapter presented the results of a student project which involved placing an urgent message in the classified section of a newspaper indicating a situation in which a 21-year-old male student gives himself three weeks to live and asks readers to respond if they can give reasons why he should not kill himself. The two primary categories from an overwhelming response centered on the notion of suicidal thoughts as universally experienced phenomena among young persons and on the human experience of loneliness during the adolescent period.

Intervention

These findings form the background supportive data for a framework, grounded in sensitivity to adolescents, for the prevention of suicide and the identification of suicidal risk, as well as for the tasks, challenges, and focus of intervention. No one is 100% suicidal. The ambivalent nature of suicide is what makes it so preventable; it is also what makes suicide the most tragic form of death. It is the expressed belief of researchers and clinicians in the field of suicidology that suicide is essentially a cry for help, an ultimate communication when other forms of cries have failed. It is a situation in which a form of tunnel vision is operating and in which alternatives are not seen by the person in emotional pain.

There are no neat little interventions or pat answers, nor is there any solid literature specific to adolescent suicide risk. As Seiden[14] noted, there are minimal substantive theories for explaining suicide and for the generation of hypotheses for clinical testing.

All there is, in reality, is you or me, coming with who I am, my life and my hopes. The point is that we are not coming to save lives as moralizers or theologians; rather we are professional persons eliciting life. In a sense, this is a kind of creativity in which each of us is involved. And, the ability to bring life to others is dependent upon our day-to-day self-creation. The invitation for the potential helper is to be creative, to vitalize.

Consider the adolescent whom we have perceived to be in distress — the signs are there. He might be in the midst of crisis, and, by definition, crisis actually provides an unusual opportunity for positive intervention, for it implies a state which cannot be tolerated indefinitely. The principal factors are the overwhelming importance of an intolerable problem and the feeling of hopelessness and helplessness in the face of it; the pressure of these feelings compels one toward some action for immediate resolution. Something must change.

So much depends on the relationship and the quality of the relationship. Each of us will need to adapt the words and find the authentic style which best speaks for us. Many advocate a humanistic and caring approach which assumes that:

1. The adolescent has within him the capacity, though it may be latent, to understand the factors in his life which cause him unhappiness and pain and to recognize himself in such a way as to overcome these; and
2. These strengths will become effective if the helping person can establish with the adolescent a relationship that is sufficiently warm, accepting, and understanding.

It should not be a relationship of words only, but one that establishes contact on a feeling level and is marked by an effort to understand. To one who feels unworthy and unloved, caring and concern are great sources of encouragement.

One of the first tasks in crisis intervention is to identify the source of distress; this may be difficult, since suicide thrives on secrecy. Relevant questions to stimulate comfortable disclosure might be:

•What has been happening to you lately?
•When did you begin to feel worse?
•What's new in your life situation?

Each of us will have to find the comfortable words to try to gain an understanding of ''Why now?'' in the adolescent's life. The potential adolescent suicide should be encouraged to diagnose the problem in his own words and to pin down as precisely as possible the precipitating stresses. This should be accomplished in an atmosphere of acceptance; the young person should feel that ''it's OK'' to express true feelings with comfort. If he is reluctant to share, one might say: ''You seem to be in pain. You seem sad and troubled. Perhaps if you could tell me how you feel I might be able to understand and to help." Accept the adolescent and his point of view; try to understand from his frame of reference, for that is what is real for him. Let him talk, and listen to his perhaps unspoken pleas for help. Do not be afraid to use the word "suicide," because frequently bringing the "dread and feared word" to the level of open communication is actually relieving to an adolescent who is carrying the burden of suicidal thoughts. You might also ask if there are important people in the adolescent's life who are not hearing him. Also, you might ask if there is any way in which you can help them to hear the adolescent; finally, ask, "Am I hearing you?"

Bearing in mind the categories of stresses that adolescents characteristically experience in situations of suicide risk (parents, peers, broken romance, pregnancy, school failure, identity concerns) and the notion of process and progression of escalating problems, you might also want to ask, sensitively, about the following three critical dimensions. Is there a long-standing history of problems? Have these problems become worse? Is the stage set for the familiar chain-reaction dissolution of meaningful relationships?

You might also ask how the adolescent has handled similar situations prior to this time, as a means of assessing coping mechanisms and discerning strengths. Try to discover what still matters, what is still available that has meaning. Who are the persons that touch his life? Are there no alternative solutions? Is there not some hope? Above all, be available, provide a lifeline, and supply direct support. Evaluate the suicidal intent and lethality or risk by determining the specificity of the suicide plan and the availability of the means. Act definitively, based on this assessment.

Troubled adolescents give clues which the sensitive person can pick up, if listening and seeing. The clues may be verbal or nonverbal and the literature is replete with examples of these, from the giving away of treasured possessions to the actual statement "I wish I were dead." Being alert to the unusual signs of depression which adolescents may reflect is strongly urged. Given the state of the clinical art in the recognition of signs, symptoms, and warning signals which seem to be the significant heralds of teenage suicide, the sensitive and informed helping professional may be the inspiriting catalyst for the adolescent's initial movements toward life choices. The adolescent within the home may present vague physical concerns which mask adolescent depression; drugs and alcohol may become an intermediate self-destructive behavior also indicating adolescent depression. The helping person also needs to be acquainted with the myths and taboos associated with suicide. He should be able to dispel these with knowledge and informed responses in order to directly and openly relate to the suicidal situation as essentially a cry for help. Since he is cognizant of the many unknowns in adolescent suicide prevention, the helping person should be alert to situations in which an adolescent suddenly becomes "different" from the usual pattern of behavior: the good student who suddenly begins to fail; the punctual and attending adolescent who becomes truant; the consistent, quiet, conscientious adolescent who suddenly becomes a behavioral problem; the adolescent who suddenly becomes sexually promiscuous.

Efforts to encourage the adolescent to talk with parents, to keep lines of communication open, should be made. Sensitive questions concerning how the adolescent's life is going might be all the adolescent needs to open the wellsprings of loneliness and hurt. The presence and interest of even one consistent and meaningful relationship in the life of the adolescent may make the critical difference in the choice for life or for death.

Given the situation of attempted suicide, the problem is out, revealed. What now? Often in the hospital emergency room or inpatient units the adolescent is subtly invited by health care professionals and others to "do it better next time," either through obvious avoidance of the person or various forms of abruptness in verbal and nonverbal communication. Perhaps this attitude comes, in part, from judgments regarding the phenomenon of suicide, judgments which are largely based on lack of information. Perhaps, too, it comes from a fear on the part of the health professional concerning questions of life and death and the mystery that still pervades the Pandora's box that is suicide: the mystery, always, Why? It would be extremely helpful for persons working with adolescents who have attempted suicide to think through some of the questions concerning their perception of the meaning of life and death. This would involve reviewing their knowledge base related to suicide study, their own hopes, and their attitudes toward—and perhaps even past experiences related to—suicide and the suicide skeletons in their own closets. It is also helpful for the person within the hospital setting to understand that the angry adolescent (a frequent manifestation in the post-attempt period) is the frightened adolescent. The ability not to become locked into the anger cycle, but to recognize that the dynamic of anger primarily involves a threat to self (esteem, competence, and control) will enable the helping person to focus upon efforts to enhance feelings of safety, understanding, and caring for the adolescent. The realization that, of ten adolescents who succeed in killing themselves, eight have previously attempted, leads to the conviction that timely intervention is imperative in the care of the adolescent attempter.

In sum, the following suggestions may be useful in focusing efforts for preventive intervention:

1. Realize that asking for psychological help is developmentally inconsistent with the adolescent's inner drives for mastery and control in the normally secretive period of growth and development; therefore, be sensitive and respond in such a way as to respect the need for privacy.
2. Familiarize yourself with the literature on adolescent growth and development and reflect on your own adolescent period. Unless we have worked through our own life experiences, we cannot deal effectively and openly with families and adolescents. Think about your own adolescent growth and development period; recall the time. It brings you close to them and facilitates genuine communication.
3. Remember the key factor of the absence of meaningful relationships and recognize that your sensitive and consistent concern may make the critical difference between life and death.
4. Be willing and ready to give information about the *normal* tasks and challenges of adolescence; it is often healing to a troubled adolescent to learn that he is normal and that adolescence is truly the "generation gap."
5. Try to assist the adolescent not only to cope with but to find meaning in crisis

and stress as opportunities to learn more about himself; help him to recognize crisis as the way in which we all grow—since, perhaps, "without a hurt, the heart is hollow."
6. Stay tuned to the dynamic that is anger and recognize it as the adolescent's way of expressing a perceived threat to self.
7. Be sensitive to masked cries for help from lonely adolescents.

Postvention: The Survivor-Victims of Suicide

The cry for help goes unheeded. The adolescent kills himself. Life is over. For the family the tragedy is just beginning. The crushing blow is a bitter experience for those left behind; they may carry it in their hearts for the rest of their lives. Who suffers more: the dead adolescent who survives only in the memory of the survivors, or the survivors who die daily in remembering?

The death of a loved one is devastating. Yet the bereaved may find consolation in believing that it was for a purpose or may accept the reality factor that there are limits to one's existence. How much more traumatic is it when loss of life is self-inflicted? Where do survivors find consolation then? Suicide may well be the cruelest death of all for those who remain. What they may believe to be the unpardonable sin has been committed. The universal taboo with its theological injuctions has been violated. For relatives and friends, intolerable feelings of guilt and grief are aroused, bringing with them the persistent and aching questions: What did I do wrong? Where did I fail? Why didn't I. . . ? And, so it goes on endlessly.

Survivors carry the stigma for life. Years after the adolescent suicide one may still be remembered as "the person whose son shot himself" or "whose daughter took an overdose" or "whose brother hung himself." Suicide seems rarely to be completely forgotten and forgiven.

But, someone has died and must be psychologically buried. The task may seem impossible—it is said that this is the most challenging of all clinical problems. Yet, there are ways to be of vital assistance to those who face perhaps the greatest tragedy and challenge of their lives.

The goals of ministering to the family of the adolescent suicide are similar to those pursued in helping other persons who face bereavement. Grief work involves the process of emancipation from the bondage to the deceased, readjustment to the environment in which the deceased is missing, and the formation of new relationships. The psychological factors which predominate in the process of bereavement for parental and sibling survivors are:

1. Guilt—a predominant feature, which may be overwhelming; the survivors experience pain because they failed to help or did not hear the cry for help; they feel that had they intervened in some way the suicide might have been prevented.
2. Denial—even in the face of concrete evidence, the parent or sibling survivor may deny that the adolescent took his own life.

3. Shame, related to the stigma of suicide.
4. Avoidance of communication about the event, which may delay the normal grief and mourning process.
5. Increased risk of suicide within the survivor group.

Herzog and Resnik[15] described a retrospective study of the families of adolescent suicides that took place during a two-year period. Within the families studied, considerable difficulty was encountered in obtaining permission for interviews with the survivors and in no family was access to the siblings of the deceased granted to the investigators. The findings of the study indicated that the parents of adolescent suicides: (1) refuse to think of the death as a suicide, preferring to consider it an accident; (2) feel hostile toward persons who designate the cause of their child's death as suicide; and (3) feel long-lasting guilt about the death of their child. Another striking observation was the frequent evidence of family disruption noted among the parents of the adolescent suicide. This, along with other implications, supports the necessity of evaluating family relationships as they were before the suicide when attempting to analyze the responses of the surviving family members after the suicide. The immediate parental and sibling response to the sudden loss of the adolescent appeared to be overwhelming hostility and denial, followed by guilt and depression. Projection of this hostility upon society as personified by the medical examiner, police, physician, nurse, or other helping professional was common. In this study, however, it was fascinating to note that the parents interviewed said that they would have appreciated having a professionally educated person to talk with immediately following the suicide. The researchers suggested that this is the best time to begin postvention with survivors so that rapport can be established before the development of barriers to entry and heightened defensive reactions.

Postvention, according to Shneidman,[16] is composed of those activities following the death of a significant other by suicide that serve to help the survivors to cope with their emotional response to the loss. The focus of postvention is directed toward bereavement as it is experienced in daily living by the survivors; thus, postvention should typically extend over the first critical year following the adolescent's death.

When assisting the bereaved, the helping person must take into account the special kind of death. What can you, the special person, bring? Your best self—neither prejudiced by outmoded prohibitions nor judgmental of the actions of the deceased or the survivors. Do not go either to justify or to censure. Conversation should be natural, interest genuine and sincere. Don't try too hard. Responsive listening and empathic discernment of what the other is experiencing from his internal—often agonizing—frame of reference is vital. The survivor is often obsessed by the thought that he should have prevented the death and often sees himself as a failure. The guilt may take the form of self-recrimination, depression, and/or hostility. One tendency is to look for a scapegoat, and often this tends to be the member of the family who is least able to bear the burden. Inwardly, the survivors may accuse themselves, but they may turn the anger outward in the attempt to cope with guilt. Minor omissions come to mind and loom as major and significant causes of death. Again and again the survivors of adolescent suicide replay the ninth inning, devising those plays that might have won the game and preserved the young life.

The concept of "postvention" borrows many elements from the process of helping: talk, opportunities for expression of feelings, reassurance, direction, and even gentle confrontation. Thus, postvention affords an opportunity for the expression of guarded emotions, especially those negative emotions such as anger, guilt, and shame. The bereaved, in essence, needs to pour out his or her heart in order that the dissolution of ties and the sharing of pleasant and unpleasant memories may be experienced. When each event is reviewed, suffering is felt at the thought that the experience will never again be repeated. As pain is felt, the individual begins slowly to dissolve the emotional ties with the dead adolescent. A gradual working through such a process is a necessary part of the mourning and is the prelude to the acceptance of suicide as a real fact. This process brings a measure of stability to the grieving person's life and at the very least provides a genuine interpersonal relationship in which honest thoughts and feelings can be expressed.

Resnik[17] further refined his concept by dividing the sequential phases of postvention, which he termed "psychological resynthesis," into three phases. The model in Table 10–1 is a redefinition of Resnik's three phases, with developed goals

TABLE 10–1. *Adolescent Suicide Postvention Model*

PHASES OF RESYNTHESIS	GOALS OF HELPING
1. Phase I: *Resuscitation* (Immediate response for support of survivors during initial 24 hours to assist in withstanding the initial shock)	a. To establish contact on a feeling level with survivors; to build a relationship b. To support during initial shock of immense loss c. To facilitate awareness of basic and normal responses at this time: confusion, guilt, blame, anger, and perhaps severe depression
2. Phase II: *Resynthesis* (Psychological rehabilitation to help survivors to learn new ways of coping with loss; may last several months during regular but unstructured contacts)	a. To formulate an agreement with the family to establish regular meeting times b. To support reintegration of the family c. To prevent perpetuation of or development of family pathology d. To foster exploration of guilt in order to dissipate gross distortions e. To assist the family to understand the dynamics of normal grieving
3. Phase III: *Renewal* (Period of forfeit of grief and attendant bondage to the adolescent suicide and substitution of new relationships and interests) (Terminated on the first anniversary of the suicide, reopening the mourning process with its pain, but only for brief period)	a. To terminate with family after time of first anniversary, with one revisit to reevaluate any continuing problems b. To counter hurt of professional termination by awareness of the importance of the date, reaffirming availability of help

of intervention for a health care professional in the postvention phase of adolescent suicide.

Additional considerations underlying intervention for survivor-victims are that:

1. Family members need to accept the adolescent suicide in their own time.
2. There is often the need to convince the family of the value of crisis intervention.
3. Family members need to learn that grief is self-limiting.
4. Family members need to learn the special and unusual ways that children grieve (e.g., regressive changes, difficulties in school, temper tantrums, and the like).

Suicidologists consistently urge that positive postvention efforts such as these will head off the schizophrenias and suicides of the next generation. In fact, survivor-victims who have not been exposed to postvention efforts have a particularly high suicide risk potential.

Postvention efforts should also be directed by the school nurse or child health associate to junior high and high school companions of the adolescent who has killed himself. There is a definite need to incorporate discussion about suicide into high school health classes or curricula which deal with social problems. Often, after an adolescent suicide in a community, the effort is made to deny its existence, to try to continue "as if nothing had happened." Curriculum content dealing with suicide is vitally needed to reduce the stigma attached to even talking about suicide. Perhaps even more importantly, it could encourage among students a discussion of two very important areas: (1) the relationship between events and emotions, and (2) sharing by students of similar, even universal, feelings of the adolescent concerning questions of life and death. In the first instance, despite our psychological sophistication, the vast majority of adolescents remain in the dark about the forces behind their volatile and ricocheting feelings. Adolescents often experience such private emotional turmoil that the young person, beset with powerful feelings, assumes not only that he or she is undergoing this in isolation, but also that the feelings are without understandable cause. A frank discussion of the roots and causes of suicide in adolescence as well as the normal pressures of adolescence leads to growth-promoting and healing self-knowledge. In the second instance, sharing dramatically reduces the sense of isolation. Though the curriculum topic may be student suicide, the content might actually focus on the importance of understanding emotions and how they influence behavior. Picture for a moment an isolated student saddled with all manner of private guilt, low self-esteem, or serious depression, who hears in a classroom—perhaps for the first time—that the classmates whom he or she has perhaps viewed as different, luckier, or better off, are beset by many of the same uncertainties and feelings and even fears. Picture this same student beginning to understand that his or her feelings have causes, that he or she is not strange, and that, though feelings may run deeper, they are nevertheless the same feelings that other classmates have, and they are *normal*. Imagine the positive impact this could have upon the isolated student.

There is also the normal tendency for a community to cover up an adolescent suicide, to pretend that it never happened, to offer excuses for its happening, or to view the family in which it happened as peculiar and unapproachable. There is no better time to discuss suicide in a classroom than after a suicide attempt or a successful suicide has taken place. It will most assuredly be talked about by the students—but otherwise in ignorance and fear. If there are siblings of the deceased student in the same school, they should be given the choice of participating or not and should be allowed to decide on the level of their involvement in the discussions. Encourage the discussion of feelings and ideas with the class. When these have been expressed, the effective school nurse or child health associate can then present in a thoughtful and sensitive manner some of what is known about the dynamics of suicide, the myths, and postvention concerns. Teachers and school nurses are often the first to detect clues to suicide; long before others become aware, they may clearly see the dramatic changes in the life style of the adolescent. Honest, open, and kind confrontation by one who cares can literally save a life.

In summary, if the helping person intervenes immediately at the time of an adolescent suicide, perhaps many of the long-term and second generational destructive effects of this difficult form of bereavement can be averted.

Summary

It is hoped that the foregoing ideas may assist those who wish to understand and lend a hand in bringing the protracted struggle of the suicidal crisis to a conclusion in which the forces of self-creation take victory over the forces of self-destruction. Most of all, we need to learn how to invite people to explore their possibilities and to try more of them, so that the invitation to live and to grow is more compelling than the invitation to die.

If at any moment an adolescent were to turn the question back to us and say, "Tell me your hopes and your dreams," how would we answer? Are we firmly founded believers in life, aware of its meaning and aware that we have ourselves received and responded to invitations to live? Perhaps the essence of preparation to be elicitors of life is to always be ready to give an account of our personal hope. For this author, the hope lies in not just a fond belief, but in the actual, repeated experience that love makes a difference.

Whence will the love come?

REFERENCES

1. Bureau of Vital Statistics. Rockville, Md.: U.S. Dept. of Health, Education, and Welfare, 1977.
2. Josselyn, F. M. *Adolescence*. New York: Harper & Row Pubs., Inc., 1971.
3. Durkheim, E. *Suicide*. Glencoe, Ill.: Free Press, 1951.
4. Freud, S. *Beyond the Pleasure Principle*. New York: Bantam Books, Inc., 1959.
5. Rohn, R. D. "Adolescents Who Attempt Suicide." *J. Pediat.* 90:636–638, 1977.
6. Niswander, G. D., Casey, T. M., and Humphrey, J. A. *A Panorama of Suicide*. Springfield, Ill.: Charles C Thomas, Pubs., 1973.
7. Shneidman, E. S., ed. *Death and the College Student*. New York: Behavioral Publications, Inc., 1972.

8. Teicher, J. D. "Why Adolescents Kill Themselves." *Mental Health Program Reports No. 4,* National Institute of Mental Health, 1970.
9. Teicher, J. D., and Jacobs, J. "Adolescents Who Attempt Suicide." *Am. J. Psychiat.* 122:1248–1257, 1966.
10. Moss, L. M., and Hamilton, D. M. "Psychotherapy of the Suicidal Patient." In Shneidman, E. S., and Farberow, N. L., eds. *Clues to Suicide.* New York: McGraw-Hill Book Co., 1957.
11. Lester, D., and Beck, A. T. "Early Loss as a Possible 'Sensitizer' to Later Loss in Attempted Suicides." *Psychological Reports* 39:121–122, 1976.
12. Jacobs, J. *Adolescent Suicide.* New York: John Wiley & Sons, Inc., 1971.
13. Frankl, V. E. *Man's Search for Meaning: An Introduction to Logotherapy.* Boston: Beacon Press, Inc., 1959.
14. Seiden, R. H. *Suicide Among Youth.* Chevy Chase, Md.: U.S. Public Health Service Pub. No. 1971, 1969.
15. Herzog, A., and Resnik, H. L. P. "A Clinical Study of Parental Response to Adolescent Death by Suicide. " In Farberow, N., ed. *Proceedings of the Fourth International Conference on Suicide Prevention.* Los Angeles: Delmar Pub. Co., 1967.
16. Shneidman, E. S. *Deaths of Man.* New York: Quadrangle/The New York Times Co., 1973.
17. Resnik, H. L. P. "Psychological Resynthesis: A Clinical Approach to the Survivors of a Death by Suicide." In Shneidman, E., and Ortega, M., eds. *Aspects of Depression.* Boston: Little, Brown & Co., 1969.

BIBLIOGRAPHY

Grollman, E. A. *Suicide: Prevention, Intervention, Postvention.* Boston: Beacon Press, Inc., 1971.
Hatton, C. L., Calente, S. M., and Rink, A. *Suicide: Assessment and Intervention.* New York: Appleton-Century-Crofts, 1977.
Jacobs, J., and Teicher, J. D. "Broken Homes and Social Isolation in Attempted Suicide of Adolescents." *Internat'l, J. Social Psychiat.* 13:140–149, 1967.
Klagsbrun, F. *Youth and Suicide.* New York: Pocket Books, Inc., 1977.
Teicher, J. D.. "Treatment of the Suicidal Adolescent—The Life-Line Approach." *Excerpta Medica,* International Congress Series No. 15, Proceedings of the World Congress of Psychiatry, Amsterdam, Excerpta Medica Foundation, 1967.

The Childbearing Adolescent

11

The Pregnant Adolescent

RAMONA T. MERCER, R.N., Ph.D.

The adolescent who becomes pregnant is faced with many decisions. She must decide whether or not she wishes to proceed with the pregnancy, whether to retain custody of the child, and, often, whether she wishes to marry the father of her child. She must also make decisions about other personal goals that relate to her education, career, and self-development.

Although adolescence is variously defined, in this section the discussion focuses largely on the teen years 13 to 19. "Teenager" and "adolescent" are used synonymously.

The scope of the problem of adolescent pregnancy is reviewed. Physiological, psychological, and sociological health risks for the pregnant adolescent are discussed, providing the theoretical base for the provision of nursing care and health maintenance in the prenatal and postnatal periods. The alternative options of abortion and adoption are discussed, along with the consequent implications for adolescent care and their special counseling needs. A discussion of the unmarried father is followed by a summary which concludes the chapter.

Scope of the Problem

Pregnancy among teenagers is an increasingly serious health and sociological problem. One in five births in the United States is to a teenager.[1] This increase in the number of teenage pregnancies is not peculiar to the United States. Throughout the world teenage mothers give birth to 10 to 15% of all babies born; a total of 12 to 18 million infants are born yearly to teenagers.[1] In the United States there are 20 million young women between the ages of 10 and 19, and one fourth of those in the 15- to 19-year bracket are sexually active.[2] Although overall rates of childbearing among teenage mothers actually declined in the early 1970s, the larger population of teenagers resulted in more infants being born to teenage mothers than ever before.[2] The fertility rate decreased less among teenagers than among older women, so that

245

the percentage of births to teenagers as compared with total births increased.[2,3] For example, in 1957 there were 13.1 million 10- to 19-year olds; 557,172 gave birth to infants. In 1975, there were 20.3 million 10- to 19-year-olds who gave birth to 594,880 infants. The greatest increase occurred in the 10- to 14-year-old group, with a rise from 6,960 births in 1957 to 12,642 births in 1975.[4] Although 57 out of every 1,000 10- to 19-year-olds became pregnant in 1975, the rate of live births was lower (about 42.5 per 1,000). More adolescents who were 14 years old and younger received abortions than had live births.[4]

Nonwhite teenagers have a much higher birthrate than do white adolescents, and the younger the teenager, the greater is the proportion of nonwhite births. The ratio of nonwhite to white births is 5 : 1 for adolescents under 14 years, but among 19-year-olds the ratio is less than 2 : 1.[2] Multiple reasons probably account for this differential by race, but a review of research from other countries lends credence to the fact that earlier sexual maturation, which in turn seems to lead to earlier sexual activity, is one contributing variable. A study of 471 adolescents under 15 years of age found that the age of menarche was significantly earlier for those mothers who had become pregnant before the age of 15 than it was in the 19- to 25-year-old control group.[5] In the United States, blacks, who make up about 92% of the nonwhite population, reach menarche at an earlier age than do whites; 21% of black girls, in contrast to 11% of white girls, reach menarche by age 11.[2]

A study of Finnish Lutheran young women seeking abortions found that they had begun menstruation and intercourse earlier than the national norm.[6] Family inter-actional patterns also seem to play a role in early pregnancy. Over one third of the young women seeking abortion were from one-parent families, and one third were from families in which fights and quarrels were frequent. Two other studies in this country found that four fifths and one third of their subjects, respectively, were from broken homes.[7,8] In most of the broken homes, the father was absent.

Some studies suggest that a disproportionate number of teenage pregnancies occur in the lower socioeconomic class. A study of all births occurring in a seven year period in Aberdeen, Scotland, found that women who had their first child while in their teens were predominantly from the lower occupational class.[9]

In many countries the customary age of marriage is during the midteens, which leads to more teenage births.[1] The number of teenage marriages in the United States is declining, however. Only 22% of 14- to 19-year-olds were married in 1976 contrasting with 32% in 1960.[10]

Rahe and associates[11] found that pregnancy occurred during periods of increasing social stress or change in social status. Both unwed and married women experienced a sharp increase in the number of stresses prior to pregnancy, suggesting that significant social change is related to either the planning of or susceptibility to conception.

In sum, these data suggest many factors that seem to contribute to early pregnancy. Earlier physiological maturation followed by earlier sexual activity, the environment of a broken home or a lower socioeconomic class, a cultural norm of marriage at an earlier age, or the experiencing of a great number of stressors within a short time all seem contributory.

Health Risks

The special risks that the pregnant adolescent faces may be grouped largely into the categories of physiological, psychological, and social risks. All of these risks are more or less interdependent, just as the young person's development in these areas is interdependent. If a person's physical self is threatened, there are concomitant psychological and social threats to the individual. Likewise, psychological and social risks threaten mental and physical health.

PHYSIOLOGICAL RISKS

Research reports are variable and are not always in agreement concerning physiological complications of teenage pregnancy. The lack of socioeconomic representativeness of the population and the lack of consistency in the ages chosen for comparison of younger and older women probably account to some extent for the conflicting data. However, upon looking carefully at various reports, some apparent risks due to immaturity emerge.

The young girl is physiologically, anatomically, and immunologically different from the mature woman: the younger the girl, the greater the differences.[12] For example, a urinary tract infection in a child may affect the entire body and result in dramatic systemic complaints—including neuroflex gastrointestinal symptoms, toxemia, and acid-base disturbances. Stimulants such as chilling or the voiding of highly concentrated urine can cause vesicle spasms in the immature bladder.[12] The increased sensitivity of the less mature bladder may account for seemingly disproportionate complaints of pain by the teenager who may have to be catheterized or who may have a bladder infection. The teenager who complains of more discomfort with catheterization than an adult in all probability experiences more discomfort.

Physiological changes of adolescence correlate more closely with menarche than with the individual's chronological age.[13] Erkan[13] found that 31.4% of the mothers who conceived 24 months or less after menarche had low-birth-weight infants (2,500 gms [about 5 pounds, 8 ounces] or less); this was true of only 16% of mothers who were more than 24 months post menarche at the time of conception. Statistics show that mothers below the age of 15 deliver 2.2 times the number of premature infants that mothers in the 20- to 24-year-old range deliver, whereas mothers aged 15 to 17 deliver 1.5 times more, and mothers 18 to 19 deliver 1.3 times more premature infants.[14] Two postulations are made about the etiology of the higher incidence of lower-birth-weight infants among the younger women.

It has been suggested that an incomplete development of the myometrium may contribute to premature delivery.[15] At a low gynecological age (chronological age minus age at menarche) the uterus may be structurally or functionally less proficient since it has had fewer cycles of exposure to ovarian hormones.[16] If the uterine vasculature is less well developed at the lower gynecological age, the ability to accommodate increased uterine blood flow during pregnancy could be affected.

Low birth weight may be due to inadequate nutrition. The teenager is growing at a rapid rate. The annual weight gain for the nonpregnant 12- to 13-year-old is approximately 12 pounds; for 13- to 15-year-olds, 9 pounds; for 15- to 16-year-olds, from 6 to 8 pounds.[17] If food intake does not meet these growth needs, either intrauterine growth retardation or premature labor could result.

The teenager's cervix and genitalia may be more vulnerable to laceration. Russell[18] noted in performing therapeutic abortions on 13- to 16-year-old girls that the cervix was tightly closed and small compared with the usual uterine size of an 8- to 10-week gestation. He found that this small, tightly-closed cervix is more easily lacerated or rendered incompetent during dilatation and curettage. King[19] also observed that the hypoplastic cervix frequently observed in adolescents places them at risk for cervical injury. Genital lacerations were observed to be the most frequently occurring intrapartal complication for teenage mothers by Briggs and associates.[20] Although Hassan and Falls noted a high rate of cervical lacerations in teenagers under 16 years of age, the control group had a higher rate.[17] The cervical lacerations were observed in the 12- and 13-year-olds, however, suggesting that the more immature girl is more vulnerable to cervical laceration.

Adolescence and a first pregnancy have been identified as two periods when there is very active metaplasia in the cervical epithelium, a fact which suggests sensitivity of the dividing epithelial cells to any mutagen in the environment, particularly herpes simplex virus type 2.[21] The potential for development of cancer is increased on this basis. The sexually active pregnant adolescent may be doubly vulnerable to herpes simplex virus type 2. Hein and associates[22] found a prevalence rate for early neoplastic changes of 35 per 1,000 in 12- to 16-year-old sexually active girls from a youth detention center in New York. Out of 403 Pap smears, 168 showed evidence of inflammation or cytologic atypia. In 14 of the smears there was evidence of early neoplastic change in the cervical epithelium.

Vaginal infections have been reported as the most frequently observed problem in teenage pregnancy.[23] The high rates of venereal disease add to the potential for a greater number of infections during teenage pregnancy. In 1975, of the 276,255 reported cases of gonorrhea in 10- to 19-year-olds, 158,552 were in females.[24] 918,000 school days are lost annually; 5,750 girls are absent from school daily because of gonorrhea.[24] The adolescent who has gonorrhea often has mixed infections of monilia and trichomonas, requiring additional treatment of the mixed infections to relieve her symptoms.[25] Possible sequelae of gonorrhea include potential scarring of the fallopian tubes, leading to infertility or ectopic pregnancy; thus future childbearing is jeopardized.

Although peak skeletal growth occurs before menarche, some individuals grow considerably taller after menarche.[26] Aiman[27] found in a comparative study that the pelvis of the average pregnant adolescent 16 years old or younger is smaller than that of the average woman older than 16 (mean 23.4 years), suggesting that growth of the pelvis is not complete by age 16. A higher incidence of contracted pelvises was also observed in the teenager 14 years old and younger[5] and 16 and younger.[28] In contrast, Semmens,[29] from his study of pregnant teenagers who were dependents of military men, deemed the teenager a physically mature obstetric patient as she nears term. Height and immaturity cannot be considered in isolation from other factors, however, since twice as many tall women were found among upper-class women as among lower-class women, in a study in which the majority of the teenage births were to lower-class women.[9] There is also the possibility that high estrogen levels of pregnancy may limit long bone growth (levels of estrone and estradiol are 100 times higher at labor than during the luteal phase of the menstrual cycle, and urinary estriol levels are 1,000 times greater).[30] Endocrine development may continue for 5 to 6 years after the menarche.[31]

Anemia is a persistent and widely distributed problem among pregnant teenagers. It is usually defined as a hemoglobin of less than 10 grams per 100 ml. The high rate of anemia may be an effect of the teenager's penchant for junk foods and "lack of time to eat," since she is involved in many activities and constantly "on the go." It may in part reflect the large lower socioeconomic group representation among pregnant teenagers. When pregnancy is imposed on an already poorly nourished adolescent, she has a low nutritional reserve for her own growth and development.[32] Particularly rapid growth occurs at two periods in life—during fetal growth in utero, and between 8 to 10 and 14 to 16 years of age.[33] The need for iron is greatly increased during these two periods; thus, the young pregnant adolescent is placed in double jeopardy for iron-deficiency anemia. Even if the youthful mother has good prenatal care, she may not take the iron prescribed for her. Webb[34] noted this to be true.

One study found that the older the young mother, the higher was her hemoglobin.[35] Although many studies have found anemia to be a leading complication for the youthful pregnant woman,[17,23,36,37,38] other studies reach other conclusions. Hulka and Schaaf[39] found no difference in antepartal anemia between mothers 15 years old and under and 19- to 21-year-old mothers, although the older mothers did have a higher incidence of postpartum anemia. Others[40] found anemia less frequently among teenagers who received adequate prenatal care than among other subjects. Coates,[41] who compared adolescents under 14 years of age with young women over 14 years, found that the precentage of mothers with anemia was somewhat higher (23.7% in contrast to 19.7%) in the group of mothers over 14 years of age.

Toxemia of pregnancy has been one of the most feared of all complications in teenage pregnancy. Reports of rates observed in teenagers range from 4.3% to 23.5%. Although by far the majority of studies of teenage pregnancy report a higher incidence of toxemia, two reports found that rates of this disease were lower for the younger mother.[20,42] Briggs and associates[20] found in two groups, one group 16 years old and younger and the other 21 years old and older, that the incidence of toxemia was 3% in the teenage group and 5.7% in the older group. All subjects in both groups were predominantly Caucasian and lived in a residential home with closely supervised antepartal care. The authors attributed the overall low incidence of toxemia to the racial group and to the close supervision of nutrition in the home. Youngs and colleagues[43] observed that hypertensive disorders occurred in 10.5% of their sample of 202 adolescents who were 17 years old or younger; 89% of the subjects were black. They saw the higher incidence of chronic hypertensive disease in the black population as contributing to the high rate of hypertension observed.

Hibbard[42] found, in surveying maternal mortality over 15 years (1957–1972) in Los Angeles County, that the average age at death due to toxemia was 27.5 years; 19% of the deaths occurred after 35 years. Of the 67 who died, 63% were members of ethnic minority groups; only 53% of the minority group members had private care, in contrast to 79% of the other groups. Since only 10 deaths, 15% of the total, were of 17- to 20-year-olds, Hibbard suggested that socioeconomic factors contribute more importantly to the prevalence and severity of toxemia than age. Jovanovic[23] observed that the incidence of pregnancy-induced hypertension increased in teenagers as maternal age decreased. High incidences of pregnancy-induced hypertension have been observed worldwide among teenagers; it is not a phenomenon found only in the United States.[1] The awesomeness of the disease is recognized not only by the physician and the nurse, but also by the youthful mother, as the following account illustrates.

Cindy, a 17-year-old black adolescent, described at one month postpartum the convulsions she had experienced antepartally:

I was having convulsions and throwing up and everything. It was terrible. I felt like I was all balled up into a knot. It was so terrible. I could feel my arms going out and my whole body felt like a knot. I couldn't do anything or stop it. I don't even like to think about it. My mamma was crying the whole time; all of this was happening at home.

Nationally, the maternal mortality rate in 1973 was lower for the 15- to 19-year-old group (11.9) than for any other group except 20- to 24-year-olds (9.2).[44] For mothers under 15, however, it was higher (46.7) than for any other age group except 40 to 44 (78.5) and 45 years or older (154.5)[44] Rates represent number of deaths per 100,000 live births.

The increased vulnerability of the pregnant younger adolescent to cervical lacerations, anemia, sexually transmitted diseases, pelvic contraction, pregnancy-induced hypertension, and higher mortality is sobering. Prevention of the pregnancy indeed seems a paramount concern for these adolescents.

PSYCHOLOGICAL RISKS

Teenage pregnancy is seldom planned. Unplanned events such as pregnancy more often than not result in conflict with other personal goals. For the adolescent these goals may be excelling in school, achieving honors in sports, or testing oneself in a particular role. Pregnancy makes it more difficult for the young woman to accept and become comfortable with her body image. Depending upon her psychological maturity, pregnancy may facilitate or impede the development of her sense of femininity. Emotional responses to interruption of the pursuit of goals by an unexpected pregnancy may include depression—depression so deep that its worst mode of expression can be suicide. A higher rate of suicide attempts was found in a group of young women who were pregnant before they were 18 than is expected in the general adolescent population.[45] The stress that lead to the pregnancy could have led to the suicide attempt. The enigma of adolescent suicide is dealt with extensively in Chapter 10.

Deutsch[46] considers the sexual permissiveness of our society to be the provoking agent leading ''specific'' individuals at specific phases of adolescence to become pregnant. Deutsch suggests that the superego and ego ideal are poorly internalized for these individuals. Psychodynamically, the girl deeply longs for a revival of the close mother-child relationship and seeks in the relationship with her partner in an intimate situation the longed-for relationship with her mother.

Over two thirds of the 30 teenage mothers in one study had intense dependency needs.[7] Over one half had poor tolerance for work, school, and frustration. One half had poor judgment, primitive defenses, and a marginal adjustment. Three psychodynamic patterns were predominant: (1) the girl's relationship to her mother—dependency versus independency, identification with and competitiveness with the mother; (2) her relationship to the father or reaction to his absence as reflected in an unresolved oedipal conflict; and (3) a need to prove oneself with peers. Most of the teenagers had weak egos, deficient superegos (minimal expression of guilt), and poorly formed ego ideals. Their ambivalent feelings toward their mothers made it hard for the teenagers to accept them as ego ideals.

A bland emotional affect and often amnesia concerning the sexual act have been observed in young, unwed mothers.[47] In some, affection for their fathers and a high occurrence of impregnation by much older men led to the postulation that the pregnancy represented a dissociation state in which the young women acted out incestual fantasies as an expression of the oepidal conflict.

These reports all suggest that psychological flaws could have been contributory to an untimely pregnancy. The mental disequilibrium usually accompanying any pregnancy, when imposed on psychologically immature persons, can be a frightening and alarming experience with varying negative effects, as is illustrated by the following account.

Pam, a 13-year-old who came to the antepartal clinic when she was three months pregnant, illustrates the awesomeness of pregnancy to such a young adolescent. She related a rape fantasy to describe her predicament. She was very depressed and stated that she did not want to have a baby. Pam said that she had been attacked while walking her German shepherd on a leash; someone had grabbed her from behind. She did not know what happened, but the next thing she knew she was back on the sidewalk walking her dog. Her stepmother refused permission for Pam to have an abortion, saying, ''If you let these young girls get away with it one time . . . '' Pam sat still and ''grinned'' throughout this discussion. Plans were begun for Pam's infant to be relinquished for adoption, however. Pam never wore maternity clothes during her pregnancy—an index of denial of her pregnant state. As the pregnancy neared term, she became increasingly overwhelmed by the thought of being cut and delivering the baby. The threat of loss of body intactness was frightening. During the eighth month of pregnancy she was preoccupied with her perineum:

How long does it take the stitches to rot out? Do they use spray or a light to put on your stitches for pain? Mamma says the baby won't be bigger than three pounds, no more than I eat . . . I watched that film on labor 5 or 6 times. The first time I saw it, I got sick. It looked awful—the baby coming out.

Pam delivered a stillborn girl one month later, following a two-hour labor. Her antepartal anxieties and fantasies were realized in her infant's death and her postpartal headaches, fever, and gonorrheal infection. She had acquired gonorrhea during her pregnancy after her initial clinic examination. She was depressed and had no appetite. What long-range psychological impact did such an experience have on this young, immature person?

Bibring and associates[48] described three psychological tasks a woman works at during pregnancy that facilitate her maturation. First, a woman must accept and incorporate the intrusion of the fetus as a representation of her partner. Second, she must recognize the baby growing within her as a separate person and prepare for the birth. Third, she must make the transition from nonmother to mother. Pam did not indicate that she achieved the first psychological task of pregnancy; she chose to deny both conception and the pregnancy. Although she fearfully anticipated the birth of the infant, her concern seemed more to be a wish to be rid of the pregnancy than a recognition of the new, unique life within her. Her thoughts centered on fears of bodily harm to herself rather than on preparation for the birth. The death of her infant in utero precluded the necessity of her moving from the nonmother to the mother role.

Rubin[49] identified four maternal tasks during pregnancy which may be viewed as psychological. The first is to seek and insure a safe passage through pregnancy and the childbirth experience for both herself and her child. The second is to find acceptance for her child by persons most meaningful to her. A third task involves incorporating the idea of a child into her self-system. A fourth task involves the giving of herself, largely to the unborn child, through food and clothing. Pam seemed to work at securing a safe passage for herself; she attended antepartal clinic regularly. She did not, however, work at the second or third tasks described by Rubin, because she did not intend to keep the child. Pam fantasized about joining the Navy. She did not work on the fourth task of giving herself to the unborn child. She crocheted vests to give to friends and to her sister during her pregnancy. She gave to others, but not to the baby. That she seemed to unconsciously "deprive the baby of food" is suggested by her comment that she ate so little her mother had said the baby would weigh only three pounds. A three-pound baby would be less of a threat to Pam's safe passage at delivery, however, than a larger baby.

Because of the rapid growth and development most young adolescent girls have experienced prior to conception, the new physical changes of puberty may not have been fully incorporated into their body images. The rapid bodily changes occurring with pregnancy may pose additional fears and threats to self which could make it difficult for the adolescent to work on the psychological tasks of pregnancy. There is a tendency for adolescent girls to overestimate body width and underestimate height.[50] Pregnancy with its increasing body girth may be highly exaggerated to the young woman.

Although pregnancy may dramatize the young woman's femininity, if she is unmarried the pregnancy may be in conflict with her personal value system. Pregnancy also threatens her ego ideal and future identity whether as a teacher, lawyer, chemist, or social worker. In interviews with 200 unwed mothers, ages 12 to 42, Friedman[51] observed a deficiency in ego functioning. All had lacked a reality-oriented awareness of and concern for their sexual lives. The adolescent mother, therefore, faced with the psychological tasks of pregnancy, is handicapped not only by the conflicts presented for her life's goals, but perhaps also by deficiencies in her ego, superego, and ego ideal. Many professionals have observed that it is characteristic of pregnant women to relax their usual defenses and to express previously repressed or unconscious conflicts with highly mobilized and highly charged material.[52,53] How does the adolescent deal with the handicaps of her immaturity and the psychic changes during pregnancy?

For the adolescent under 15 the psychological tasks of pregnancy may be impossible, if she has not acquired the cognitive capacity to think logically and to reflect critically on abstract thought. Cognition encompasses both emotion and thought constantly interacting.[54] Placed within the context of Erikson's[55] psychosocial developmental tasks, the pregnant adolescent is working on generativity before she has accomplished a sense of identity or achieved the task of intimacy. Her sex act resulting in pregnancy may be pseudointimacy "in which sexual behavior becomes the symbolic expression of intimate interpersonal contact that, in reality, does not exist" (p. 118).[54] Unresolved pseudointimacy leads to passiveness, alienation, or rebellion.[54]

SOCIOLOGICAL RISKS

The sociological risks for the pregnant adolescent have an impact as great as, or greater than, other kinds of risks. There are no conflicting research reports about sociological risks for the pregnant adolescent. She is more likely to have additional children while she is still an adolescent, which, in turn, increases the physiological risks for both herself and her infant. She will have difficulty pursuing her education; without an education, she is at an increased risk for dependence on others, making it difficult for her to achieve independence or to maintain an optimal standard of living and health care. If the youthful mother marries, she is at increased risk for divorce and is faced with the additional adult task of assuming the role of wife, a task for which she is ill prepared. Ballard and Gold[56] summarized the risks of the unmarried mother as the "adolescent trap." (See Figure 11–1.)

Waters[57] coined the phrase "syndrome of failure" in describing the young pregnant adolescent. The syndrome of failure includes failure to: fulfill functions of adolescence, remain in school, limit size of family, be self-supporting, and have healthy infants.

While it is helpful to delineate special sociological risks for the pregnant teenager, it is well to acknowledge something of the interactive process between society and the teenager! Four problems within American society are suggested by Klerman[58] as having serious impact on our youth. First, the apparent lack of the kind of societal purpose that was present in our earlier history, as World War II. Absence of societal goals may lead to the selfish pursuit of individual pleasures. A lack of a meaningful role for the young person presents another problem. This was discussed in Chapter 1. The traditional narrow view of the role of women is a third problem for the adolescent girl. The lag between sexual practice and social attitude is a fourth problem; premarital sex was widely practiced for several years before states began enacting laws affecting couples who live together without marrying.

Unwed Versus Wed Mothers: Social mores have sufficiently relaxed within the last

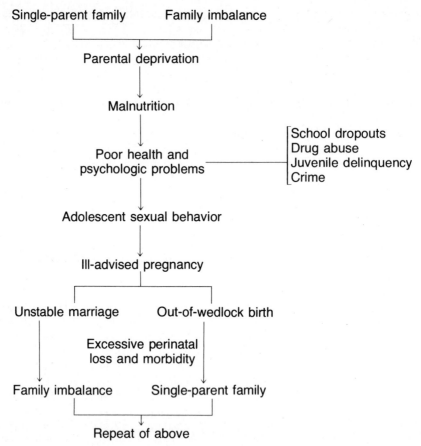

Figure 11–1. The adolescent trap. Reproduced with permission of the author, W. M. Ballard, and the publisher Harper and Row Pubs., Inc., from "Medical and Health Aspects of Reproduction in the Adolescent," *Clinical Obstetrics and Gynecology* 14(2):353, 1971.

one and a half decades so that the social stigma is not as great for the unwed mother or for her child as it once was. Concomitantly with this acceptance or tolerance by society more young mothers are electing to retain custody of their infants. Today's single adolescent mother as a rule is very reality-oriented about the additional tasks inherent in traditional wife roles, and of the additional handicaps she would face in a premature marriage. The youthful mother often states that it would hold her back if she married the father of her baby. Sixteen-year-old Pat openly commented, "Because I made one mistake, I don't need to make another." Furstenberg[59] noted that participants in his study did not wish to marry the father of the child if he was not capable of supporting a family.

Although alliance with the father seems to enhance the quality of parenting for the child, since parenthood is perceived as less stressful when the mother receives emotional support from a mate, one study found that the single mother fared better contraceptively, educationally, and usually vocationally.[60] This supports what many young mothers have observed and determined by themselves.

LaBarre[61] observed that marriage and pregnancy sometimes made it easier for the teenager to achieve a firm feminine identity and a definite role and status. However, other teenagers merely transferred their dependency on parents to their husbands, without ever achieving adult feminine identity and independence. The husband was used as a ''good father'' whom they were seeking.

A comparative study of prenatal anxiety in 15- to 27-year-old unwed and wed mothers found higher levels of anxiety in the single women, which suggested greater stress.[62] Over one half of the single subjects had experienced an upsetting change in the environment just prior to the pregnancy, such as the death of a close relative, dating problems, or a significant change in their family. These changes may have precipitated both their experienced anxiety and their pregnancies.

Both teenage marriages and premarital pregnancies have decided odds against them. Divorce rates are high across all age groups, but teenage marriages are more likely to end in divorce than marriages occurring among older persons. Teenage American women who marry between 14 and 17 have a 72% chance of divorce; those who marry at 18 or 19 have a 46% chance.[10]

Often, teenagers who marry are already pregnant. Feelings of entrapment and resentment of the loss of either adolescence, education, or social position have been observed among premaritally pregnant married couples.[63] Premaritally pregnant couples were found to have substantially less earning power and to possess fewer assets than other couples at the end of four years.[64,65] Husbands had less education, and there was only a fifty-fifty chance that the man would complete high school. These disadvantages can lead to decreased self-esteem. Male head-of-household characteristics and family income continue to provide major cues for self-placement in our society.[66]

The young woman who begins bearing children in her teens has an increased chance of having a second or third child while she is in her teens.[57,67] Intensive programs with extensive follow-up for the youthful mother seem to help reduce the incidence of repeated pregnancies.[68] Young mothers who married following delivery were found to have a higher pregnancy rate within one year than those who remained single.[69]

The pregnant adolescent's choice of whether or not to get married is a serious one. Viewed from the perspective of the higher divorce rate for youthful marriages and the observed socioeconomic and developmental disadvantages, the nursing practitioner and other health professionals are indeed challenged to encourage the young couple and their families to examine all options available to them and to weigh the various alternatives in terms of what the option means for each involved person's long-range growth and maturation.

School Dropout: Pregnancy has a crippling effect on educational pursuits. Furstenberg[59] observed that half of the pregnant teenagers finished high school, in contrast to 90% of a comparative group who did not become pregnant.

Waite and Moore[70] used data from the 5,000 subjects sampled from 1968 to 1972 in the National Longitudinal Study of the Labor Market Experiences of Young

Women to determine differences in educational attainment at ages 18, 21, and 24 between those who had become mothers and those who had not. They found that the younger the female when she became a mother the less schooling she had completed. Further, those having children at a young age did not catch up with the educational attainment of their childless peers as they matured. The white adolescent who had a first birth at 15 or younger had twice the educational decrement that the black adolescent had; at all ages the effect of the first birth was smaller for blacks. A higher family status measured by the father's education contributed to educational attainment for early childbearers. The youthful mother needs an extensive support system to continue in school.

Violet, a 14-year-old mother, illustrates some of the difficulty the pregnant teenager faces: "I have to go back to school. Otherwise it's always going to be like this. I won't be able to do anything but have babies and clean house. I can't stand it any more." Unfortunately, she dropped out of school after reentering, and was pregnant when her son was seven months old. Attempts to help her achieve her goal failed when she refused to stay in a facility where she would have had the help that would have enabled her to attend school. Situations like Violet's reflect Menken's[71] observation that the unwed girl who has an infant before 16 "has 90 percent of her life's script written for her."

Alternative Choices in Pregnancy

The teenager, like any other woman, is faced with what Juhasz[72] refers to as a chain of sexual decision making. (See Figure 11–2.) Once pregnancy occurs, however, available options include delivery or abortion. Once delivery occurs, options are to keep the child or to relinquish the child. The mother may opt to stay single or to marry in either of these instances. Inherent in decision making is the *right* to know all of the options and to weigh possible consequences.

Lieberman[73] proposed a unique approach to reduce the number of handicapped children resulting from unwanted pregnancies. He suggested that persons should become parents only with their "informed consent," which is analogous to informed consent for medical procedures. All potential parents would be told their chances of producing and rearing a healthy child; information about genetics, nutrition, prenatal care, and child-rearing would be easily available and would be introduced in school. Only parents who were committed to rearing a child and who really desired a child would continue a pregnancy if a contraceptive mishap occurred. They would be free to choose an abortion. The adolescent should benefit from informed consent both prior to pregnancy and following an unplanned pregnancy.

COUNSELING THE PREGNANT ADOLESCENT

Many persons of varying professional backgrounds are in the position of counseling pregnant adolescents. Mace[74] emphasized that a counselor's major work is to support the woman nonjudgmentally in her struggle to make a decision and to

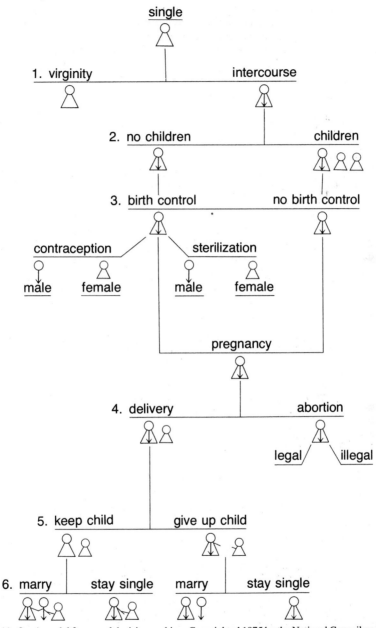

Figure 11–2. A model for sexual decision-making. Copyrighted 1975 by the National Council on Family Relations. Reprinted by permission of the National Council on Family Relations and the author, Anne McCreary Juhasz, from "A Chain of Sexual Decision-Making," *The Family Coordinator,* 24(1):45, 1975.

assist her in coping with the crisis "in such a way that it can become for her, despite its misery and anguish, an experience of personal growth and discovery." This is the philosophical stance that the term "counseling" incorporates in discussions in this chapter. "Counselors" include nurses, social workers, physicians, teachers, or clergymen.

Baldwin[75] accurately calls attention to the major conflicts that a woman with a problem pregnancy is experiencing. She usually experiences a basic cultural conflict, in that what occurred is not condoned, and a personal conflict that relates to her ambivalence about the pregnancy and her life's goals. In helping a young woman to move to a decision that is acceptable to her, the counselor needs, in addition to interviewing and self-awareness skills, a knowledge base that includes reproductive physiology, the legal implications of adoption and abortion, and the availability of resources within the community to help the woman meet her needs and goals.

Counseling for a woman who is exploring her alternatives in a problem pregnancy is also time-limited—both in terms of the length of the contact with the counselor and in the time available for making a decision—i.e., abortions are not usually done after 20 weeks gestation, and many pregnant adolescents wait a considerable time before seeking help, if they do seek it at all.

What skills do counselors need? A sensitivity to their own responses in any situation and an ability to withhold personal judgments and emotional responses to what seem like devastating circumstances are crucial. Counselors must constantly analyze their own emotional responses so that their interpretations of what the client is saying are not biased. What is threatening or devastating to one individual may be less threatening to the next individual because of the enormous diversity in cultural conditioning and in support systems for individuals.

Baldwin[75] offers specific suggestions for information exchange in alternative counseling. The counselor collects all of the information possible, through careful listening and observation, that is relevant to the young woman's specific situation. After gathering substantial information, the counselor's responsibility is to carefully analyze the information that has direct bearing on the adolescent's problem and to share this information with her. This may be done in the manner that seems most acceptable to her. The counselor's summary and reflection help to clarify whether the summarized information accurately reflects the adolescent's perception of the situation. The reflective analysis may enable her to select from the available alternatives the one that seems most feasible for her.

Another approach is to have the client summarize those factors which seem to be most relevant in her decision making. If there is an omission of an item that she mentioned earlier that seems important, this item may be an area of conflict for her. The counselor might explore it further by saying, "A comment was made earlier that the father of the baby was a very protective and caring person . . ." Sometimes the woman will respond to the open-ended approach immediately, or she may offer reasons for omitting the father in choosing among her alternatives, or she may suggest that it would be a good idea for her to consult with him.

The pregnant woman is the only person who can weigh the impact of each potential decision in relation to *her* life's goals. The counselor cannot expect to know the client's defenses, coping ability, personality predispositions, level of maturity or independence, support systems, inner conflicts, and cultural conditioning within a short time. Glimpses of each facet may be obtained, but the knowledge that is necessary to make such far-reaching decisions comes from the client.

ABORTION

Abortion has been a viable choice for women since the 1973 Supreme Court ruling that a state may not intervene in the decision that a woman and her physician make regarding an abortion during the first trimester of pregnancy. More than one fifth of all single women end their pregnancies by abortion.[76] The white single teenager chooses abortion seven times more frequently than does the black single teenager.[76] Figure 11–3 shows percentages of teenage abortions compared with those of births during 1974.

Pregnancy and abortion both have the potential to arouse or to deepen the conflict between being mothered and being a mother that any adolescent may be experiencing.[77] This conflict is also a part of the adolescent's move from dependence to independence. Schaffer and Pine[77] were able to predict which adolescents would regress, progress, or move in less decisive directions by observing their interactions with their mothers. The girl who regressed allowed her mother to discover the pregnancy and to make the decision for the abortion; she remained passively mothered. The girl who progressed sought support from others in the social system; thus in a sense she mothered herself, which seemed to strengthen her nurturing qualities. She discovered her pregnancy, made the decision about what action to take, and sought the abortion and made the arrangements herself. The young woman whose personal maturation was less advanced was less decisive; she had only reached the midpoint in her mastery of the developmental task of shifting from a passive position of being mothered to a more active mothering position. She enlisted her mother's help and sought outside help. Although she assumed a somewhat active role in making decisions, her actions remained within the context of a mother-child relationship.

Hatcher[78] observed from research and from clinical practice that "the tomboyish early adolescent girl, the oedipally activated and rebellious middle adolescent girl, and the 'almost adult' late adolescent" were easily distinguished by their responses to pregnancy and to abortion. The early adolescents were the only ones in her study who did not have a basic knowledge of conception and contraception; neither were they receptive to this information. The early adolescent's subconsious motivation for becoming a mother was to become closer to her mother, yet she had a strong wish to remain her mother's baby. The early adolescents used much denial throughout, maintaining that they did not know who had impregnated them because they were either "high" or "blacked out" at the time. Thirteen-year-old Pam, whose case was presented earlier, fits this picture; e.g., she "didn't know" what had happened except that she was "grabbed from behind" and then found herself "back on the sidewalk walking her dog."

Although Hatcher observed that the middle adolescent usually had more knowledge about contraception, she placed the blame on the male father figure who

Percentage of pregnancies

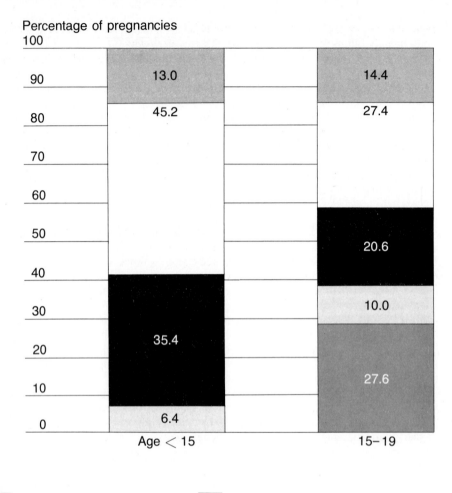

Age < 15   15–19

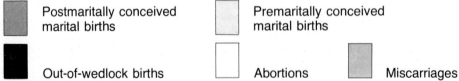

Postmarritally conceived
marital births

Premarritally conceived
marital births

Out-of-wedlock births

Abortions

Miscarriages

Figure 11–3. Outcome of pregnancies to teenage females, United States, 1974. Reprinted with permission from *11 Million Teenagers: What Can Be Done About the Epidemic of Adolescent Pregnancies in the United States*, published by the Alan Guttmacher Institute, New York, 1976.

impregnated her. The middle adolescent's underlying fantasy of knowing how to interact with her father better than with her mother often resulted in the fantasy's being carried out through impregnation by an older or a married man. She also seemed to be moving out to test her autonomy, in a beginning search for her identity; consequently, she strongly desired something of her own.

In Hatcher's study, late adolescents were more realistic about their pregnancies and were nearest to attaining a mothering ego. Because of this, the decision to have an abortion was more difficult for them to make. The same developmental level of personality functioning continued following an abortion. All of the young women were extremely sensitive to the hospital environment, including roommates, nurses, and physicians. One older adolescent was observed recording the length of time a nurse took to answer her requests as opposed to those of her roommate, who had delivered a baby. Noting that the nurse took longer to meet her requests, the adolescent perceived herself as stigmatized and as considered unworthy of the nurse's attention. This finding has much relevance for nurses. Although the nurse may have judged that the new mother needed more help with her own and her infant's care, the other young woman, after an abortion, had needs as great or greater, of a different kind. The woman who has had an abortion is resolving conflict about her willful decision to end her pregnancy and is grieving for her lost pregnancy. The newly delivered woman perhaps dramatizes this loss for the woman who has had an abortion.

Because of the three very different and distinguishable developmental levels of adolescents, Hatcher stressed that the consequent counseling needs of each level are very different.[78] In her study, Hatcher found that the early adolescent rebelled against one-to-one counseling, maintaining that she "didn't need to talk about such things with an adult." Therefore, group counseling and teaching seemed more effective with this age level, and attendance improved significantly in small groups where peer pressures were greatest.

The middle and older adolescent profited from one-to-one counseling. However, it is very important that the adult be nonthreatening and nonjudgmental in working with the usually rather angry middle adolescent. The older adolescent affords positive reinforcement to the counselor; she expresses her appreciation for help, and her insight is such that she profits most quickly from intervention.[78]

As was stated in Chapter 1, the three developmental levels of early, middle and late adolescence are not necessarily synchronous with age. The counselor must be aware that an 18- or 19-year-old's personality development may reflect middle-adolescent behavior and that a 16-year-old may be quite mature.

In an effort to determine differences between those young women who choose to deliver and those who choose to abort, Fischman[79] interviewed 151 black urban adolescents who decided to deliver and 78 who had an abortion. Those adolescents who chose to deliver had better relationships with their mothers and had more support from the family. They had higher self-esteem and had had longer relationships with their boyfriends. The boyfriend was more frequently working full-time and planned to help support the baby. Poverty seemed to precede pregnancy for the subjects, but one half of the women who chose to deliver lived in a home on welfare. The deliverer's mother had completed fewer years of school than the aborter's mother and more often tended to have an unskilled job. In spite of poorer environmental circumstances, only 17 of 151 deliverers (11%) were unhappy about becoming pregnant. Fischman postulated that in the milieu of poverty and poor education, childbearing is one of the few acceptable roles available to girls who feel unable to achieve in the social world. Educational attainment and socioeconomic status seemed to be interrelated and there was a positive relation between education and more liberal attitudes toward abortion.[80]

The young woman's potential for growth, as well as situations in which she needs more intensive counseling and supportive help before making such an important decision for her life must be recognized by the health care worker. Martin[81] found that 19% of the unwed teenage girls who had difficulty adjusting following an abortion felt guilty, were in poor mental health prior to the abortion, had no close friends, had been considerably involved with their pregnancy, were unhappy about their decision, and felt worse following the abortion. They had little knowledge about sex prior to pregnancy, poor relationships with their mothers, no support from the fathers of the babies, no one to take their problems to, and, often, medical complications following the abortion. Typically, this young woman felt that she would not make the decision to have an abortion again and that others viewed her less favorably for having had the abortion. The converse was true for the 77% who had no difficulty adapting after the abortion. The adjustment for 4% of the subjects was not clear.

Barglow[82] observed that the developmental immaturity of the teenage woman contributed to her ambivalence about an abortion, and that almost all young women experienced the procedure as frightening, dangerous, punitive, and, many times, overwhelming. Although 21 of 25 who could be contacted for follow-up one to three months later felt that the procedure had been positive and beneficial, all had experienced symptoms of the grief process. Four subjects had conscious regrets and two were severely depressed.

Bracken and associates[83] found that about 40% of two groups of single, never-married women, those who chose to deliver and those who chose an abortion, had changed their minds about their decisions at least once. Adoption was not an important option for this group. Only 2% of those delivering thought they might place the infant for adoption. Half of the women planning to deliver had had a previous abortion, and half of the aborters had had an infant. The researchers concluded that the decision for the outcome of a pregnancy depended on the situation more than on the characteristics of the woman.

These research studies demonstrate the importance of counseling that enables the young woman to make her decision with knowledge about all of the facts and *without any pressure* — societal, familial, or professional. No matter how clearly events seem to indicate that abortion is the only workable solution to the young woman's problem, the professional must check any impulse to use persuasion. The young woman's goals for her life must be determined by her. Although family members or partners may be helpful, the nurse or counselor must reflect reality objectively: Who will support the child? Who will care for the child? Who will assume responsibility for the child? It helps the young woman to have her *choices* emphasized, so that she can make responsible decisions. Through responsible decision making she can help improve her self-concept and see herself as having control over her life. There are situations in which the young adolescent may be unable to make these decisions—e.g., that of an unemancipated minor/or a mentally retarded adolescent. In these instances, the client and her family or legal guardians all consult with health care and legal professionals in making a decision.

It is important for the young woman to deal with her feelings about her mother and about the father of her baby. In her view, to what extent are these two persons entitled to be involved in her decision making? What right, legally and morally, does each have in the decision making? Open-ended interview questions can direct the woman toward thinking about the roles of other persons in her decision-making process.

Since a young woman may have made the decision to have an abortion during a time of initial fear and panic, often amidst family accusation, shouting, and namecalling, she needs to explore her alternatives in a safe, neutral setting. Only in a neutral setting can she objectively view and elaborate on the pros and cons of each alternative and the problems inherent in each pro and con—from her unique perspective at this time and at this place in her life. This means that she must reexamine her goals for her life and the implications that her decision will have for her goals.

Because we know that some young women experience difficulty in adjusting after an abortion, an attempt should be made to ensure continued follow-up care when possible. Follow-up interviews are sometimes difficult because the young woman may have deliberately sought an abortion outside of her home state or city either to avoid the risk of encountering persons who know her or for legal reasons. Researchers in one study found that almost one half of the teenage subjects did not return for the follow-up interview because they felt they had "talked too much" previously.[77] Some were so distressed because of information they had given that they requested that all of the records be destroyed. They stated that they had felt "terrible" and "naked" after the interview. Apparently the exposure was too threatening to the adolescents. As was stated earlier, a woman during pregnancy is able to permit much more of her id, or unconscious desires and feelings, to emerge than when she is in a nonpregnant state.[52] Perhaps the teenager with a less strong ego cannot cope with these feelings or with exposure of these feelings. This raises a question for the counselor. How much information does the adolescent need to share for her decision-making process in order that necessary questions may be directed to her for her consideration? This is a very important factor for the counselor to consider. *Legal Implications:* The question of the legality of a minor's giving consent for an abortion without her parent's consent or knowledge is rightfully raised. The Supreme Court affirmed the rights of minors to abortion without parental consent in a July 1976 decision on a case that involved a Missouri statute requiring parental consent for abortion for minors. The Court noted in this ruling that the interest of the parents and the interest of the minors may not be the same.[84]

In the first chapter, it was pointed out that the development of abstract reasoning, conceptualization, and problem solving during adolescence usually occurred at approximately 15 years of age, with variation from individual to individual. The counselor working with adolescents seeking an abortion is wise to consider the adolescent's capability of giving informed consent. Holder[85] suggests that consent for abortion is obtained on the same basis of comprehension as that shown by an individual in any nonemergency procedure. It is necessary to become familiar with the statutes and rulings in the state in which one works because of variations in both age limits and substantive provisions; the age limit ranges from 14 to 18 years for consenting to ordinary or nonemergency medical treatment. Some statutes permit a pregnant minor to give her own consent for any medical treatment, since pregnancy seems to constitute a priori emancipation. An emancipated minor is no longer subject to her parents' control or supervision, usually does not live with her parents, is self-supporting, and makes major decisions about her life.[85] As a rule, young people become emancipated when they get married, regardless of their age. During the last 20 years no decisions in which a parent recovered damages for treatment of a child over 15 without parental consent have been found.[85]

Regardless of the client's age, informed consent is an important right of every individual. This means that the client must be informed about possible complications and expected or unexpected results of any treatment. If a client does not understand the risks and benefits inherent in any given intervention, informed consent does not exist. Obviously, if the adolescent seeking abortion does not understand her alternatives, as well as the risks and possible complications of the abortion procedure, she cannot give informed consent, and parental consent or a court order is warranted. In any situation in which the minor does not object to her parents' knowledge of her condition, it is wise to seek parental consent.

The minor who has a right to consent to treatment also has the right to refuse treatment. This is particularly relevant in situations in which parents do not wish their daughter to have a baby and request an abortion against the girl's wishes. A physician who performs an abortion on a minor against her wishes can be sued for assault and battery when the minor comes of age at 18.[85] The importance of careful and skillful counseling prior to abortion cannot be overstressed; at no time should counseling be such that it could be interpreted as coercion at a later date.

ADOPTION

The adolescent who relinquishes her infant for adoption has not been the focus of much research. Research seems to have been centered largely on the young mother who chooses to have an abortion. Many reasons probably account for this. A primary reason may be that the young woman who relinquishes her infant for adoption often seeks temporary residence away from her home, and, once she has delivered, wishes to sever all contact with those who know her "secret" and to resume her life anew. Such was the case of 16-year-old Joan. Her father applied for and received a temporary job transfer, and the entire family moved to a distant state until the birth of Joan's baby. A second reason may be the decline in the number of infants released for adoption by teenage mothers. The number of mothers choosing adoption decreased considerably from 1966 to 1971; with the increased option of abortion, the number will probably continue to decrease. The decline in the number of infants released for adoption by single mothers may also reflect society's more accepting attitude toward (and tendency not to stigmatize) the illegitimate child and legal actions taken by courts—both leading to less coercion by parents. Gill and associates[9] observed that adoption was less often considered by members of lower occupational classes, who seemed to accept early pregnancy as inevitable and to accept care for the baby without consideration of alternatives. This description of lower occupational class attitudes suggests that this group perceived their lives as being externally controlled. The externally controlled individual believes that reinforcement or reward in life is contingent upon luck, fate, or the external forces in the environment, whereas the internally controlled individual believes reinforcement to be contingent upon his own action.[86]

Health professionals are obligated to present viable options to the teenage client to facilitate her decision making so that she realizes she has some control over her life. One of the most important considerations is for the health professional—nurse, social worker, physician—to realize that circumstances in the young person's life may alter considerably from the time of conception until the end of her child's first year of life. Decisions that are made under one set of circumstances may not hold in another set of circumstances. Consequently, the young mother who decides during the last few months of her pregnancy to retain custody of her infant may later be faced with a situation in which her boyfriend disappears, none of the promised support money is forthcoming, and she is unable to find a babysitter so that she can either continue school or work. In her frustration she may batter her child, either physically or psychologically or both. Or the youthful mother, once she is faced with the reality of the demands and needs of a helpless infant, may realize that this was not what she had bargained for. In such situations, the young woman needs help in considering viable alternatives. Is there a residential home where she may live and where child care will be provided while she continues her schooling? Does she now wish to relinquish the child for adoption? Does she desire temporary foster care for her child or for herself?

On the other hand, there is the young woman who decides to relinquish her infant for adoption during pregnancy but who changes her mind following the infant's birth. Such was the case with 19-year-old Carol. Her 19-year-old husband was in trade school and did not feel he was ready for the responsibilities of a child. Carol and her husband, through counseling with the social worker and the public health nurse, decided to proceed with adoption plans. Carol and her husband did not share their plans for the adoption with family members who became increasingly excited about a prospective first grandchild. The youthful husband actively coached and supported his wife during labor and the delivery. He became engrossed with his daughter shortly following her birth, and he soon felt that being a father was really "neat." On the second postpartal day, the parents decided to drop the adoption plans. Carol confided later that their earlier decision to proceed with adoption plans had been difficult, but they had felt it was important to base their decision on what they saw as best for the two of them and not on what others wanted. As it turned out, they felt that they could resolve the strains imposed on their financial and educational plans by their daughter without resorting to adoption. They were both pleased with their daughter and were attached to her very soon after birth. Counseling enabled them to change their minds without stress, and their families never knew of their earlier decision. This young couple and their daughter matured over the first year, to the extent that Carol commented, "I wouldn't trade this experience for anything. It's been a great experience."

When the young mother makes the decision to relinquish her infant, she should be consulted about the amount of contact she wishes with her infant following delivery. Some health practitioners seem to continue to cling to the idea that the young mother should not be allowed to see, hold, or feed her infant. They withhold the child from the mother in an almost punitive or all-knowing way, either because they feel that the mother "doesn't deserve" to interact with her child or because they wish to "protect her from the pain" of attachment and subsequent separation. Giving up a child that has grown within one's body is analogous to giving up a part of the self; a grief process follows. Even though the youthful mother relinquishes her child because of an inability to provide him with a stable home, or for family reasons, she usually wonders what her child looks like at birth, and at one, two, three, or four years, as she watches other children at play. She may still wonder 35 years later, even though she may have married and successfully reared other children. It is painful, and the pain cannot be erased for her. Empathic support can be given, and sources of compatible counseling can be provided for her, however.

Because every young parent has many fears and fantasies, seeing her child seems to help increase the mother's self-esteem; the knowledge that she indeed produced a normal, healthy, pretty baby confirms that her body functioned perfectly and her infant was not punished by her untimely pregnancy. Many mothers express relief on seeing their child: "I never thought he would be so pretty," or "I never thought he would be so strong." The kind of reassurance that comes from seeing the child and ascertaining its normality helps to enhance her self-concept in a situation that departs from normality. If the mother is not permitted to see her child, she fears her worst dreams have come true—the infant is deformed, or was injured at birth, or is dead. One young single mother very happily told the father of the baby via a long-distance telephone call, "He is perfect in every way. He is a beautiful baby. It is a relief to know nothing is wrong with him."

The grieving process seems to be facilitated when the young parent has a mental picture, a concrete image of her infant. Seeing the infant seems to bridge the gap from the small being inside "who kicked more when he was hungry," or "kicked more listening to music" to a real baby with visible, unique characteristics. Mothers attribute many behaviors to the infant in utero, but his or her appearance and sex are all pure fantasy until the birth. Although it may be more painful initially for the mother to hold or feed her baby, her grief process can be facilitated by grieving for the loss of a real, normal baby, rather than for a fantasy and/or the perceived inability to produce a normal baby.

When possible, follow-up counseling is necessary to ensure that the grief process is proceeding normally and that the young woman is adapting to school, her work, and her continuing adolescent development. Adolescents like Joan, who was mentioned earlier, often prefer no follow-up, however.

Decision making and the assumption of responsibility for the consequences of decisions involve a high level of independent functioning. The adolescent may need help in practicing the making of decisions; she might begin with factors involving immediate and short-term effects during the pregnancy before proceeding to decisions on matters having a permanent impact, such as whether to have her child adopted or not. From a legal perspective, a pregnant teenage girl is considered emancipated in that she has the legal authority to make this decision.[84]

The Unmarried Father

The tendency to overlook the father and to view him askance when he is considered, has been difficult to overcome, even among health professionals. In one very comprehensive program for the teenage mother, a 19-year-old father said:

> If someone had just indicated some interest in me. Everyone was running around asking her what she needed and how she felt, and she was referred to all sorts of people for counseling, but no one ever asked me how *I felt* or what I was worried about. The father is always treated as the outsider that caused all the trouble, and I felt bad enough about everything, and needed someone to talk to. If only there were a male counselor or male doctor to talk to. Sure there are nurses and groups, but you don't get at your intimate feelings in a group, not when you don't know the people in the group.

This young husband, who married his 16-year-old wife when she was four months pregnant, has probably expressed what many young fathers have felt. A glance at the published literature reveals that very little attention has been directed to the unmarried father.

One writer cautioned that including fathers in programs for school-age mothers should be studied carefully since the couple's being together could lead to another pregnancy and data are unavailable as to whether the delay of subsequent pregnancies is more important for future health than providing a father.[58] If the young woman chooses to maintain contact with the father, the school program has little impact on her choice. The major problem may be when and where to include the father in the teaching program.

Supreme Court decisions since 1972 have ruled favorably in protecting the rights of single fathers whose infants were adopted without their knowledge.[87] Ignoring the father could have legal implications if the single father chose to pursue the question of his rights to the child, especially if the child is adopted.

Pannor and Evans[87] succinctly outlined steps for the counselor to take to involve the single father in counseling sessions. A first step for those who counsel single parents is to become comfortable about asking the young woman to name the father of her baby. There may be several reasons for her to deny this knowledge initially. However, after she has had an opportunity to examine her reasons for not disclosing the father's name, and after better rapport has been established, she may be asked again. The young woman may be helped to look at her reasons for either naming or not naming the father through various counseling methods, such as paraphrasing and restatement, and by recognizing her feelings and responding to them at a level that is comfortable to her. The mother profits by recognizing or accepting positive feelings that she had for the father, especially if she had a long relationship with him. Her denial of positive feelings toward the father may reflect initial anger and could preclude a valuable positive support person both at the present time and in the future. Apart from the mother's feelings, there are some practical reasons why adoptive parents need some information about the biological parents. The biological father's family history may help to rule out the possibility of hereditary disease at some later date, and if the child has some information about his father as an individual rather than a fantasy figure who ran away or deserted his mother, he may grow up with more positive feelings about himself.[87] The legal implications of failing to name the father vary from state to state; these should not be overlooked, yet should be presented in a nonthreatening manner and in a realistic framework. A realistic framework would include eligibility for state or federal aid and the single father's legal right if adoption is a considered option.

Once the mother names the father, early and active enlistment of his involvement is a next step for the counselor.[87] In dealing with the father, just as with the mother, the initial approach should emphasize the social aspects of help for him; the father's involvement is enlisted by assuring him that help is available to him and that he can be of help to the child and the mother.[87] All attempts should be made to involve the father in a positive manner before resorting to discussion of local legal statutes. Although the child's welfare is a paramount consideration, the interests and legal rights of all three persons should be carefully considered to afford optimal growth for all.

Robbins[88] found, in a comparative analysis of single unwed fathers, wed fathers, wed-unwed fathers (married to one woman and fathered infant by another woman), and bachelor non-fathers, from 14 to 27 years old (mean 19.6 years), that unwed fathers were more likely to be illegitimate themselves than were the other men. They were not from homes with unhappy parents or homes in which the mother was dominant in a family setting with both parents present. Although the men approved of contraceptives, they did not use them. Although they approved of abortion, they did not approve of abortion for women whom they impregnated, yet they would not choose to keep the child if the mother did not!

All of the men in all groups had poor information about all aspects of sexuality and reproduction, and all had received inaccurate information from their parents and peers. The majority of the fathers felt some responsibility to the mother and the child, and most had known the mother for about two years at the time of the birth. Three out of five fathers still had contact with the mother when the child was one year old. The men had an accepting attitude about premarital and extramarital sexual relationships; they would not hesitate to marry a woman with illegitimate children and they saw nothing wrong if their own children should become unwed parents.

Ethnic, socioeconomic, educational, or psychological factors did not distinguish the unwed father.[88] There was no evidence of unconscious motivation for the pregnancy. The young men felt that their maleness was demonstrated by their ability to impregnate and they wanted to continue the line for generations, to reproduce themselves, to gain recognition, to prove potency, to have a baby and a home, and to form a bond—all very conscious reasons for becoming a father.

Rothstein[89] found that there was a "striking lack of knowledge" about contraception and abortion among men accompanying their partners for elective abortion and that they did not ask questions. They indicated later by questionnaire that they would have liked more information, however.

These research studies have strong implications in counseling the young couple. The father has the same need as the mother for accurate, intensive teaching in areas of reproduction, sexuality, and contraception in order for the couple to have control over the future directions and goals of their lives and to make responsible decisions about their sexual behavior. That the young men had conscious reasons for becoming fathers speaks to the potentially strong support, both emotional and psychosocial, that is possible through the young man's involvement with the pregnancy. The young men's desire for fatherhood also suggests that the father must learn about the physiological, and sociological risks to the adolescent mother and her infant in order to ensure his cooperation in preventing frequent future pregnancies during her adolescence.

Summary

Vital statistics verify that the problem of adolescent pregnancy is extensive. By sheer numbers alone, the problem warrants our most empathetic and creative efforts at intervention, our best tools and skills. The numbers of our population facing the problem of pregnancy at an immature age are perhaps less dramatic than is the potential impact of the problem on the future quality of life in our nation. In 30 years the teenage parents of today will be major contributors to the social system from both economic and political, as well as other qualitative, aspects. We cannot afford *not* to prepare them for that role.

Data are not in agreement regarding the physiological handicaps of premature pregnancies for young women. However, there is agreement that a small nulliparous cervix is easily lacerated and damaged by dilatation for abortion. What does this mean when the young woman, upon reaching an ideal time in her life to become a mother, finds that she has an incompetent cervix and cannot meet her goals for that time of life? The younger the teenager the more dramatic her physiological response to systemic insults, either infectious or mechanical. Depending upon the developmental stage of her bone growth there is the added potential of pelvic contraction due to immaturity.

General agreement seems to exist that pregnancy-induced hypertension is an omnipresent threat during the pregnancy of the youthful adolescent. Iron-deficiency anemia, because of the accelerated demands of iron both for her own body growth and for fetal growth, is a threat.

No conflicting data were found about the psychological and sociological risks of the youthful pregnancy. Cultures within our United States society as a whole have not trained or prepared young people in their early teens for parenthood. The social support system at this time in our history is not developed to a sufficient degree of proficiency to help the youthful parent overcome the handicap of premature interruption of her or his preparation for adulthood. Adolescents are more likely to remain financially and educationally handicapped for years following childbirth in their teens. Psychologically, the immature ego may have difficulty in dealing with the usual emotions resulting from the hormonal changes of pregnancy. Inability of the young woman to identify with and not separate from her mother poses additional problems. In addition, the status of the adolescent's cognitive development and the range of understanding needed for true informed consent must be recognized and dealt with accordingly, and consideration of the local legal statutes regarding the minor's right to give consent for self must be considered.

Decision making, or choosing from viable alternatives, has the potential of promoting the pregnant adolescent's sense of independence and self-esteem. Enabling the adolescent to gain an understanding of herself and to regard her striving for independence as a healthy, maturational behavior rather than a destructive, antisocial force, can allow her to see strengths and good in herself that foster self-reliant and dependable adult behavior.

The young man has received the same cultural shaping as the young woman; therefore, his maturation and development are equally important. It is indeed folly to assume that a young woman can be so thoroughly grounded in knowledge and can become so sophisticated in decision making that her changed behavior alone can alter future statistical trends in unwed pregnancies, repeated teenage pregnancies, and unstable youthful marriages! A young woman learns her feminine and mothering role in interaction with the masculine and fathering roles. The young man with whom she interacts is, and will usually always remain, a powerful influence on her decision making and her behavior. Why we have chosen to ignore this for so long in attempts to ameliorate the conditions caused by untimely teenage pregnancies is an enigma.

The health care and counseling for adolescents who become pregnant in their teens has to be the most skilled, the most intensive, the best we have to offer, if we are to have a large number of our future citizens emerge in their most productive years in sound mental and physical health.

The next chapter deals with prenatal care for the adolescent who chooses to deliver her baby.

REFERENCES

1. *Population Reports,* Series J, No. 14, March 1977. Washington, D.C.: George Washington University Medical Center.
2. Baldwin, W. H. "Adolescent Pregnancy and Childbearing—Growing Concerns for Americans." *Population Bull.* 31(2):2–34, 1976.
3. Klein. L. "Early Teenage Pregnancy, Contraception, and Repeat Pregnancy." *Am. J. Obstet. & Gyn.* 120(2):249–255, 1974
4. Eddinger, L., and Forbrush, J. *School-Age Pregnancy and Parenthood in the United States.* Washington, D.C.: The National Alliance Concerned with School-Age Parents, 1977.
5. Deunhoelter, J. H., et al. "Pregnancy Performance of Patients Under Fifteen Years of Age." *Obstet. & Gyn.* 46(1):49–52, 1976.
6. Widholm, O., et al. "Medical and Social Aspects of Adolescent Pregnancies" *Acta Obstet. Gyn. Scand.* 53:347–353, 1974.
7. Babikian, H. M. "A Study in Teen-Age Pregnancy." *Am. J. Psychiat.* 128(6):755–760, 1971
8. Boyce. J., and Benoit, C. "Adolescent Pregnancy." *New York State J. Med.* 76(6):872–874, 1975
9. Gill, D. G., et al. "Pregnancy in Teenage Girls." *Soc. Sci. & Med.* 3:549–574, 1970
10. *Intercom* 6(2):10, 1978.
11. Rahe, R. H., et al. "Social Stress and Illness Onset." *J. Psychosomat. Res.* 8:35–44, 1964.
12. Nesbitt, E. L., Jr., in Altchek, A., ed. "Sexual Revolution Poses Dilemmas in Pediatric, Adolescent Gynecology." *Contemp. OB/GYN* 9(1):90, 1977.
13. Erkan, K. A., et al. "Juvenile Pregnancy Role of Physiologic Maturity." *Maryland State Med. J.* 20:50–52, 1971.
14. *11 Million Teenagers: What Can Be Done About the Epidemic of Adolescent Pregnancies in the United States.* New York: The Alan Guttmacher Institute, 1976.
15. Donnelly, J. F., et al. "Fetal, Parental, and Environmental Factors Associated with Perinatal Mortality in Mothers Under 20 Years of Age. " *Am. J. Obstet. & Gyn.* 80(4):663–669, 1960.

16. Zlatnik, F. G., and Burmeister, L. F. " 'Low Gynecologic Age': An Obstetric Risk Factor.'' *Am. J. Obstet. & Gyn.* 128(2):183–186, 1977.
17. Hassan, H. M., and Falls, F. H. "The Young Primipara." *Am. J. Obstet. & Gyn.* 88(2):256–269, 1964.
18. Russell, J. K. "Pregnancy in the Young Teenager." *Practitioner* 204:401–405, 1970.
19. King, T. M., in Altchek, A., ed. "Sexual Revolution Poses Dilemmas in Pediatric, Adolescent Gynecology." *Contemp. OB/GYN* 9(1):86, 1977.
20. Briggs, R. M., et al. "Pregnancy in the Young Adolescent." *Am. J. Obstet. & Gyn.* 84(4):436–441,1962.
21. "Herpesvirus and Cancer of Uterine Cervix." *Brit. Med. J.* 1(6011):671, 1976.
22. Hein, K., et al. "Cervical Cytology: The Need for Routine Screening in the Sexually Active Adolescent." *J. Pediat.* 91(1):123–126, 1977.
23. Jovanovic, D. "Pathology of Pregnancy and Labor in Adolescent Patients." *J. Reproductive Med.* 9(2):61–66, 1972.
24. *VD Fact Sheet 1976*. Atlanta, Ga: U.S. Dept. of Health, Education, and Welfare, Center for Disease Control. DHEW Pub. No. (CDC) 77–8195.
25. Buchta, R. M. "It is Important to Search for Mixed Vaginal Infections in Sexually Active Young Women with Endocervical Gonorrhea." *Clin. Pediat.* 16(11):1001–1002, 1977.
26. Faust, M. S. "Somatic Development of Adolescent Girls." *Monographs of the Society for Research in Child Development* 42(1), 1977.
27. Aiman, J. "X-Ray Pelvimetry of the Pregnant Adolescent Pelvic Size and the Frequency of Contraction." *Obstet. & Gyn.* 48(3):281–286, 1976.
28. Bochner, K. "Pregnancies in Juveniles." *Am. J. Obstet. & Gyn.* 83(2):269–271, 1962.
29. Semmens, J. P. "Implications of Teen-Age Pregnancy." *Obstet. & Gyn.* 26(1):77–85, 1965.
30. Lane, M. E. "Contraception for Adolescents." *Fam. Plann. Perspectives* 5(1):19–20, 1973.
31. Widholm, O. "The Need for Gynaecological Services During Adolescence." *Ann. Chirurg. & Gyn. Fenniae* 60:68, 1971.
32. King, J. C., et al. "Assessment of Nutritional Status of Teenage Pregnant Girls. I. Nutrient Intake and Pregnancy." *Am. J. Clin. Nutrition* 25:916–925, 1972.
33. Committee on Nutrition of the Mother and Preschool Child. *Iron Nutriture in Adolescence*. Rockville, Maryland: U.S. Dept. Health, Education, and Welfare, 1976.
34. Webb, G. A. "Care of the Pregnant Adolescent." *Pediat. Ann.* 4(1):99–109, 1975.
35. Israel, S. L., and Woutersz, T. B. "Teen-Age Obstetrics." *Am. J. Obstet. & Gyn.* 85(5):659–666, 1963,
36. Aznar, R., and Bennet, A. E. "Pregnancy in the Adolescent Girl." *Am. J. Obstet. & Gyn.* 81(5):934–940, 1961.
37. Osofsky, H. J., et al. "A Program for Pregnant Schoolgirls." *Am. J. Obstet. & Gyn.* 100(7):1020–1027, 1968.
38. Scher, J., and Utian, W. H. "Teenage Pregnancy—An Inter-Racial Study." *J. Obstet. & Gyn. Brit. Commonwealth* 77:259–262. 1970.
39. Hulka, J. F., and Schaaf. "Obstetrics in Adolescents: A Controlled Study of Deliveries by Mothers 15 Years of Age and Under." *Obstet. & Gyn.* 23(5):678–685, 1964.
40. Efiong, E. I., and Banjoko, M. O. "The Obstetric Performance of Nigerian Primigravidae Aged 16 and Under." *Brit. J. Obstet. & Gyn.* 82:228–233, 1975.
41. Coates, J. B. III. "Obstetrics in the Very Young Adolescent." *Am. J. Obstet. & Gyn.* 108(1):68–72, 1970.
42. Hibbard, L. T. "Maternal Mortality Due to Acute Toxemia." *Obstet. & Gyn.* 42(2):263–270, 1973.
43. Youngs, David D., et al. "Experience with an Adolescent Pregnancy Program." *Obstet. & Gyn.* 50(2):212–216, 1977.
44. Stickle, G. "Pregnancy in Adolescents: Scope of the Problem." *Contemp. OB/GYN* 5(6):85–91, 1975.
45. Gabrielson, I. W., et al. "Suicide Attempts in a Population Pregnant as Teen-Agers." *Am. J. Pub. Health.* 60(12):2289–2301, 1970.
46. Deutsch, H. *Selected Problems of Adolescence*. New York: International Universities Press, Inc., 1967.
47. Kasanin, J., and Handschin, S. "Psychodynamic Factors in Illegitimacy." *Am. J. Orthopsychiat.* 11:66–84, 1941.

48. Bibring, G. I., et al. "A Study of the Psychological Processes in Pregnancy and of the Earliest Mother-Child Relationship." *Psychoanalytic Study of Child* 16:9–61, 1961.
49. Rubin, R. "Maternal Tasks in Pregnancy." *Mat.-Child Nurs. J.* 4(3):143–153, 1975.
50. Halmi, K. A. "Perceptual Distortion of Body Image in Adolescent Girls: Distortion of Body Image in Adolescence." *Psycholog. Med.* 7:253–257, 1977.
51. Friedman, C. M. "Unwed Motherhood: A Continuing Problem." *Am. J. Psychiat.* 129(1):117–121, 1972.
52. Caplan, G. *Concepts of Mental Health and Consultation.* Washington, D.C.: U.S. Dept. Health, Education, and Welfare, 1959.
53. Loesch, J. G., and Greenberg, N. H. "Some Specific Areas of Conflicts Observed During Pregnancy: A Comparative Study of Married and Unmarried Pregnant Women." *Am. J. Orthopsychiat.* 32:624–636, 1962.
54. Barnett, J. "Dependency Conflicts in the Young Adult." *Psychoanalytic Rev.* 58:111–125, 1971.
55. Erikson, E. H. *Childhood and Society.* 2nd ed. New York: W. W. Norton & Co., Inc., 1963.
56. Ballard, W. M., and Gold, E. M. "Medical and Health Aspects of Reproduction in the Adolescent." *Clin. Obstet. & Gyn.* 14(2):338–366, 1971.
57. Waters, J. L., Jr. "Pregnancy in Young Adolescents: A Syndrome of Failure," *Southern Med. J.* 62(2):655–658, 1969.
58. Klerman, L. V. "Adolescent Pregnancy: The Need for New Policies and New Programs." *J. School Health* 45(5):263–267, 1975.
59. Furstenberg, F. F., Jr. "The Social Consequences of Teenage Parenthood." *Fam. Plann. Perspectives* 8(4):148–164, 1976.
60. Smith, P. B., et al. "Selected Aspects of Adolescent Postpartum Behavior." *J. Reproductive Med.* 14(4):159–165, 1975.
61. LaBarre, M. "Pregnancy Experiences Among Married Adolescents." *Am. J. Orthopsychiat.* 38:47–55, 1968.
62. Everett, R. B., and Schechter, M. D. "A Comparative Study of Prenatal Anxiety in the Unwed Mother." *Child Psychiatry & Human Devel.* 2(2):84–91, 1971.
63. Dame, N. G., et al. "Conflict in Marriage Following Premarital Pregnancy." *Am. J. Orthopsychiat.* 36:468–475, 1966.
64. Coombs, L. C., and Freedman, R. "Pre-Marital Pregnancy, Child-spacing, and Later Economic Achievement." *Population Studies* 24:389–412, 1970.
65. Coombs, L. C., et al. "Premarital Pregnancy and Status Before and After Marriage." *Am. J. Sociol.* 75:800–820, 1970.
66. Felson, M., and Knoke, D. "Social Status and the Married Woman." *J. Marr. & Fam.* 36:516–521, 1974.
67. Oppel, W. C., and Royston, A. B. "Teen-Age Births: Some Social, Psychological, and Physical Sequelae." *Am. J. Pub. Health* 61(4):751–756, 1971.
68. Currie, J. B., et al. "Subsequent Pregnancies Among Teenage Mothers Enrolled in a Special Program." *Am. J. Pub. Health* 62(12):1606–1611, 1972.
69. Graves, W. L., and Bradshaw, B. R. "Early Reconception and Contraceptive Use Among Black Teenage Girls After an Illegitimate Birth." *Am. J. Pub. Health* 65(7):735–740, 1975.
70. Waite, L. G., and Moore, K. A. "The Impact of an Early First Birth on Young Women's Educational Attainment." *Social Focus* 56(3):845–865, 1978.
71. Menken, J. "The Health and Social Consequences of Teenage Childbearing." *Fam. Plann. Perspectives* 4(3):45, 1972.
72. Juhasz, A. M. "A Chain of Sexual Decision-Making." *Fam. Coordinator* 24(1):43–49, 1975.
73. Lieberman, E. J. "Informed Consent for Parenthood." *Am. J. Psychoanal.* 34(2):155–159, 1974.
74. Mace, D. R. Foreword. In Wilson, R. R., ed. *Problem Pregnancy and Abortion Counseling.* Saluda, N.C.: Family Life Publications, 1973, p. vii.
75. Baldwin, B. A. "Problem Pregnancy Counseling: General Principles." In Wilson, R. R., ed. *Problem Pregnancy and Abortion Counseling.* Saluda, N.C.: Family Life Publications, 1973, pp. 1–19.
76. Zelnik, M., and Kantner, J. F. "The Resolution of Teenage First Pregnancies." *Fam. Plann. Perspectives* 6(2):74–80, 1974.
77. Schaffer, C., and Pine, F. "Pregnancy, Abortion, and the Developmental Tasks of Adolescence." *J. Am. Acad. Child Psychiat.* 11(2):511–536, 1972.

78. Hatcher, S. L. "Understanding Adolescent Pregnancy and Abortion." *Primary Care* 3(3):407–425, 1976.
79. Fischman, S. H. "The Pregnancy-Resolution Decisions of Unwed Adolescents." *Nurs. Clin. N. Am.* 10(2):217–227, 1975.
80. Fischman, S. H. "Delivery or Abortion in Inner-City Adolescents." *Am. J. Orthopsychiat.* 47(1):127–133, 1977.
81. Martin, C. D. "Psychological Problems of Abortion for the Unwed Teenage Girl." *Genetic Psychol. Monographs* 88:23–110, 1973.
82. Barglow, P. D. "Abortion in 1975: The Psychiatric Perspective with a Discussion of Abortion and Contraception in Adolescence." *JOGN Nurs.* 5(1):41–48, 1976.
83. Bracken, M. B., et al. "Abortion, Adoption, or Motherhood: An Empirical Study of Decision-Making During Pregnancy." *Am. J. Obstet. & Gyn.* 130(3):251–262, 1978.
84. Pilpel, H. F. "Legal Implications of Adolescent Pregnancy." In Bogue, D. J., ed. *Adolescent Fertility.* Chicago: University of Chicago Press, 1977. pp. 72–74
85. Holder, A. R. *Legal Issues in Pediatrics and Adolescent Medicine.* New York: John Wiley & Sons, Inc., 1977.
86. Rotter, J. B. "Generalized Expectancies for Internal Versus External Control of Reinforcement." *Psycholog. Monographs: Gen. & Applied* 80(1):1–28, 1966.
87. Pannor, R., and Evans, B. W. "The Unmarried Father Revisited." *J. School Health* 45(5):286–291, 1975.
88. Robbins, M. *The Dynamics of Unwed Fatherhood.* Doctoral dissertation, University of California, Davis, 1975. Ann Arbor, Mich.: Xerox University Microfilms, Number 75–22, 858.
89. Rothstein, A. A. "Men's Reactions to their Partners' Elective Abortions." *Am. J. Obstet. & Gyn.* 128(8):831–837, 1977.

12

Prenatal Care

RAMONA T. MERCER, R.N., PH.D.

The section on nutrition counseling was contributed by Yolanda Gutierrez, M.S., the author of Chapter 4.

One of the recurrent findings in research studies is that inadequate prenatal care contributes heavily to poor outcome for the pregnant teenager. Multiple personal, developmental, sociological, and environmental factors are interacting that inhibit her seeking and following through with good prenatal care. The greatest challenges facing the health care system are to recruit pregnant adolescents early for care and to render a high quality of care once they are recruited. Although all health care professionals have important roles in providing prenatal care for the adolescent, much of this chapter focuses on specific roles for the nurse. This discussion centers on assuring quality care, the adolescent's initial antepartal visit, antepartal counseling and teaching, and important considerations for monitoring maternal and fetal health.

Assuring Quality Care

The nurse is responsible for promoting a high quality of care for the pregnant adolescent. Some research findings indicate that with excellent prenatal care the morbidity and mortality rates for pregnant adolescents do not differ significantly from those of mothers in their twenties.[1,2] The overall goal for the adolescent who chooses to deliver her baby is that she will grow as a result of her experience, maintain optimal health in doing so, and deliver a healthy infant. The entire prenatal period may be viewed as a learning and maturational experience. To ensure a high quality of care, the adolescent needs early confirmation and assessment of her health state, early enrollment in a comprehensive health program, attention to her physical, social, and psychological needs, and an opportunity to increase her knowledge of sexuality, reproduction, and contraception. Mothering activities, child development, and child care information should be offered if the teenager is ready or interested.

During pregnancy it is difficult for the adolescent to deal with anything other than her body image changes, impending labor and delivery, the laboratory tests and examinations, and the care of her body and fetus. Unless she indicates an interest or readiness to learn about child care or child development such information may not be heard or absorbed. Following delivery she needs help in reentering activities that have been interrupted or help in pursuing new goals, such as entering college or vocational school. This means that she needs day care for her child and special educational counseling and assistance for herself.

The youthful woman often uses denial during early pregnancy, so that she may be well into the second trimester of her pregnancy before she seeks medical help. She may also be afraid to tell her parents that she is pregnant and may postpone telling them until her parents ''discover'' the fact of her pregnancy.

Once the adolescent enrolls in an antepartal program, steps must be taken to ensure that she is conscientious about maintaining her return visits and in adhering to the regimen prescribed. Is the waiting room attractive? How long does she have to wait? Is there a good selection of the kinds of magazines that teenagers enjoy? Sixteen-year-old Susan commented, ''I might as well come at noon for a ten o'clock appointment.'' When she finally saw the doctor and he told her to return in one week instead of two, as the visits were previously spaced, she asked the nurse, ''What will the doctor do next week when I come?'' When told that he would do essentially the same thing that he had done this week, but that more frequent checkups were needed to ensure her health during the last month, she said, ''I have to come all the way from (a nearby suburb). I have to get a streetcar to town and then a bus from town to Fifth Avenue, and then I have to walk the rest of the way.'' Many of the young women who do not drive need careful explanations and the prospect of receiving some benefit to motivate them to take such extensive journeys to the clinic that literally take the better part of a day.

If waiting periods are unavoidable, the time may be utilized effectively for special teaching or counseling sessions with the nurse, social worker, or psychologist, instead of scheduling such sessions after she sees the physician. Effort should be made to ensure that the adolescent does not face ''empty'' or ''wasted'' time. When audiovisual tapes on contraceptives, reproduction, breastfeeding, and infant care are available, the young woman may review them as she feels the interest and need. She may use these aids to clarify questions she has but has been unable to articulate in one-to-one or group counseling, or to reinforce information she has received. Some teenagers view such visual aids each time they come to the clinic.

A carefully integrated continuous recording method is important so that all vital information is accessible to all of the health professionals caring for the teenager and each is not asking for the same information. Personal histories need not be repeated; if the social worker usually gets a complete family history and history of interrelationships in the family, the nurse does not need to repeat these kinds of questions for the nursing history. If the nurse takes a complete sexual history, then the information should be recorded so that the psychologist does not need to repeat the same interview. There are times, such as when information is scanty or incomplete or rapport with one member of the health team is better than with others, when parts of an interview need to be repeated. But, as a whole, repetition should be avoided as much as possible. Young people are very sensitive to the seeming insensitivity of others. If they share information that is vital to their health, then they assume that those needing the information have it. It is important to explain how the information obtained through the interview will be utilized. It is the adolescent's right to know how the information will be used and who will have access to it.

Confidentiality is as important to the teenager as it is to older clients and must be adhered to along the same principles. If the teenager requests that information be withheld from parents or other persons, it is important to respect this request. If for some other reason it later seems propitious to share information with parents or others, permission must first be sought from the teenager. Permission should always be obtained before relaying information to third parties. Parents have access to school records of unemancipated minors; therefore, information that is relayed to schools may become a part of a school record and become accessible to parents. Exceptions to maintaining confidentiality that apply to adults also apply to the teenager—for instance, if she has a contagious disease that can infect others, or if her health or life is in imminent danger, i.e., if she is believed to be on the verge of suicide.[3]

In any program of prenatal care for the teenager it is the responsibility of the nurse clinical specialist or the nurse who is managing the clinic to evaluate the outcome of the projected goals for the program of care. Careful records should reflect the outcome for both the mother and her infant so that this can be measured against the projected goals. If the goals were not reached, why weren't they reached? What are the gaps? Do the adolescents return on a regular basis for prenatal and postpartal care? If not, what seems to be inhibiting their return? Are more appointments not kept during the second trimester than in the third? What are the incidences of complications? Is the young woman able to continue her activities, such as school, that are unrelated to the pregnancy? These are just some of the questions which should be considered during the evaluation of care.

When the outcomes do not meet the desired goals, timely action is warranted to bridge the gap.

THE INITIAL VISIT TO THE CLINIC OR PHYSICIAN

The young woman approaching a clinic or physician on her first antepartal visit is usually quite frightened and tense. Sixteen-year-old Paula illustrates some of the fears of a very typical adolescent as she describes her first visit to the clinic:

I was scared to death the first day I was up here [clinic]. I was in a cold sweat. I'd never have come up here if my mamma hadn't made me come, and brought me. Then I saw this big old—nurse—like a monster. I said, "uggh, uggh, forget it. If they have nurses like *that.*" They are all so big and old; they look so mean. I hate hospitals. I had to go to the emergency room when I was 8 once when I broke my arm. This big old nurse, must have weighed 180—big and fat, sat on kids to hold them down. I was scared she would sit on me, and I screamed and my daddy came running in there and held me and said he wouldn't let her sit on me. But I got her, I really bit her. She held her arm in front of my mouth and I let her have it but good. I bit her as hard as I could.

Paula's first visit to the clinic aroused earlier fears that she had experienced in hospitals and with nurses, whom she saw as big, old, fat, mean monsters. The pervasive theme is that of one who is small, young, and helpless in the hands of monsters.

The young woman on her first visit to the clinic is also faced by a barrage of instructions and numerous places to go. On top of all of these confusing encounters, she may be facing her first pelvic examination. Is it any wonder that she appears uncommunicative? She is, most likely, in a state of shock in the midst of a busy setting in which she sees that she has little or no control.

Because of the many persons that a young woman is meeting for the first time and because many of the experiences are intrusive, it is probably best to obtain a detailed nursing history at a later visit. The nursing history is a detailed personal and social history that provides information needed in planning care during the prenatal and postpartal periods. It is important for the adolescent to develop trust in the adult who is caring for her and to understand why any information she gives is important for planning her care. Therefore, the nurse may have to begin assessment and intervention with data that the teenager volunteers on her first visit.

An overview of all of the interviews, tests, and examinations, with the rationale for each, should be shared with the young woman during the first few minutes of contact. This needs to be done pleasantly and positively and should focus on the young woman's desires and needs, so that she sees they are considered central in planning her care. Although, because of her anxiety, she may not hear everything initially, explaining something about each person's interest in her care at least begins to teach the young woman something about the multifaceted nature of the care and concern that are offered for her and her infant. The social worker's services should be described briefly so that the young woman can make some mental notes and prepare for that interview. The interview in the business office (if one is done) should be described beforehand, so that the young woman does not feel threatened by the possibility that she may be deprived of care if her answers or financial status are ''incorrect'' or unfavorable.

Visits to the psychologist, dentist, and nutritionist—if these professionals are routinely involved in the teenager's care—should be carefully explained; she should be told the reasons for their involvement and something about the kinds of help that each has to offer. Sixteen-year-old Paula made the following observations about the psychological testing that she had experienced:

> I ain't about to take no more of those dumb tests. I was in there last week. I was in there the first time I came up here. Those are stupid questions. ''Are you sad all the time, are you blue all the time?'' He'd say, ''Which is the most like you,'' and I'd say, ''None of them.'' He'd say, ''Isn't one more nearly like you?'' and I'd say, ''No.'' And stupid questions like, ''What would you recommend someone else to wear when they're pregnant?'' . . . Anybody would know what to wear.

Paula's response indicates that little was learned about her true feelings and that she received little help in the interaction.

A barrage of ''don'ts'' can be very upsetting to a teenager who is already rebelling against the parental "don'ts" in her home. For example, Susan, a 16-year-old, illustrated the ineffectual "don't" method of counseling in response to the question, "What did you learn from the nutritionist?": "Oh, I don't know. *Don't* eat this, *don't* eat that, and that and that. I didn't pay no mind to her. I ate it anyway. I'll eat what I want to."

Many clinics provide dental care for adolescent clients. The importance of dental care and the visit to the dentist needs careful interpretation. The need to avoid infection from decayed teeth from the perspective of promoting her health and that of her infant might be one approach. The adolescent's routine dental checkups are important in order to detect cavities, whether she is pregnant or not. If the adolescent has not completed her bone growth, the additional demands of this along with fetal growth increase her calcium requirements. The dentist can reassure her that her edematous gums, which bleed when she brushes her teeth, are a temporary change due to pregnancy, and he can reinforce the importance of her nutrient intake to avoid calcium depletion during pregnancy. Many folk beliefs inhibit proper dental care during pregnancy: e.g., "A tooth for every baby," and "Pulling a tooth during pregnancy will mark the baby." Whenever possible, extractions of impacted wisdom teeth should be delayed until the young woman becomes comfortable with the clinic setting. Observations indicate that the pain, edema, and inconvenience of extracted impacted wisdom teeth constitute a very negative experience for the teenager as she comes back for suture removals and has to avoid solid, chewy foods for a period of time. She often perceives this intrusive surgery as punishment. There may be some who would argue that punishment provides a catharsis, so that one begins a new slate with less defensive energy expelled, but in all fairness to a young woman, it is important that she should have established a sense of trust and acceptance of the health team before she experiences such traumatic procedures as the extraction of uninfected wisdom teeth.

The blood work that is required at the first visit frequently evokes in the teenager repressed feelings about earlier experiences of "receiving shots" or being stuck, or of being hurt when she was a child; it is a procedure that adolescents fear. Thus, explaining the rationale for all of these intrusive procedures is imperative. Because of the teenager's newly acquired logic and her penchant for intellectualization, knowing a reason for or having some degree of understanding about what is happening to her gives her some measure of control, which is badly needed in her struggle for independence.

The warmth of this milieu, which often appears extremely busy and confusing, may determine the teenager's continued future use of the facility. Actively involving the teenager while teaching her about the various components of her health care helps her to become a part of the health team as a responsible person who can assume responsibility for her own and her baby's well-being. Following the overview of services, perhaps with the exception of the physical examination and laboratory work, she can be given the choice of whom she wishes to see on this first visit, as opposed to a later one.

Once the teenager has an overall idea of the health care facility, she should be asked what she has heard about the physical examination. The youthful mother-to-be avidly collects information from a variety of sources. If she is attending a special school for pregnant teenagers, the grapevine is even more extensive, and often the information is highly exaggerated. Depending upon the young woman's response concerning her knowledge of the examination, the nurse or physician can prepare her accordingly. For example, if she replies that she was told by peers that a huge instrument was "shoved up" in the vagina, it may be helpful for her to see or hold a speculum, so that she can see how it opens to allow visualization of the vaginal vault and thus makes it easier to get cervical and vaginal smears. A colleague* suggests that if the adolescent continues to be particularly resistant to the examination, the nurse practitioner, midwife, or physician may wish to allow her to insert the speculum herself, explaining that it may be inserted "like a tampon." Although the younger adolescent may be turned off by this approach, the middle and older adolescents usually like to view their own genitalia, especially the cervix. A hand mirror should be handy for this. In situations where modesty is the issue rather than fear of the examination per se, it is important that the nurse or physician convey understanding of the client's feelings and recognition that the position is an awkward and embarrassing one for her. It may be helpful to mention that the pelvic examination is a regular part of every woman's life and is an important part of her health care since it provides information the clinician needs in assessing her health status. If the clinician is a woman, she may add that she also has regular pelvic examinations. It is vital for the clinician to reassure the client that every step in the examination will be explained to her as well as sensations that she may feel during the process, and that if the examination becomes painful to her, he will stop and wait for her to tell him to resume. Allowing the young woman this control usually increases her tolerance level for the discomforts involved.

For the youthful teenager who is extremely tense, agitated, and fearful, it is important to make every attempt possible to gain her cooperation through empathic concern and conversation in order to help her to relax. Very little information is obtained from a pelvic examination when the young woman is hysterical and tense and scoots up the table. Punitive admonishments that she has already separated her legs for something larger than two fingers or the instrument are demeaning and cruel and will further increase her anxiety, as well as her distrust of and discomfort with persons in the setting. Such admonishments are, unfortunately, not rare. Some young women who are extremely upset have been sexually abused by the partners who impregnated them; for those young women the pelvic examination may arouse fears and fantasies of a "rape scene."

In the initial interview, the young woman should be asked how much involvement she wants and expects from her mother, the father of the baby, or from others. Nurses have frequently observed that the pregnant adolescent may be quite talkative and may share her concerns freely, but when her mother enters the room, all conversation ceases. Careful assessment of the mother-daughter relationship needs to be made in planning supportive care for her. In order for the young woman to develop trust in all who work with her, it helps to clarify what information she wishes shared with whom, and this trust must not be violated. When it becomes necessary to

*Appreciation is expressed to Connie Stockdale, M.S., C.N.M., for these suggestions about methods that she has found helpful in her practice.

share information with a parent, the youthful client must be approached forthrightly: "If it's OK with you I'd like to talk to your mother about your blood pressure. You need much more rest, and unless your mother understands the importance of this rest she may keep asking you to do the housework for her."

Upon completion of the initial examination, the teenage client should be acquainted with the usual procedures for subsequent visits. Some clinics have comic books describing their services, teaching about venereal disease and contraception, etc. If the young woman receives a "gift" as she departs, she may feel better about the service; the book is also a tangible reminder about the return visit.

PARENTS' RESPONSE TO PREGNANCY

A teenager's discovery that she is pregnant and the consequent telling of her family usually constitute the first and most intense emotional crisis the pregnant teenager faces.[4] Parents feel overwhelming guilt that they have not been good parents, and the evidence is there for everyone to see. In their guilt they blame each other and the daughter, and often angry words and accusations are a part of the "telling" scene.

Two studies have focused on this crisis from the perspective of the pregnant adolescent's mother. Bryan-Logan and Dancy[5] observed that three phases occur in the interaction between the pregnant daughter and the mother. A "silent phase" occurred first in which there was no admission or discussion of the pregnancy. The mother often said that she knew the daughter was pregnant but was waiting for her to share her concerns. During the second phase of "question-denial," the mother hinted that the daughter was pregnant with indirect statements such as "Is something wrong?" The daughter denied anything was wrong. The second phase continued—both women knowing of the pregnancy yet denying it until it could no longer be denied. The "accepting phase" then began; the adolescent's mother rationalized about the pregnancy and opened negotiations for resolution of the problems presented. The first negotiation was with the expectant father and his family, and finances were a primary concern. Interestingly, the adolescent's mother usually handled these negotiations alone. Marriage was a second issue that was negotiated. This negotiation took several forms: the future grandmother approached the expectant father's parents; the expectant father approached the future grandmother with the desire to marry her daughter; both expectant parents approached the young woman's mother; or all parties involved made an agreement—both sets of future grandparents and the expectant parents. Sometimes the future prospective grandmother negotiated the daughter's relationship with the expectant father. The daughter's care had to be negotiated; what could they afford? The expected child's mothering was also negotiated.

Smith[6] described seven phases in the pregnant adolescent's mother's transition to the grandmother role. The first phase was the "informing process," in which the mother learned about the pregnancy; her expectations for her daughter indicated how early she learned of her daughter's pregnancy. Although the daughters concealed their pregnancies as long as possible, mothers who had expectations that their daughters would become pregnant usually had kept records of their menstrual cycles and knew of the pregnancy very early. Smith's "informing process" phase seems to incorporate Bryan-Logan's and Dancy's "silent" and "question-denial" phase. A "period of disequilibrium" followed in phase two, in which the prospective grandmother worked at resolving the asynchronization of her premature advancement to the grandmother role. A period of restoration of normality occurred in phase three. Decisions about abortion and possible adoption were considered during this phase, and other normalizing efforts resembled the negotiations described by Bryan-Logan and Dancy.

During the fourth phase, Smith noted a "taking on of the grandmother role," in which the future grandmother began active preparations and bought gifts for the baby. A "period of reality" occurred in the fifth phase, when physical changes during the last trimester dramatized the reality of the coming baby for both the mother and daughter. Phases six and seven occurred following the birth; this period was marked by a "three generational confusion stage," in which the daughter did not feel like a mother nor the grandmother like a grandmother, and there was a shifting of role expectations for each. Until the daughter had a clear identity as a mother, the grandmother was unable to internalize her role for the seventh phase.

These research findings have implications for both the prospective grandmother and her daughter's care during the antepartal period. Although much hostility may be evident when the young woman first presents herself to the clinic, it may represent the "period of disequilibrium" that will be followed by negotiation, rationalization of the situation, and, finally, a period of normality. It may be helpful to share these phases that have been observed with both mother and daughter. Empathic understanding that this is a difficult time for both of them, because both are frightened and worried, can be helpful. With supportive help, they can begin resolving many of the problems.

The mother is often the major support person for the teenager, especially the very young girl under 16. Smith[6] observed that the mothers often delayed telling the fathers as long as possible. Many pregnant teenagers report that their mothers "took it better than their fathers." Whether the mother's role as major support person to the pregnant adolescent is acquired by default or by choice is not known. The health professional can observe the phases of adjustment as they occur and can encourage the relationship between the mother and daughter along positive lines. In situations where the adolescent's mother kicks her out of the home, the prospective grandmother may deny her role transition and/or take years to internalize the role. The adolescent in this situation benefits from having an older, caring woman as a mother surrogate.

In some cases the adolescent's mother may feel excessive guilt; or her husband may project blame onto her to such an extent that the stability of the family is threatened and she may need psychological or family counseling. The question, "How are things going at home now?" may help to elicit information that indicates whether the family needs help, and, if so, the kind of help needed.

Antepartal Counseling, Teaching

Over the approximately seven months that the teenage client receives antepartal care, her mental health and maturation are noted as well as her physical health. During these months, sexual, contraceptive, and reproductive teaching and counseling are just as important as maternal and fetal monitoring tests and examinations for physical care. Ideally, the young woman is continuing in school. In some areas she continues in the regular high school. In other areas special programs are available which provide special classes or schools for pregnant girls.

There are advantages and disadvantages in both instances. When the pregnant girl continues in a regular high school, the awkwardness of her enlarging abdomen and gait of pregnancy may be even more depressing to her as she constantly contrasts herself to her svelte and fashionable peers. Classes are not shortened in accordance with her fatigue level at regular schools, and there may not be as many opportunities for special classes focusing on pregnancy and child-craft. In special schools with educational programs designed for the pregnant adolescent, she has numerous role models; everyone is in the same boat as she. She learns from those who are a few months ahead of her and teaches those who are a few months behind her. Classes may be held in the morning so that she can nap following lunch. In some schools, nurses conduct special classes that focus on her specific needs. One disadvantage of the special educational programs is that separate educational facilities may not be equal to those of the regular high school. If special educational programs are held in old, unattractive buildings that are difficult to heat, or where educational equipment is lacking, it is difficult to motivate the young woman to attend regularly. Consequently, she misses many school days in addition to the couple of weeks she misses for delivery and postpartum, making her reentry into the regular high school even more difficult.* Also, once the young mother has delivered, she typically dislikes the school for pregnant teenagers. One 14-year-old said she didn't want "to go back to that old school with all the big stomachs." She was finished with pregnancy, wanted no reminders, and was much happier when she returned to a regular high school. This is a very personal matter; it might be better for many of the young women to go back to a regular school rather than the special school to finish the semester. The special schools usually have accommodations for the infants and are paced for adequate rest for the mother during the first six weeks postpartum, however.

It is important that teaching programs in the antepartal clinic be designed specifically for the pregnant teenagers. Many have observed that the pregnant teenager is uncomfortable, and therefore responds less freely and openly, around women who are her mother's age.[7,8] Teenagers are reluctant to reveal their "not knowing," and have a tendency to ask fewer questions when in classes with older women. Research also indicates that the teenager needs a more extensive knowledge base. Adult women sometimes do not hide their disapproval of the young woman's plight, or sometimes they are overly sympathetic. The young woman wants neither

---

*The reader who wishes further information about educational programs for school age parents is referred to the May 1975 issue of the *Journal of School Health* 45(5), which focuses on problems and risks of school age parents and the special kinds of programs provided.

response. A 16-year-old stated, "We don't speak the same language; even the women in their early twenties have different interests and are of a different era."

NUTRITION COUNSELING

Yolanda Gutierrez, M.S.

The special nutritional needs and problems of the pregnant adolescent were discussed in Chapter 4. Optimally, nutrition counseling begins long before a young woman experiences pregnancy, since, to a large extent, food habits and nutrient stores from childhood determine the nutritional status during pregnancy.

The nutritional status and diets of many pregnant women continue to receive insufficient attention in routine prenatal care despite research studies demonstrating the ill effects of maternal malnutrition on both the fetus and the mother. Since adolescents often do not seek prenatal care until late in pregnancy, their vulnerability for nutritional risk is increased. For example, one of the most consistently noted complications among pregnant adolescents is toxemia. Maternal mortality from toxemia is associated with the state's per capita income; "the lower a state's income, the higher the maternal mortality from toxemia" (p. 11).[9] Although the etiology of toxemia remains an enigma, the fact that toxemia tends to occur more frequently in pregnant women of low socioeconomic status, who consequently have poor diets, deserves consideration. Many teenage pregnancies occur in low income families where there is the least money to purchase food and the least understanding of the importance of the nutritional needs of pregnancy, and where prenatal care and adequate counseling often come too late to prevent many complications.

Nutritional counseling during pregnancy has a triple purpose: achievement of an optimal nutritional state favorable to the adolescent's continued growth; achievement of an optimal nutritional environment for fetal development; and the establishment of sound food practices for the future. The same approaches and Food Guides described in Chapter 4 for general nutrition counseling are to be used in counseling throughout pregnancy, including both the formal dietary history and the individual nutritional assessment that every pregnant woman should have.

The pregnant adolescent is facing the most dramatic changes in her entire life; she is undergoing the physiological stresses of pregnancy along with her normal adolescent development. Therefore, the counselor should keep the following factors in mind when counseling her:

1. Maintenance of emotional and psychological stability
2. Promotion of optimal height and weight gain
3. Prevention of iron-deficiency anemia
4. Promotion of optimal environmental factors
5. Consideration of ethnic or cultural background

An analysis of her attitudes towards her adolescence, her pregnancy, and her acceptance or rejection of the baby, will help health care practitioners to determine the goals of the counseling. An appeal to the teenager to eat properly for the sake of the growing fetus may be futile if she does not want the pregnancy or if she is obsessed with the idea of remaining slim. She may use food as an outlet for her emotions. Often she selects foods that are rich in calories but low in nutritional value. To motivate her to practice better nutrition habits, the counselor may need to talk in terms of the adolescent's own well-being.

The emotional and psychological stability of the pregnant adolescent may be influenced by her attitudes about her body image in relation to weight gain during pregnancy. It is important for the pregnant adolescent to realize that the desirable weight gain during pregnancy is 11.2 to 13.5 kilograms (24 to 30 pounds) and that the weight gain should be steady and gradual. As was stated in Chapter 4, on the average, 0.9 to 1.8 kilograms (2 to 4 pounds) are gained during the first trimester. About 454 grams (1 pound) a week is desirable during the remainder of the pregnancy. This weight gain is imperative for the mother's continued good health and for the normal development of the fetus. One must consider that this *average* recommended weight gain reflects the normal *range* for most healthy women. The total number of pounds gained in pregnancy will vary among individual adolescents, depending upon age and growth needs. An evaluation of the adolescent's weight status at conception, as well as her usual dietary practices and activity patterns, are necessary in order to determine the weight gain that will be best for her. The obese and underweight pregnant adolescent present specific nutritional problems. Both are encouraged to gain the desirable 11.2 to 13.5 kilograms (24 to 30 pounds) during pregnancy. Weight loss or no gain during pregnancy presents serious risks for both the mother and the unborn infant.

The health care practitioner can more effectively encourage the young prospective mother to eat the necessary foods for optimal nutrition by explaining that the gained weight is distributed largely to the growing fetus for his environment and maintenance. Table 12-1 illustrates this point.

In counseling the obese pregnant adolescent it should be emphasized that this is not the time for her to lose weight; rather it is the ideal time for her to establish good eating habits. She should learn the nutrient and caloric values of foods, the amounts and kinds of food needed during her pregnancy, and the importance of regularity in meal patterns. If the assessment of the obese teenager indicates that she is gaining too much, too rapidly, because of an excessive intake of calories, predominantly in the form of carbohydrates, she should be advised that fat deposition not only accelerates her obesity but also fails to provide nutrients for fetal development. It should also be pointed out that if her protein intake is low her own lean body mass will be consumed to support the fetal tissue growth.

The underweight pregnant adolescent presents a critical situation. If she is bothered by nausea and vomiting and is unable to tolerate food, dietary counseling should include the importance and special value of frequent, small meals. It is helpful for her to try dry foods first and to have liquids between meals. Also she should avoid foods that aggravate the situation, such as fatty and highly seasoned foods. She needs close supervision throughout pregnancy.

The adolescent who was underweight prior to pregnancy was found to have a greater risk for poor pregnancy outcome by Hollingsworth,[10] who studied 400

TABLE 12–1. *Weight Gain During Pregnancy*

(Weights are Approximations)

Baby	7 1/2	lbs	3 1/3	kg
Placenta	1 1/2	lbs	2/3	kg
Uterus	2	lbs	1	kg
Increased maternal blood volume, interstitial fluid, and amniotic fluid	8 1/2	lbs	4	kg
Body changes for breast feeding	4 1/2	lbs	2	kg
TOTAL	24	lbs	11	kg

Source: Adapted from "Your Weight and Weight Gain," prepared by California Department of Health, Carol G. Corruccini, M.S., Nutrition Consultant.

adolescents who were pregnant for the first time. There were 29 in the thin group (below normal weight), 318 in the normal weight group, 34 in the moderate obesity group, and 19 in the significant obesity group; all had comparable weight gains during pregnancy, from 11.9 to 12.2 kilograms (26 to 27 pounds). The thin group had twice the fetal loss that the normal group had: 10% in contrast to 5%. The moderately obese group had a 3% fetal loss and the significantly obese group had a 5% fetal loss; 62% of the moderately obese group and 55% of the thin group had normal pregnancies. The moderately obese group had the greatest number of large babies, but no infant weighed over 4,000 grams (8 pounds 13 ounces) in the significantly obese group. The thin group had the highest incidence of infants weighing less than 2,500 grams (5½ pounds). The thin group had a mean placental weight of 586 grams (1 pound 5 ounces); the normals, 679 grams (1 pound 9 ounces); the moderately obese, 679 grams (1 pound 9 ounces); and the significantly obese, 575 grams (1 pound 4 ounces). Preeclampsia was observed as often in the thin group as it was in the moderately obese group: it occurred in 17% of the thin group, 9% of the normal group, 18% of the moderately obese group, and 21% of the significantly obese group. Hollingsworth's study dramatizes the importance of nutritional counseling from childhood.

Because of both the adolescent's and her fetus's increased needs for iron, the pregnant adolescent is at special risk for iron deficiency anemia. In addition to the recommended supplements, certain nutrients involved in hemoglobin formation require special attention: protein, Vitamins B-12 and B-6, and folacin. For food sources of these nutrients see Chapter 4, Table 4–2. The reader is encouraged to refer to the sections on pregnancy, dietary habits of adolescents, and nutrition counseling in Chapter 4 for background information needed in counseling the pregnant teenager.

The California Department of Health has published a revised Daily Food Guide suggested for nutrition during pregnancy and lactation (Table 12–2). This guide is helpful in the evaluation of diet adequacy. However, it should be pointed out that the guide provides the number of servings required by the *adult* pregnant woman. As it is, the Guide provides the RDA for all nutrients except iron and folacin, which require the usual recommended supplementation. Energy needs are not met by the recommended number of servings of the Food Guide; approximately 400 additional

TABLE 12–2. *Revised Daily Food Guide*

FOOD GROUP	NUMBER OF SERVINGS		
	NON-PREGNANT WOMAN	PREGNANT WOMAN	LACTATING WOMAN
Protein foods			
animal*	2	2	2
vegetable†	2	2	2
Milk and milk products	2	4	5
Breads and cereals	4	4	4
Vitamin C rich fruits and vegetables	1	1	1
Dark green vegetables	1	1	1
Other fruits and vegetables	1	1	1

* 1 serving is 2 oz. (60 g).
† should include at least 1 svg. legumes.

Source: Reprinted from "Food Guides: Their Development, Use, and Specific Changes Suggested for Nutrition During Pregnancy and Lactation," published by the California Department of Health, Maternal and Child Health Branch, June 1977, p. 5.

calories are needed to fulfill the energy requirements of any pregnant woman. For the pregnant adolescent, the additional calories needed can be provided by the ingestion of an extra serving of milk and by the addition of fats and oils to the food groups which are not included in this revised form. Additional calories can be obtained from increased servings of the food groups. It is strongly recommended that the pregnant woman include at least one serving of legumes (beans, lentils, garbanzos) in her selection of recommended vegetable proteins—legumes provide Vitamin B-6, folacin, iron, and zinc in good amounts.

The use of the Food Guide in counseling is also a valuable tool for ensuring an average intake of essential nutrients that will meet the metabolic needs of the pregnant woman. A wide variety of food patterns, menus, and number of meals can be developed using the guide. Teaching the pregnant teenager and her family how to use the Food Guide is an essential factor in achieving the purpose of nutrition counseling during pregnancy.

Nutritional consideration should be given to the lactating teenager, since her nutrient demands are even higher than during pregnancy (see p. 77). During lactation the most significant increases of nutrients are recommended for protein and energy.

SEXUALITY COUNSELING

Because the adolescent developmental task of achieving feminine identity will be attained earlier or later by some, the pregnant adolescent may fluctuate between various stages of internalizing the feminine role and may possess differing levels of sexual knowledge. Both individual and group sessions are important to facilitate optimal maturation and growth. The young woman may have very little knowledge about conception, sexuality, and reproduction, and even less knowledge about her anatomy and her sexual feelings during pregnancy. This is especially true of the teenager who yearned for a closer relationship with her mother; sexual intercourse with her boyfriend was primarily to please him, because it offered a feeling of closeness that she desired, however temporary. The young woman who has a partner with whom she is continuing a relationship may need a quite different kind of counseling. Guidance should be aimed at enabling her to grow in her ability to maintain an intimate relationship and to promote her health and that of her infant.

The nurse who counsels the adolescent about various aspects of sexuality needs to have not only a sound, accurate knowledge base in these areas, but must also be comfortable with her own sexuality. She must be aware of her own values and attitudes and of how these affect her relationships with others. The nurse who has difficulty dealing with premarital intercourse, mechanical contraception, etc., will be less effective in helping the pregnant teenager to explore her feelings about why she became pregnant and to make choices for the future. This is especially true if the teenager's basic philosophy differs considerably from the nurse's. If the nurse is uncomfortable about certain areas of sexuality, and if specific questions cause extensive facial blushing or blanching or other nonverbal cues, the teenager is immediately informed that the nurse cannot help her look objectively at all facets of the situation, and will withdraw.

The adolescent's social milieu is an essential consideration when teaching about any aspects of sexuality. Probably more cultural taboos and regulations are associated with childbirth and sexuality than with any other area of human concern. Without knowledge of the client's cultural beliefs, values, and attitudes, much of the nurse's teaching may appear irrelevant or inapplicable to her, and may "turn her off."

Many times the teenager states that she will not be engaging in sexual relations in the future and that her pregnancy was due to a chance happening or a one-time "forced" type of situation. It is important to respect her decision, although information about conception, pregnancy, and contraception should continue to be given throughout her care. Contraceptive counseling should not be forced with the idea that since she got pregnant once, sexual intercourse is inevitable for her. The knowledge about contraception may be helpful for her in the future, however. Continuing to offer contraceptive information is especially important for the early adolescent who is at the concrete level of cognitive functioning. Planning ahead and abstracting about consequences of her behavior are often beyond her level of functioning.

Pregnancy is an optimal time to review knowledge of conception and enlarge upon this knowledge. Reproduction is always an interesting topic to the teenager, but the pregnant young woman particularly enjoys knowing about and following her infant's development. Violet, a 14-year-old, became very excited while looking at a birth atlas with her nurse. She pointed out the size of her baby, compared the current size to the expected size the next month, and noted that fingernails would soon appear. While teaching about anatomy and pregnancy, contraceptive knowledge can be incorporated quite naturally. The teenager's knowledge of contraception can be obtained by a question such as, "What will prevent the spermatozoon from fertilizing the ovum?" (This follows, of course, after she has learned the meaning of "spermatozoon'' and ''ovum.'') Teaching can be followed up in the group process and intensified according to individual need and interest. Visual aids and models are essential tools in teaching the teenager, particularly the early teenager, who is unable to think abstractly.

Teenagers often use slang terms for body parts and functions. The nurse, after interpreting the correct terms, should use them correctly as a role model.

The timing for contraceptive counseling during pregnancy is important. It is best introduced during the first two trimesters. When a teenager is queried a few weeks before her due date about the contraceptive method she plans or wishes to use, her response may be quite negative. All of her energy at that time may be directed toward the labor and delivery that she will soon face. Her need to learn more about labor and delivery and what will happen to her at that time may preempt thought about avoiding future pregnancies. This is variable, however. One high school class of pregnant teenagers continued to raise questions about contraceptives at almost all special classes with the author, despite the topic planned for class. As some of these younger and middle adolescents faced the increasing bodily discomforts of pregnancy, they were intensely interested in contraception: ''I don't want to go through *this* again any time soon.'' The same questions were repeated week after week, which suggests some difficulty in comprehending the content. They found it particularly difficult to believe that approximately 250 to 350 million spermatozoa are in each ejaculate. The high school group forced individuals to face reality in a very helpful way. One 17-year-old who was living with her boyfriend maintained she would avoid pregnancy by avoiding intercourse. The group rejoined, ''You think he's going to stop wanting it just like that after all this time?''

A 14-year-old argued that drugstores were not open, or available, at midnight when a contraceptive was needed. An explanation that a condom and an applicator of foam could be kept in her purse for such circumstances was countered with, ''He doesn't like rubbers.'' A firm reply, ''If you don't want to have another baby right away, and a rubber is the only way he can have sexual intercourse, he will like it,'' met with general agreement from the group. The ability of a young adolescent to stand firm in such a decision might be reinforced by group consensus that this is her right to demand. The reader is referred to Chapter 5 for more specific content on contraceptive counseling.

Masturbation is a common practice; at the same time, it is often associated with many myths and it is wise for the nurse to introduce the topic. Whether the teenager has a sexual partner or not, she needs to know that masturbation during pregnancy is not harmful except in situations such as threatened premature labor or threatened abortion, when orgasm is contraindicated. To ensure her understanding of the different modes of release of sexual tension and the acceptability and harmlessness of masturbation, it should be part of her learning about her own sexuality and sexual needs.

Although coitus, conception, contraception, venereal disease, and masturbation are relevant topics for sexual counseling, the teenager is often hesitant to initiate the conversation in these areas of sexual concern.[11] Once the nurse introduces the topics, however, the young woman usually begins to ask questions and to discuss these concerns.

For all adolescents, but especially for those with a partner, factual knowledge about coitus during pregnancy is very important. When there are no complications during the pregnancy, intercourse usually may be continued up until the time of delivery. Intercourse is contraindicated in the presence of vaginal or abdominal pain, ruptured membranes, bleeding, threatened abortion, or threatened premature labor. It is usually contraindicated if there is an infection of the genital tract, if the baby is low in the pelvis, if extensive vulvar varicosities are present, or if there is a history of spontaneous abortions.[11] Discussion about alternative ways of providing sexual release for her partner is appropriate if she has to avoid intercourse and/or orgasm for any of those reasons.

The teenager may be particularly naive about positions for intercourse other than the common "missionary position," (man superior). Alternative positions of intercourse may be presented with a discussion of why each position may be more comfortable during pregnancy. The client should be encouraged to try any position that is comfortable for her as long as excessive abdominal pressure and deep penile penetration are avoided.[11]

A vital part of the health maintenance program during the teenager's pregnancy should include increasing her knowledge about venereal disease and the impact it could have on her health and that of her baby. Myths abound concerning venereal disease—how the diseases are contracted, how they are avoided—and it is not uncommon for a teenager to possess the naive belief that once she has been cured of a venereal disease, she is immune to it.

PREPARATION FOR LABOR AND DELIVERY

The teenage client is particularly fearful of labor. She needs classes preparing her for labor as well as an opportunity to talk about labor. A tour of the hospital labor and delivery rooms is especially helpful. During the last trimester, and particularly in the last month of pregnancy, many of the adolescent's thoughts center on what labor and delivery will be like for her. The young woman has collected data on what it has been like for numerous others. Remarks made by 17-year-old Alison at 37 weeks gestation, while on a tour of the labor and delivery unit, reveal the fears of the teenager and some sources of her data. She related the following to the nurse who was with her:

My insurance man told me I might die. But he was trying to sell insurance. He said people were more apt to die when they had babies than at any other time. I'm scared of labor. . . . [At this time, the nurse and Alison entered the labor unit and Alison's eyes opened wide.] You mean this is all there is in the labor room? I thought there must be lots and lots of beds, 50 in a labor room. How else could people be talking about all the people next to them screaming and yelling? And they told me you were penned up with bars around you. [The bed rails were demonstrated, and the explanation given that they added security in a narrow bed.] How do you get to the delivery room? When do you move? My girlfriend said her baby's head came down and the nurses kept making her pant like a puppy while they fooled around getting the doctor, and she nearly died with the head down there trying to come out. How do you get over to the table? You move over all by yourself? Where are the other rooms? [The nurse and Alison walked by other labor rooms; the door to one room was partly open and a patient was inside. Alison stretched her neck to look in as she passed the door. When asked if she felt like going to see the delivery room, she promptly said, "I feel like it." Both gowned, put covers over their shoes, and went into the delivery room. Alison's eyes looked as if they would pop out.] I'm scared of labor, but they tell me I'll hurt so bad that I'll not think to be afraid. [While she was looking at the delivery table, her attention was called to the mirror. She leaned over and looked at herself in the mirror.] I don't want to watch. How many people will be in here when I have my baby? . . . This doesn't look like I thought. They're so light. The labor rooms are so light. I don't know why, but I thought of them as being dark. I just imagined both of them as being real dark. What is the other room like? [Another delivery room.] Don't they put your legs up in something? . . . I'm still afraid of labor. [They went to the postpartal unit.] I don't like it up here. . . . Will I have to be in a room with all those *old* women? Do you have 40-year-old women who have babies?

This tour of the labor and delivery suite did not allay Alison's fear of labor significantly. But it helped dispel the fear that she would be in a dark room penned behind bars with several women who were "screaming and yelling." The fear of death which her insurance man reinforced would remain until the delivery was over and she saw that she had survived.

Since the purpose of the classes is to decrease anxiety and to avoid increasing anxiety, the nurse faces a challenge in preparing the adolescent for labor and delivery. Paula illustrated some of the fright that a 16-year-old has about delivery when the doctor asked her about the kind of anesthesia she wanted for delivery: "I want to be asleep. I do not want to see anything." She adamantly rejected saddle block or epidural anesthesia, which he carefully explained, saying, "I don't want to see anything. My mamma won't sign for me to have anything else." This concluded their pursuit of this discussion.

In special education high school programs, preparation for childbirth classes may be more accessible for teenage clients. Community childbirth classes usually have largely couples attending, which inhibits the single unmarried mother's participation or attendance. Because of this, classes probably are more effective and reach a larger number of teenage clients if they are held in the clinic or facility in conjunction with antepartal care. This poses a problem for those who plan to have a mate as labor coach who is working or attending school during daytime hours. Therefore, it is helpful if classes are offered during both daytime and evening hours to enable selected labor coaches to attend.

Various modes of teaching may be used to present information that the teenager needs without adding to her anxiety. One method of determining a young teenager's knowledge of the labor process is to mold a hollow uterus, using modeling clay, and place an oval form (representing a baby) inside. The teenager is then asked to demonstrate how the baby gets out during labor. A small sock with an elastic top and a tennis ball may also be used in a similar way. Some understanding of cervical effacement and dilatation may be gained through the use of these concrete examples. Explanation of changes in contractions at different phases of labor and of a woman's physical and emotional feelings at these phases may provide knowledge to help her remain in control. It is helpful to stress the individual variation in labor patterns.

Ample time is needed for answering and exploring questions. Sketches and such practical devices as the sock and tennis ball or clay models may create less anxiety than do films. If the young woman becomes highly anxious about trauma to her body, she may not hear what is being taught about the labor process and how to cope with contractions. It has been this author's experience that many very mature women in their twenties or older turn away from films when the actual delivery occurs.

Frequent informal group discussions accompanied by refreshments of cookies and fruit juice or milk at regular clinic visits may result in more successful learning for some. Hearing her peers express feelings and questions that are similar to hers can allay some of her anxiety. She may then pose questions that she was uncomfortable about raising in a one-to-one situation.

PREPARATION FOR INFANT CARE

Because so much of the young woman's energy is directed toward her body changes and her concerns about labor and delivery, antepartal preparation for the infant's care is difficult. Also it is hard for the adolescent, who is present-oriented, to anticipate the infant and the potential needs of the infant. Hatcher[12] observed that the early adolescent in the "draw a baby" test viewed the fetus as an "it" and drew a lifeless stick figure image which was not supported (by cradle or arms). The middle adolescent drew a baby that was highly exaggerated and more conspicuous than drawings of adults, suggesting that she fantasized the pregnancy and fetus as power with which to compete or manipulate. The older adolescent drew mother-infant scenes or placed the infant in a crib. These findings indicate that the middle and older adolescent could be more actively involved in learning something about infant care and development than the early adolescent.

During the second trimester, the pregnant teenager may begin to role play for the mothering role. If she cannot find a babysitting job with an infant or toddler and desires contact with small children, she may be directed to a local day-care center. Volunteer work at a day-care center or church nursery, preferably one that has infants enrolled, can afford her the opportunity for role rehearsal in changing diapers, in feeding and playing with an infant. This kind of role playing is especially helpful to the young woman who has no younger siblings or who has had no contact with small children.

It is helpful in ascertaining the young woman's expectations for her infant and it is sometimes also fun for her to prepare a collage that is described as illustrating something about what life will be like after the baby arrives.* Groups may particu-

* Appreciation is expressed to LaVahn Josten, R.N., M.S., who is a consultant in maternal and child health with the Minneapolis Health Department, for this suggestion. She has found that she derives much helpful information for counseling in this manner.

larly enjoy doing this. A good supply of old magazines for clipping pictures is important. Some of the girls choose pictures of older children to represent their infant. Single girls often include a father playing with the infant. Foods and toys are included as well as mothers involved in various activities with their infants. Something is learned about the young woman's fantasies, perceptions of parenting, and knowledge of babies in this exercise.

The adolescent may express her perceptions of what it will be like after the baby arrives in a game such as "The Pregnancy Game."[13] Such a game is especially good for both of the partners, but if the prospective mother has no partner, the game may be played with two prospective mothers as partners. This particular game has questions on cards which are drawn by players such as, "Your baby is fussy, feels warm, and refuses to eat; what would you do?" and "What are some fun things you and your partner can do with your one-month-old?" The counselor can learn much about the adolescent's expectations and about areas where intensive help will be indicated through a game like this.

In group sessions, young mothers are usually more attentive and enthusiastic when they are focusing on concerns and questions that they have introduced. Baby bath demonstrations, infant care, and such tasks may come across as "dullsville" if they are unsolicited; some pregnant teenagers have helped care for younger siblings and are competent in caretaking tasks. Informal opportunities to teach developmental knowledge should be utilized whenever possible. If the adolescent is not ready to learn infant care antepartally, close one-to-one work is begun with her upon the birth of her infant. The frequent concreteness of the very young adolescent's thinking may make it more difficult to practice an infant bath on a doll; it may be too close to her earlier doll play so that such practice seems "silly" to her.

One 13-year-old primigravida on a tour of the postpartal unit was visibly upset at seeing an infant brought out for a bath demonstration. The nude, squirming baby seemed to create anxiety, and the young woman backed away saying, "I didn't know she meant they would bring the baby in *here*. It's too *cold*." She demonstrated none of the curiosity or amazement that one observes among older women who usually want to move closer to "peek at the baby." She was not ready to identify the fetus growing within her with the actual, active baby she viewed, and she seemed to feel threatened by the overwhelming reality facing her.

Monitoring Maternal and Fetal Health

The professional nurse, as a key figure in providing quality care for the pregnant adolescent, is ipso facto the key figure in monitoring the health of the maternal-fetal unit. The nurse in this pivotal role needs the special knowledge about the young woman that is obtained through a detailed nursing history. Ongoing nursing assessment to keep the nursing history data updated is vital. Life is dynamic, and this dynamic quality of life is very apparent throughout the course of pregnancy. A discussion of the nursing history and ongoing assessment and of the nurse's monitoring for pregnancy-induced hypertension, anemia, and vaginal infections, three of the more common complications in adolescent pregnancy, follows.

NURSING HISTORY

A complete nursing history is taken on a subsequent visit if the milieu was not conducive to this at the initial antepartal visit. If a particular institution requires that all assessment forms be completed at the initial visit, it is helpful to review these and to note gaps. During a second or later visit, the needed information may be obtained. Usually each institution has developed its own standard history and health record forms. There are, however, areas in which knowledge seems helpful in providing quality nursing care for the teenager, and if standard forms do not have space for these areas, an additional page may be added.

In order to establish good communication with the adolescent client, it is important to ascertain her level of understanding and communication skills. Knowing her grade level in high school and whether she is in school provides some knowledge of a baseline both for obtaining further data and for counseling.

Ascertaining the client's knowledge of reproduction, contraception, and pregnancy and the extent of her preparation for the baby produces essential information both for teaching in groups and for individual counseling or counseling for the couple. If the client has had high school biology, she can grasp reproductive concepts more easily. This needs to be established early, so that the young woman is not "talked down to" and yet understands all that is being discussed.

Information is needed about the client's parents—where they live and their marital status (often the parents are separated or divorced and have remarried). A complete family history is important in order to determine the complexity of the household, its socioeconomic status, its stability, the occupations of various members, and the physical and mental health of its members. Hereditary conditions come to light while the family health history is being taken, and indications for special counseling with parents may be identified.

In particular, it is important to determine the client's relationship with her mother or primary caretaker. Is her mother available and willing to help her during the pregnancy and afterward? What does her mother do, if she is employed? How does the adolescent feel about her mother? Does her mother reflect qualities the client would choose in a role model and ego ideal? If the mother is an alcoholic or chronically ill, a foster home or a residential home, such as the Salvation Army or Florence Crittenton centers, may be preferable to her usual home environment. The girl's relationship with her mother affects her assumption of both a feminine and a mothering identity; when the mother cannot fulfill this function, a mother surrogate is needed for the young pregnant girl. If the teenager lost her mother during her early years, this has implications for the kinds of dependency needs that may be expected and that will need to be met during pregnancy and following delivery, if she is to mature and learn to mother.

Next to the parents, the father of the baby has been observed to be the person most supportive of the teenage mother.[14] Therefore, knowledge about the client's relationship with the father of the baby, his response to the pregnancy, the impact of the pregnancy on him, whether they plan to marry, how they are helpful to each other, and her acceptance of his involvement with the pregnancy, labor, and delivery are all important in supervising her care.

If the young woman is continuing the relationship with the partner, with her permission the partner should be invited to participate in counseling and teaching sessions. As was noted in Chapter 11, his knowledge about sexuality and reproduction is no greater than hers. An individual interview with the man will ascertain any special referrals that he feels might be helpful to him; for example, he may prefer a male counselor or he may wish to talk to a social worker or have legal counsel if the couple are unwed.

The client's and her partner's sexual habits are important. The majority of the young women choosing to deliver babies have stable monogamous relationships,[15,16,17] but some may have had many sexual contacts. If so, and if this practice is continued, the client needs more frequent smears and serological tests for venereal disease.

The teenager's hobbies and recreational activities are important. The nine-month wait during pregnancy seems forever to a teenager. Sixteen-year-old Susan illustrated the difficulty of a middle adolescent during this long wait when she was at 26 weeks gestation:

> For all I care, he could come *today*. He moves so much I don't even pay any mind to him anymore. Except when he kicks me up under the ribs. And it hurts me. He kicks so hard. I'm ready to get *rid* of this. I've been sick all month; I haven't even been to school the past two weeks. I couldn't even walk for days, and I can't eat anything. It makes me sick.

Her remarks were related in a very hostile tone and with a very sulky expression. To be pregnant and large and to feel sick is especially miserable for any 16-year-old. Knowing that Susan in this example enjoyed crocheting, the nurse encouraged her to think about items she could crochet. She crocheted booties for her baby and for gifts for her friends at her school who were expecting.

Hobbies may need to be introduced for a deprived adolescent who has not previously been exposed to creative outlets. Hobbies not only offer release of tension, but are also a valuable creative outlet; being able to make something can increase the person's self-esteem. Success in making something may increase her enthusiasm about "making a baby."

An important part of the nursing history is to learn whether the young woman has used or has been exposed to chemicals—either drugs, alcohol, cigarettes, or chemicals where she has worked. Clients who are on drugs or alcohol may also be in an especially poor nutritional state. The adolescent may not be aware of the dangers that threaten infants whose mothers smoke cigarettes and/or drink moderate amounts of alcoholic beverages—i.e., smaller birth weight[18] and mental retardation,[19] respectively. Just as adults continue to smoke despite warnings about hazards to their health, some pregnant adolescents may not quit smoking. Group sessions are a good place to discuss the hazards of cigarettes, alcohol, and other chemicals because peer pressure is probably more effective than the health care worker's strong urging. Long-range effects should be discussed, as in the example of cigarettes; the smaller-at-birth babies resulting from maternal smoking also tend to have more health problems during infancy, possibly because of their initial stunted growth and inhaling their mothers' smoke after birth. Baric and associates[18] stress that in order to change the smoking habits of pregnant women the credibility of existing knowledge must be increased and health education must stress that the absence of ill effects from smoking in previous pregnancies does not guarantee absence in future pregnancies.

Substance abusers (both drugs and alcohol) face increased morbidity for both themselves and their infants. If the method of drug use is injection, the mother is vulnerable to diseases such as hepatitis, endocarditis, thrombophlebitis, abscesses, tetanus, and pulmonary complications, to name a few. Pregnant addicts complying with a methadone treatment program have fewer complications than women on street drugs. Their infants, however, may experience withdrawal symptoms just as infants of mothers on heroin do. Withdrawal symptoms may appear anytime following birth up to two weeks of age; the majority appear within 72 hours.[20] The incidence of infant withdrawal is decreased if the woman does not abuse other drugs or alcohol while she is in a special counseling methadone program that enables her to reduce the dosage to 20 mg or less daily before delivery.[20]

ONGOING NURSING ASSESSMENT

It is essential to obtain information about all of the above items for the nursing history. At each subsequent antepartal visit, the ongoing nursing history and assessment are carried forward by expressing interest in the teenager: ''What are your concerns now?'' ''What has happened since your last visit?'' ''What changes in your body have you noticed in particular?'' ''How do you feel with your changing body?'' ''Does the baby move a lot?'' ''What do you do to get comfortable?'' ''What do you do to relax?'' ''How do you manage your rest periods?'', etc. Questions that focus directly on the teenager and her welfare let her know that you are concerned about her physical and mental health as well as that of the baby. If such questioning as that described above does not fit the client's or the nurse's own styles, the same information may be obtained by the opening phrase, ''Tell me about . . .''

Allowing dependency while encouraging independence as a maturational step is an important facet of prenatal care.[21] Involving the teenager in some of the routine monitoring during pregnancy gives her a sense of independence and control. She may, for example, weigh herself as she comes into the clinic, check her own urine, and record these findings directly on her chart. In most clinics client charts are placed in the examining room, opened to the page for recording these findings. When the young woman is allowed to record directly on the chart an atmosphere of trust is fostered; seeing the chart gives her the feeling that it is not a ''sacred preserve of secrets'' about her but a factual recording of her health status during pregnancy. Most adolescents are anxious to weigh themselves, and head for the scales immediately upon arriving at the clinic.

The fundal height measurements can be shared with the teenage mother, and this knowledge, along with her weight gain, assures her that the baby is growing. When the fetal heart tones are audible, having her listen to them is a very positive reinforcement, just as it is to any mother. When palpating for fetal position, having her feel the head and rump is often exciting to her and reinforces what she may have already surmised. This sort of involvement lends credibility to the idea that a real baby is growing within her—a fact that is sometimes very hard for any woman to really absorb.

The impact of the bodily changes of pregnancy on a young teen who has perhaps only had breast development and pubic hair for a couple of years is profound. The change from a thin body with small, developing breasts to a body with heavy buttocks and thighs, an abdomen covered with striae, and larger breasts with darkened areolae is a startling event that is hard for her to comprehend and accept. Seeing her friends running around in skin-tight jeans and halter tops makes the teenager tend to want to stay home more because she "looks so bad." Withdrawing from activities results in less exercise, which in turn leads to her feeling worse and possibly gaining more. This adolescent needs very sensitive, supportive encouragement from clinic personnel. Involvement in exercise groups practicing for labor and delivery is helpful.

As the teenager becomes more comfortable in the prenatal setting, it is wise to acquaint her with some of the frequently used methods of fetal monitoring. Later if she has to collect urine for a 24-hour estriol excretion, or has to have an oxytocin stress test, she may not be quite as anxious.

PREGNANCY-INDUCED HYPERTENSION

The terms "toxemia of pregnancy" and "pregnancy-induced hypertension" are used interchangeably; pregnancy-induced hypertension is used more often in recent literature. The reason for this may be to differentiate more clearly between hypertension induced by pregnancy and hypertensive disease. Toxemia, or pregnancy-induced hypertension, is one of the unsolved mysteries of obstetrics. Hypotheses about its etiology have included uterine ischemia, hormonal imbalance, nutritional deficiency (amino acid deficiency), placental toxin, climate (high temperature, high humidity, and low barometric pressure), and emotional factors. It seems to be a greater threat in some regions of the United States than in others; for example, the southeastern states continue to have a higher incidence than do the western coastal states. This probably reflects per capita incomes in states rather than regional differences.[9] Termination of the pregnancy continues to be the only cure for the disease. Zuspan[22] demonstrated that increased amounts of epinephrine and norepinephrine are associated with pregnancy-induced hypertension, which indicates that the adrenal gland and sympathetic nervous system are altered. Other factors that may be involved include: "activation of coagulation mechanisms with deposition of circulating fibrin aggregates in the glomeruli, decreased inactivation of pressor amines, and salt and water retention due to renal damage and hormonal changes" (pp. 418–419).[23]

Although hypertension may seem to appear suddenly at an antepartal visit, researchers have shown that the disease is chronic in development.[24] Gant and Worley[24] observed that in 192 primigravid women 16 years old and younger, those who later developed hypertension became increasingly sensitive to angiotensin II fusions as indicated by baseline diastolic blood pressures earlier in their pregnancies. The authors developed a very simple screening test that the nurse can perform, however, the results of which correlate with the presence or absence of angiotensin II. This screening test, called the "rollover test," when done between the twenty-eighth and thirty-second week of pregnancy can identify a potential preeclamptic client as much as three months in advance of symptoms. This is an important preventive aspect, since both mother and fetus are adversely affected several weeks prior to the appearance of hypertension. Persons with positive "rollover tests" developed pregnancy-induced hypertension 76% of the time, and 92% of the persons with negative "rollover tests" maintained normal blood pressures during their pregnancies.

To conduct the "rollover test" the client is placed in a lateral recumbent position, and the diastolic blood pressure is recorded until it appears stable, or for a minimum of 15 minutes. The client is then asked to roll over on her back, and the blood pressure is taken at one and at five minutes. A positive "rollover test" is indicated by an increase in diastolic blood pressure of 20 mm Hg or more.

The Gant and Worley studies suggested that severe pregnancy-induced hypertension, salt restriction, diuretics, and antihypertensive drugs all decrease uteroplacental perfusion. These data reflect the basis for discontinuing the treatments that were common in the 1950s and 1960s for preeclampsia. Salt restriction and diuretics were routinely prescribed in the fifties, and after antihypertenisve drugs were discovered in the sixties, they were added to the treatment regimen.

When a client has a positive "rollover test," steps may be taken either to delay the onset of the disease or to reduce its severity.[25] Bed rest in the lateral recumbent position increases renal blood flow and aids in the elimination of edema.[26] The client with a positive "rollover test" may be advised by her physician to rest for periods each morning and afternoon, and to decrease her activities.

Toxemia of pregnancy has three stages in the disease process: mild preeclampsia, severe preeclampsia, and eclampsia. Mild preeclampsia is characterized by a 30/15 increase in blood pressure noted on two or more occasions six hours apart, or a blood pressure higher than 140/90; edema, weight gain greater than 5 lb/wk (or 2.3 kg), and proteinuria of 0.3 gm/L or more on two occasions six hours apart.[26]

Severe preeclampsia is defined as the presence of one of the following symptoms: blood pressure greater than 160/120; oliguria (24-hour urinary output less than 600 ml); cyanosis or pulmonary edema; visual symptoms (spotting or blurring vision) and/or epigastric pain; and proteinuria greater than 3 to 4 plus on a catheterized urine specimen or more than 5 grams per 24-hour urine specimen.[24] Babson and associates[26] list a blood pressure of 160/110 or greater as being a symptom of severe preeclampsia.

Eclampsia is characterized by convulsions (tonic and clonic) or coma and/or hypertensive crisis or shock following the presence of signs of severe preeclampsia.[26]

Careful monitoring of the teenage client is warranted to observe for edema, sudden weight gains, hypertension, and proteinuria. Gant and Worley[24] advise that the primigravid woman should be admitted to hospital at the first sign of hypertension (any blood pressure over 140/90 in a previously normotensive woman). For the teenage client a lower blood pressure may indicate hypertension. For example, her normal blood pressure may be 90/50, and an increase of 30/15 or over may indicate hypertension. Gant and Worley have observed that proteinuria and edema decrease and the majority are normotensive after one week of decreased activity in the hospital.

A frightening aspect of pregnancy-induced hypertension is its seemingly rapid development to severe preeclampsia with fetal growth retardation or fetal jeopardy. Fetal growth retardation is suggested when sequential growth is not observed and the mother has not gained weight or has lost weight after the thirty-fourth week of pregnancy.[24] A small-for-gestational-age infant may be born, however, when weight gain has occurred. As was pointed out earlier, this may happen if the mother was underweight at conception[10] or smoked heavily.[21] Diagnosis of fetal growth retardation is confirmed by serial ultrasound examinations of fetal thoracic and biparietal diameters.* Meconium-stained amniotic fluid (obtained by amniocentesis) or a positive oxytocin test indicate fetal jeopardy.

The teenager particularly may be very frightened by the required examinations and may need additional, careful interpretation. Her response may be one of anger, hostility, and uncooperativeness if she does not understand the sincere interest in her well-being. An account of an 18-year-old primigravida with hypertension and a four-pound weight gain in one week illustrates the difficulty encountered in working along with the hostility in order to obtain the desired cooperation.[27] To exercise some control, the young woman refused to be admitted directly to the hospital, but chose to go the next day; she demanded that she be given cab fare and be admitted at 1:00 P.M. rather than 9:00 A.M. She seemed to be testing the physician's true interest in her as well as attempting to maintain independence. A lack of understanding on the young woman's part prevented her from seeing the seriousness of her condition, and the physician's concern for her and her infant's life probably overshadowed his understanding of the young woman's strong need for self-esteem and independence at this point in her life. The clinic nurse has an important role in interpreting and clarifying the concerns of both parties in these kinds of situations.

ANEMIA

Periodic monitoring of the hemoglobin helps to verify whether the young woman is taking her iron pills and whether she is eating adequate protein. An indirect way of checking on whether she is taking her iron pills is afforded if she is obtaining the pills at the clinic. If she does not need a new supply at the projected time, she more than likely is not taking the iron. Another method is to ask what color her stools are; if they are not black, she is not taking her iron.

Lynn, a 13-year-old, commented about the iron pills, "They are a little hard to go down sometimes. They get caught right here [points to throat]." Although the pills were difficult for Lynn to swallow, she did take them, as was evidenced in the

---

* Carol Howe, M.S., C.N.M., has observed in her practice that the adolescent fixates on the word "retardation" and it is very difficult to convey that one is referring to "growth retardation." By using the term, "the baby is small," as the reason for a sonogram, less anxiety seems to be evoked in the young woman and her family that the infant is "mentally retarded."

rise of her hemoglobin. Other youthful mothers, however, may balk at taking the iron pills which may make them nauseated and sometimes constipated.

Collaborative efforts with the nutritionist to have the client increase iron intake in the diet are important. If a nutritionist is not available, the nurse counsels the young woman about her food habits.

The finger sticks to check the hemoglobin are viewed as threatening and intrusive by young people and often precipitate anxiety related to fears previously experienced in hospitals or doctor's offices earlier in life. Lynn commented, "They stuck my finger like that when I was in Children's Hospital when I was 8 and had a high fever."

INFECTIONS

The health care worker must maintain openness, trust, and comfort with the client, if an atmosphere is to be achieved in which the adolescent can share her most intimate concerns. Vaginal discharge may be an especially threatening occurrence to the adolescent.* The pervasive odor of a vaginal infection is disturbing and may affect her sexual relationship. The vaginal discharge may be profuse and may leak at inappropriate times, emphasizing her lack of control over a bodily secretion. Often she fears she has a venereal disease and may be hesitant to tell the clinician about a discharge. A statement to the effect that "during pregnancy vaginal infections occur frequently and often have annoying symptoms such as an increased discharge and itching or burning," may facilitate the adolescent's reporting these symptoms. Since the adolescent is highly narcissistic and at the same time hates to be different from others, it is reassuring for her to know that the distasteful occurrence of a vaginal infection is commonplace.

It is important that smears and cultures be made for all complaints of vaginal discharge. The high incidence of gonorrhea, monilia, and trichomonas found among nonpregnant teenagers warrants this practice.[28,29] Venereal disease can be present in the absence of symptoms, however. Mumford and associates[30] found an incidence of 2.4% cases of gonorrhea from smears and cultures from the cervical os of 740 pregnant adolescents aged 10 to 19 years. Virtually none of them had any symptoms, even after intense questioning following the positive smears. If infection occurs during pregnancy, the importance of adequate treatment may be incorporated into teaching about the growth of the fetus during pregnancy. At each phase of fetal development, it can be pointed out which drugs as well as which diseases affect the fetus.

The health care provider must keep in mind that even if the teenager's smears were negative when she first came to the clinic, she may become infected later in her pregnancy. Depending upon her sexual history, smears for gonorrhea may need to be

---

*Two extremes are observed in response to vaginal discharge: No vaginal discharge is visible, and the adolescent asks, "What is that terrible discharge?"; or the vaginal vault is filled and the vulva and legs are chafed, and in response to the practitioner's query, "How long have you had this discharge?" the young woman asks, "What discharge?" Vaginal discharge seems to present extra threat to her body image. (Carol Howe)

repeated later during pregnancy. Gonococcal salpingitis is not a problem after the third month of pregnancy because the chorion laeve fuses with the decidual parietalis and seals the endometrial cavity between the cervix and the oviduct.[31] However, the pregnant teenager may have an asymptomatic infection of the lower genital tract, urinary tract, vagina, or rectum, and if the infection is not detected and treated, the newborn can contract gonorrheal ophthalmia during delivery.[31]

When a syphilis infection occurs during pregnancy, it may go unnoticed if the primary lesion is inside the rectum or vagina since pelvic examinations are not usually repeated during the first two trimesters. Treatment of syphilis during pregnancy usually eliminates the chances of disease in the child.[32] The fetus rarely becomes infected before the 18th week, so adequate treatment before that time prevents infection of the fetus.[31] With untreated syphilis, the infant may be stillborn or born with congenital syphilis. False positive serologic tests in pregnancy are not uncommon; however, a *Treponema pallidum* immobilization test and Reiter's protein complement fixation test should be done and the client's partner should be tested as soon as possible following any positive test so that active treatment may be begun if necessary.[32] It would be well for the nurse to inform the client whose history seems to preclude the possibility of infection with syphilis about the occurrence of false positives and the necessity for follow-up, however. Some women have become so angry at being told their serologic test was positive that they changed physicians, or quit coming to the clinic.

Summary

The teaching and counseling needs of youthful parents-to-be are extensive and have great potential impact on their futures. Good nutritional habits may be learned during pregnancy, important knowledge about sexuality may be gained, and new or additional contraceptive knowledge offers adolescents some measure of responsible control over their future lives. With help from the social system to allow them to remain in school, they can continue the education they will so badly need for economic independence.

Careful monitoring of the health of mother and fetus helps assure a safe outcome for both. Establishing good rapport and communication with the pregnant adolescent is critical in providing quality health care. Both are crucial for obtaining the detailed nursing history and ongoing assessment that provide a basis for interventions.

REFERENCES

1. Semmens, J. P. "Implications of Teen-Age Pregnancy." *Obstet. and Gyn.* 26(1):77–85, 1965.
2. Webb, G. A. "Care of the Pregnant Adolescent." *Pediat. Annals* 4(1):99–109, 1975.
3. Holder, A. R. *Legal Issues in Pediatrics and Adolescent Medicine.* New York: John Wiley & Sons, Inc., 1977.
4. LaBarre, M. "Emotional Crises of School-Age Girls During Pregnancy and Early Motherhood." *J. Am. Acad. Child Psychiat.* 11(2):537–557, 1972.
5. Bryan-Logan, B. N., and Dancy, B. L. "Unwed Pregnant Adolescents: Their Mothers' Dilemma." *Nurs. Clin. N. Am.* 9(1):57–68, 1974.

6. Smith, E. W. "Transition to the Role of Grandmother as Studied with Mothers of Pregnant Adolescents," *ANA Clin. Sessions 1970.* New York: Appleton-Century-Crofts, 1971, 140–148.

7. Dickens, H. O., et al. "One Hundred Pregnant Adolescents, Treatment Approaches in a University Hospital." *Am. J. Pub. Health* 63(9):794–800, 1973.

8. Graham, E. H. "Young Parents' Group." *J. Nurse-Midwif.* 20(1):15–19, 1975.

9. National Academy of Sciences. *Maternal Nutrition and the Course of Pregnancy Summary Report.* Rockville, Md.: U.S. Dept. Health, Education, and Welfare. DHEW Pub. No. (HSA) 75–5600, 1970.

10. Hollingsworth, D. R. "Teenage Pregnancy and Weight Gain." *Briefs* 42(4):55, 1978. Abstracted from "Underweight in Teen Before Pregnancy is Riskier to Fetus," *Ob. Gyn. News* 13(3):43, February 1, 1978.

11. Russell, L. K. "Sexual Counseling: An Approach to the Integration of Sexual Counseling into the Antepartal Management of Teenagers." *J. Nurse-Midwif.* 20(1):24–30, 1975.

12. Hatcher, D.L. "Understanding Adolescent Pregnancy and Abortion." *Primary Care* 3(3):407–425, 1976.

13. Rosenfeld, G., et al. *The Pregnancy Game Resource Book and Rules.* George and Jean Rosenfeld, 5730 River Oak Way, Carmichael, Calif. 95608.

14. Mercer, R. T. "Teenage Motherhood: The First Year. Part I, The Teenage Mother's Views and Responses." *JOGN Nurs.* In press.

15. Lorenzi, M. E., et al. "School-Age Parents: How Permanent a Relationship?" *Adolescence* 12(45):13–22, 1977.

16. Fischman, S. H. "Delivery or Abortion in Inner-City Adolescents." *Am. J. Orthopsychiat.* 47(1):127–133, 1977.

17. Bracken, M. B., et al. "Abortion, Adoption, or Motherhood: An Empirical Study of Decision-Making During Pregnancy." *Am. J. Obstet. & Gyn.* 130(3):251–262, 1978.

18. Baric, L., et al. "A Study of Health Educational Aspects of Smoking in Pregnancy." Perinatal Reprint Series. New York: The National Foundation March of Dimes. Reprinted from *Internat'l J. Health Educ.,* Supplement to 19(2), April–June 1976.

19. Streissguth, A. P. "Maternal Drinking and the Outcome of Pregnancy: Implications for Child Mental Health." *Am. J. Orthopsychiat.* 47(3):422–431, 1977.

20. Kaufman, E. "How Drug Abuse Causes Complications for the Mother and Neonate." *Contemp. OB/GYN* 11(6):32–47, 1978.

21. Frye, B. A., and Barham, B. "Reaching Out to Pregnant Adolescents." *Am. J. Nurs.* 75(9):1502–1504, 1975.

22. Zuspan, F. P. "Pregnancy Induced Hypertension." *Acta Obstet. Gyn. Scand.* 56:283–286, 1977.

23. Wilson, D. R. "Renal Function in Pregnancy." In *Perinatal Medicine.* Baltimore: Williams & Wilkins Co., 1976.

24. Gant, N. F., and Worley, R. J. "The Clinical Management of Pregnancy-Induced Hypertension," In Goldstein, A. I., ed. *Advances in Perinatal Medicine.* New York: Stratton Intercontinental Medical Book Corp., 1977, 185–196.

25. Gant, N. F., and Worley, R. J. "Prospective Laboratory and Clinical Studies of Pregnancy-Induced Hypertension," In Goldstein, A. I. ed. *Advances in Perinatal Medicine.* New York: Stratton Intercontinental Medical Book Corp., 1977, 61–76.

26. Babson, S. G., et al. *Management of High-Risk Pregnancy and Intensive Care of the Neonate.* St. Louis: C. V. Mosby Co., 1975, 155–157.

27. Bomar, P. J. "The Nursing Process in the Care of a Hostile, Pregnant Adolescent." *Mat.-Child Nurs. J.* 4(2):95–100, 1975.

28. Buchta, R. M. "It is Important to Search for Mixed Vaginal Infections in Sexually Active Young Women with Endocervical Gonorrhea." *Clin. Pediat.* 16(11):1001–1002, 1977.

29. Hein, K., et al. "Cervical Cytology: The Need for Routine Screening in the Sexually Active Adolescent." *J. Pediat.* 91(1):123–126, 1977.

30. Mumford, D. M., et al. "Prevalence of Venereal Disease in Indigent Pregnant Adolescents." *J. Reproductive Med.* 19(2):83–86, 1977.

31. Hellman, L. M., and Pritchard, J. A. *Williams Obstetrics,* 14th ed. New York: Appleton-Century-Crofts, 1971.

32. Dwyer, J. M. *Human Reproduction: The Female System and the Neonate.* Philadelphia: F. A. Davis, Co., 1976.

13

The Adolescent Experience
In Labor, Delivery,
and Early Postpartum Period

RAMONA T. MERCER, R.N., PH.D.

The teenager in labor may be handicapped psychologically, cognitively, and physiologically because of her developmental level. The younger adolescent, under 15 years of age—because of her tendency to use denial and her beginning level of problem solving and conceptualization—is usually unprepared for active participation in the labor process. Further, the closer she is to puberty or the age of menarche, the less physiologically mature she is apt to be.

Middle and older adolescents who have had good prenatal care and careful preparation for labor seem to fare better. The adolescent who is 16 and older has the potential to be better prepared psychologically and, because of increased cognitive development and more practice with problem solving, may have a better and more realistic grasp of the situation.

The teenager's preconceived notions about labor and delivery are strongly influential and are intertwined with her emotional and psychological preparation for the experience. Whatever the cultural background of the young woman, she has grown up with some expectations about the childbirth experience. Her responses to pain, to childbirth, to the hospital, doctors, and nurses, are all culturally shaped to some extent. Although it may be quite foreign to her, it is important for the nurse caring for the laboring woman to recognize and respect the client's cultural context. The nurse may learn from the laboring family about their perceptions of, their interpretation of, and their goal for the experience. Only in this sort of sharing context can the childbirth experience proceed as a meaningful, enriching, and growing process for all who are privileged to share it.

The risks the adolescent faces are viewed in the light of research reports, from cultural, psychological, and sociological perspectives. Clinical cases of the young, middle, and older adolescent in labor are presented and the implications for their nursing care are discussed. Because of her intimate role with the laboring family throughout the labor and delivery process, the nurse is a major advocate for the youthful mother and her support system. The nurse also has a major role in the coordination of the new mother's care during the early postpartum period and upon discharge from the hospital. The special needs of the adolescent mother during the postpartum period are discussed within the context of providing the most meaningful and helpful nursing care to assure the health of the young family.

The Adolescent's Labor and Delivery Experience

Research findings were discussed that documented physiological risks for the pregnant adolescent and her infant in Chapter 11, The Pregnant Adolescent, and in Chapter 12, Prenatal Care for the Adolescent. These physiological risks are discussed in relation to the psychological and sociological factors that are interacting with the labor and delivery experience and that affect the risks perhaps even more than does age. Cultural variations, ethnic anatomic differences, and socioeconomic status are all interacting and will have an impact on the nature and outcome of the adolescent's labor and delivery experience. The special risks for both the adolescent and her infant are discussed and are related to the psychosocial stressors that any woman in labor experiences.

QUALITY AND LENGTH OF LABOR

While no differences between the labor of the younger mother and that of the older control subjects were observed in two studies,[1,2] uterine dysfunction has been observed to be significantly higher in the youthful mother 14 years old and younger.[3] Jovanovic[4] observed an increased rate of uterine hypertonia in the mother 17 years old and younger. Prolonged labor was observed in the "juvenile" mother under 14[5] and under 17 years of age.[6,7,8]

In another study of over 12,000 teenagers 13 to 19 years of age, both extremes in labor were observed.[9] A large number of mothers had precipitous labors (less than three hours) and a large number had prolonged labor (longer than 20 hours). For subjects under the age of 15, the incidence of prolonged labor was double that of the general population, encompassing all ages. A large number of the adolescents were multiparas (2,955 in the 15- to 19-year-old group); 30% of these 15- to 19-year-old multiparas experienced a labor that was under three hours for all three stages. Subjects in this large study were all military dependents. They represented every social level; 99% were married, and 10% were black.[10]

In general, prolonged labor seems to occur more frequently in the younger adolescent, 12 to 14 years of age. The younger adolescent is probably more anxious, has less understanding of the process over which she has no control, and has a less sophisticated mode of adaptation than does the older adolescent.

Prodromal or false labor often occurs late in the third trimester; these contractions are the usual Braxton Hicks contractions that occur throughout pregnancy, but they have become more painful and dystonic.[11] The teenage primigravida, like any other gravida, may experience prodromal labor, which results in very slow cervical effacement.[11] This advance cervical preparation may explain some of the precipitate labors observed.

CONTRACTED PELVIS

As was discussed earlier on page 248, the greater the adolescent's age beyond menarche, the more likely it is that the pelvis is fully mature for childbearing. A higher incidence of contracted pelvises was observed in studies of teenagers 14 years old and younger,[12] and 16 years old and younger.[7] Aiman[13] controlled for both socioeconomic status and race in his study of the adolescent's pelvic size and the frequency of contractions. He found that the transverse dimensions (inlet transverse, interspinous, and intertuberous) of the 16-year-old and younger adolescent's pelvis were almost always significantly smaller, and that the pelvis was contracted with a greater frequency than the pelvis of the older woman. This was true for both the black and the white adolescent.

Two studies with African black teenage subjects suggested differences in the size and the angle of inclination of the pelvises of black and white teenagers; these findings should be considered when viewing differences in teenagers.[14,15] A high angle of pelvic inclination was observed in the black subjects.[14] The fetal head was rarely engaged in the black teenagers prior to labor, and fetal engagement prior to onset of labor was not a prerequisite for vaginal delivery. These reports show the importance of controlling for ethnic background when comparing the adolescent's and the older woman's pelvises.

CESAREAN BIRTH

Aiman[13] cautioned that the adolescent's smaller pelvic size did not mean she could not deliver vaginally; vaginal delivery is influenced by fetal size, position, flexion and molding, and the efficacy of uterine contractions. Although Deunhoelter and associates[12] observed that the adolescent under 15 had a smaller pelvic inlet than the older woman and that a larger number were delivered by cesarean section (49:33), the difference was not statistically significant. There were twice as many midforceps deliveries in the age 14 and younger group than in the older group (20:10). In Coates's[3] study the percentage of primigravidas over 14 years of age who delivered by cesarean section was higher than those 14 and younger (5.4%:4.4%), although the diagnosis of contracted pelvis was higher for the 14 and younger group (15.3%:11.3%). In a study of 100 unwed adolescents 17 years old and younger, 19% had cesarean deliveries, and 8% had midforceps deliveries.[16] Ninety-five percent of the sample were nonwhite and from low socioeconomic backgrounds.

Writers have conjectured about whether there is less of a tendency to do a cesarean delivery on a very young primigravida who has many childbearing years ahead of her. The disproportionate amount of anxiety that the teenager probably experiences could result in a prolonged labor that does not require abdominal delivery. A comparative study by Smith and associates[17] of the impact of a comprehensive antepartum psychosocial educational program on medical outcome supports this concept. A sample of 126 adolescents enrolled in weekly group classes beginning at the second trimester had a lower frequency of cesarean births than a matched control group who had not attended the special classes. The researchers suggested that the classes and demonstrations concerning labor and delivery led to more efficient labor with less dystocia. However, with the improved technology of fetal monitoring during labor and increasing knowledge about the potential of neurological damage to infants during difficult forceps deliveries, the number of cesarean births among teenagers will probably increase in proportion to the number occurring among older women.

ABRUPTIO PLACENTAE

Because of the increased rate of pregnancy-induced hypertension in the young primigravida it is not surprising that one study of 1,104 mothers 16 years old or younger found a higher than expected rate of abruptio placentae with hypofibrinogenemia as a complication.[18] An earlier retrospective study found a higher rate of abruptio placentae in a population of women who were over 20, even though preeclampsia occurred at a higher rate in the population who were under 20.[19] Placenta previa was almost totally absent from the under-20 population. Despite the conflicting reports, vigilance must be maintained in the care of the pregnant adolescent so that symptoms of pregnancy-induced hypertension are treated promptly and untoward complications such as severe toxemia and abruptio placentae are avoided.

GENITAL LACERATION

Briggs[8] observed that the most frequently occurring intrapartal complications for teenage mothers were genital lacerations (14.4%), but an 11.5% incidence of midforceps and forceps rotations was observed. All lacerations observed among young teenagers by Hassan and Falls[1] were cervical. In a study reported by Kreutner and Hollingsworth,[20] 42 percent of 394 consecutively delivered adolescents suffered lacerations during delivery (14.2 percent 3rd degree, 13.5 4th degree, 7.4 urethral, and 3.1 cervical). The teenager's genital tract appears to be more vulnerable to laceration than the more mature woman's.

RISKS TO THE INFANT

Prematurity and low birth weight (2,500 grams [5 pounds 8 ounces] or less), and perinatal, neoonatal, and infant morbidity rates are all higher for infants of teenagers than for infants of women over 20.[21] Although the risk of fetal loss is not particularly high for the teenage primipara, it increases greatly for the teenage multipara.[21] Low birth weight contributes not only to higher mortality rates, but also to higher neurological defects, mental retardation, and retrolental fibroplasia. Prematurity is the leading cause of neonatal deaths for all infants, regardless of maternal age.

Although Semmens[9] found no differences in the rate of premature birth between teenagers and the general population, he observed a 100% increase in perinatal mortality in mature infants of mothers under 15. Semmens, however, did *not* have a predominantly lower socioeconomic sample, in contrast to samples of most studies done in county and university clinics. All 12,137 subjects were dependents of military personnel. In lower socioeconomic levels of society, both the concomitant state of malnutrition and environmental factors may account for prematurity and the increased rates of perinatal morbidity and mortality more than does maternal age. One study found that although the incidence of low birth weight was not observed to be consistently higher for the younger age group, it was higher in short women and in lower-class women.[22] Conclusions about prematurity rates among teenage mothers should be based on carefully controlled samples having comparable socioeconomic levels and comparable prenatal care. Prematurity was shown to vary little according to maternal age when women were classified by family income group, although a much larger proportion of women under 20 had low incomes than did older women.[23]

The discussion on prematurity in Chapter 11 suggested that physiological immaturity, including incomplete development of the myometrium, may contribute to the premature birth rate.[19,24] The physiological factors related both to immaturity and to nutrition seem to be interacting with sociological factors in accounting for high rates of prematurity and low birth weight among adolescents.

Menken[23] noted that biological factors play a large role in neonatal death rates and environmental factors play a large role in infant death rates. If the teenager is under 15 years of age, her infant is 2.4 times more likely to die during the first year than the infant born to a mother 20 to 24 years old; if the mother is 15, her infant is twice as likely to die in the first year as an infant born to a mother 20 to 24 years old.[20]

In one study, when weights were averaged, black infants weighed less than the white infants by 96 grams, or about three and one half ounces.[6] This raises the question of whether black infants may have a lower average birth weight, and whether, in the studies with high rates of prematurity, the babies may be small but not necessarily premature. Dott and Fort[25] observed that infants of teenage mothers who were white and married were at greater risk than infants of mothers who were black and single. Could a factor contributing to the increased risk for the white infant be that the black infants may have been more mature? Dott and Fort found that the adolescents' infant death rate was higher when prenatal care was poor or limited for both races. Smith and associates[17] observed that adolescents enrolled in a special intensive educational program delivered infants with higher birth weights than adolescents not enrolled in the program. The infants of mothers under 16 in the special educational program had higher Apgar scores. Antepartal class participation probably leads to better utilization of all health services and to better health care practices, both of which are crucial to the young mother and her infant.

PSYCHOSOCIAL STRESSORS IN LABOR AND DELIVERY

Almost every woman facing labor and delivery has some fear and anxiety about what faces her, particularly if she is having her first child. She fears possible mutilation or injury, and even possible death, for herself. She is concerned about injury to her baby or whether the baby will be normal and free of defects. She has fears about her ability to cope with many unknown factors—the pain, the labor process, the hospital environment, and her ability to maintain control in the situation. The pregnant adolescent experiences the same fears, but perhaps to a greater extent, and she has less ability to verbalize them. In Chapters 11 and 12 some clinical examples of fears expressed by adolescents approaching labor were given.

One's ability to cope with the labor process is dependent upon one's usual coping mechanisms, level of psychosexual development, cultural supports and cultural conditioning, and attitudes and feelings about the pregnancy. Because she has had less experience, the adolescent has less sophisticated coping mechanisms. The labor process has the potential of imposing varying degrees of trauma according to the individual's psychosexual development or level of ego functioning. Yet the labor experience also has the potential of facilitating psychosexual development and increasing self-esteem. If cultural supports are available to the youthful mother, if she has been culturally shaped or prepared for an early parenting role, the labor experience will more readily enhance her development. If the adolescent's pregnancy aroused much anger and discord in her family, and there is little acceptance for her child, the labor experience may be more traumatic for her.

PSYCHOSOCIAL CHANGES AND BEHAVIORAL RESPONSES DURING LABOR

Psychosocial changes occur in the woman as labor progresses. There is an increasing constriction of her ego, or self, so that toward the end of labor only the present moment and concern for her survival are within her perceptual field of focus.[26] Her level of functioning becomes increasingly dependent on and interdependent with others as labor progresses.[27]

During the latent phase of labor (from onset of contractions to 5 centimeters dilatation), the woman experiences a surge of energy and activity; she is both happy and relieved that she is finally in labor. Her anxiety level is mild; she is very alert, however, as she sees, hears, and grasps more. She is able to use her increased sensitivity for learning so that this level of anxiety facilitates the learning process.[28] As the latent phase nears its end, her anxiety level increases and her perceptual field narrows, although she still focuses with direction. Her autonomic responses to the increasing stress of advancing labor include flushing or pallor, deeper respirations, nausea and vomiting, dry mouth, and diaphoresis.[28]

During the active phase of the first stage of labor (from five to seven centimeters dilatation) the woman's anxiety level increases to moderate or severe levels of anxiety with a rapid reduction and possible distortion of her perceptual field.[28] She is increasingly dependent on others to maintain ego control. Her ego adaptive mechanisms may include depression, hostility, anger, withdrawal, and regression.[28]

During the transitional phase of the first stage of labor (from eight to ten centimeters dilatation) the woman's anxiety level usually reaches severe or panic levels.[28] She may dissociate from reality to prevent panic, as is indicated by her irrational mumbling and general lack of awareness of the environment. The severe pain she experiences contributes to her death fears. She cannot make decisions at this time, and she fears that she will be abandoned. Her autonomic reactions include beads of perspiration over her lip or abdomen, shaking, chills, and nausea and vomiting.[28] She is increasingly more withdrawn and amnesic, and she feels that she cannot go on.

During the second stage of labor (from complete dilatation until birth of the baby) her severe to panic level of anxiety may continue.[28] She may feel as if she is tearing or ripping and may have an intense desire to have a bowel movement yet fear she will soil everything involuntarily. She experiences a burning sensation as her perineum stretches to allow passage of the infant's head. She responds with aggressive, grabbing behavior at anyone within reach in her last attempts to maintain ego function.

During the third stage of labor (from delivery of the baby until delivery of the placenta) her anxiety level usually decreases to mild or moderate levels.[28] Any pain she experiences may be intensified by her perceived threats to self, by any critical remarks or behaviors from others, or by feelings of alienation experienced during labor.

THE TEENAGER'S RESPONSE

Anxiety and fear may account for much of the variability in the labor patterns that have been observed in the youthful mother. *Any* woman entering the labor and delivery suite experiences some anxiety and feeling of threat; for the teenager, because of her inexperience and lack of independence, anxiety and feelings of threat are greatly enhanced. The teenager probably has greater fears about damage to her body (via being cut, torn, bruised, or otherwise mutilated) and about what this will mean for her future health, than the older woman who has experienced a mature anatomical size for a longer period of time. Feelings of anxiety or helplessness about possible physical damage reinforce feelings that much of what lies ahead in the birth process is out of the realm of her control. Adaptive behavior in any threatening situation involves acquiring sufficient information, maintaining internal organization, and possessing autonomy.[29] The teenager without adequate information, who has an immature ego, and who feels helpless, will experience more difficulty in adjusting to the labor process.

The adolescent's higher degree of anxiety has its physiological sequelae: the autonomic nervous system's fight or flight mechanism is triggered by the release of adrenalin into the bloodstream which causes vasoconstriction of the blood vessels. Adrenalin (epinephrine) activates both alpha and beta receptors. Alpha receptors contract muscle fibers, whereas beta receptors relax or inhibit the contraction of muscle fibers. Experimental intravenous injections of epinephrine in term gravidas in early labor depressed uterine tonus initially; uterine tonus increased following the injection.[30] Infused epinephrine diminished uterine activity in both spontaneous and oxytocin-induced labors; increased tonus occurred after the infusion was discontinued in the spontaneous labors.[31] Epinephrine can cause vasoconstriction in uterine blood vessels and uterine ischemia. Studies have also demonstrated that bradycardia and acidosis occur in the monkey's fetus when the mother is subjected to stress.[32] These examples demonstrate the degree to which anxiety and fear have the potential of decreasing the blood flow to the fetus and of depressing or increasing the tonus of the uterus. After a vaginal examination, a frightened 16-year-old may experience diminished uterine contractions for a time, followed by hyperactive contractions, if she secretes sufficient epinephrine in her frightened state.

Friedman observed four particularly stressful periods during parturition: false labor or prodromal stress, transposition stress, transition, and the stage of expulsion.[11] The teenager's stress would also be expected to be exacerbated during the same four periods. Friedman observed that the psychological stress of the transposition phase, when the woman leaves her warm, comfortable, and familiar surroundings, often causes uterine contractions to become erratic or to cease; or, the severity of the pain experienced may be out of proportion to the intensity of the contractions. This observation supports findings about the effect of systemic release of epinephrine during anxiety.

Animal studies with mice have demonstrated that disturbances during labor and delivery or following the birth of a first pup (rotating from familiar cage to a cage without shelter and contaminated with cat urine; or holding the laboring mouse between cupped hands) resulted in prolonged labor and an increased number of stillbirths.[33,34,35] These findings led the researchers to raise the question of whether the disturbances that the poverty-stricken mother faces in laboring away from her familiar environment in a strange hospital could account for higher infant mortality rates in this group. Does the high anxiety of a teenage mother during her labor experience contribute to the observed prolonged labor and higher infant mortality rates?

Pain also increases anxiety during labor. Perceived pain, whether it was either less or worse than expected, was observed to be directly proportional to the length of labor.[36] Although the stimulus for labor pain—dilatation and pressure—is similar for each woman, her perception of the pain varies according to her past experiences, attitudes, judgments, mood, fatigue, emotional status, and the importance or significance attached to pain itself. Pain is a unique subjective and sensory experience that an individual describes variously according to motivational, affective, and cognitive functioning.

Pain tolerance has been observed to vary according to age, sex, and race.[37] In this study by Woodrow and associates, it was found that pain tolerance decreased with increased age, men tolerated more pain than women, whites had a higher pain tolerance than blacks, and Asians had the lowest pain tolerance.

A woman's cultural background influences her attitudes and feelings about pain, how she will respond to it and how she will cope with it. Culture also dictates the kind of help a woman receives in labor and whether birth is seen as an illness or a normal occasion, an open sexual event or one to be kept quiet and secret.[38] The pregnant woman's ritualistic and/or coping behaviors often conflict with those of the nursing staff. Moans or screams, acceptable expressions in many cultures, may not be tolerated, and the laboring woman will most likely be told, "You will soon have a sore throat and exhaust yourself." If the woman has been taught, and believes, that "a knife under the bed cuts the pain," why not permit a knife under the bed? Some cultural beliefs do not interfere with or in any way impede excellent maternity care; these should be respected and worked with. For example, in the Hispanic culture, common beliefs about labor suggest several expectations that a teenager in this culture might have:

> If a pregnant woman goes outside during the eclipse of the moon, the eclipse will cause either an abortion, a deformity of the baby, or a stillbirth.
> If labor occurs during a full moon, the birth will be fast and easy, and the infant is more likely to be a girl.
> If labor occurs during the new "thin" moon, the labor will be long and hard and can last as long as three days, and the infant is more likely to be a boy.
> In the absence of a full or new moon, male infants usually lead to an early and fast labor, but females are more likely to be late and give a long, hard labor.
> Pregnancy and labor are viewed as an "illness." When a person is ill many persons gather in the room because spirits of the well give strength to the spirit of the ill person.*

The position that the laboring woman customarily assumes is culturally defined. Propped or upright positions have been proven to be advantageous in shortening the length of labor.[39,40] In many cultures the laboring woman may pull on a rope or an assistant and rock her trunk while her pelvis remains steady. A hundred years ago, black women living in the southeastern United States were observed to choose the kneeling posture; with their buttocks on their heels, they glided forward and backward during labor.[41] Has medical interference with a cultural practice of upright position resulted in prolonged labors for this group of people who perhaps have a different pelvic plane and different pelvic measurements?

Formal education and preparation for childbirth contribute to a more satisfying and a less difficult labor. Persons who have reached higher levels of education frequently also have higher incomes, and usually seek an individualized type of care and preparation for childbirth. The woman who attends Lamaze classes has been observed to be better educated,[42,43,44] to be more internally controlled,[42,44] to be more aggressive in late pregnancy,[42] to view childbirth as a positive experience, to breastfeed more frequently, and to have the father of the baby in the delivery room.[42] We can conjecture about the adolescent's placement in these categories. Often, the adolescent does not have a senior high school level of education. Jovanovic's observation that hypertonic uterine activity was a common problem in teenagers who had little or no prenatal care suggests the importance of all facets of preparation in labor.[4]

All negative antecedent factors in a woman's life history or self-concept and any

*Peggy Goebel, R.N., M.S., recorded these beliefs while working with mothers in the San Francisco area and Guatemala.

negative experiences during pregnancy have an impact on her childbirth experience.[45] What about the adolescent who has been deprived emotionally, or financially? How has the trauma of telling her parents about the pregnancy and resolving the initial crisis, as was discussed in the last chapter, conditioned her for her experience in childbirth?

The teenager's mother, relatives, and friends also play an important role in her expectations. Negative experiences related by others often lead to negative expectations for self and a negative labor experience.[46] The special psychological and sociological risks of the pregnant teenager all have relevance here.

Nursing Care of the Adolescent During Labor and Delivery

This section is approached by presenting clinical examples of the early, middle, and late adolescent in labor. Nursing care is discussed along with each case. Focus should be directed to the individual response to labor and whether the physiological or behavioral response seems related to age.

THE EARLY ADOLESCENT

The early adolescent is not only more vulnerable to increased risks during labor and delivery, but she has less sophisticated mechanisms for coping with and adapting to stressful situations. Her fantasies about her infant are unrealistic. Her expectations of labor and delivery perhaps are equally unrealistic.

Lucy

Lucy became pregnant and delivered when she was 14 years old. She was a tall, large-framed, Caucasian, and looked as if she were 18 or 19. Her grandmother was her only family support. Her mother had kicked her out of the house after she had refused to have an abortion, and she went to live with her grandmother. Lucy had no prenatal preparation for childbirth.

Lucy entered the labor suite at 3:00 A.M., in early labor; she was 2 centimeters dilated, 90% effaced, with the fetal head at 0 station. She had mild contractions every ten minutes, and her membranes were intact. Her aged grandmother came to the hospital with her. At 6:30 A.M., Lucy told the nurse, "I was scared to come to the hospital. I've never been sick enough to be in the hospital and didn't know what was going to happen." Lucy related some of her history:

> I lived with my Mom and older brother before I moved in with Grandma. I was skipping school and running around a lot. I was just sick of school. I started running around with older fellows. I didn't even worry about missing periods. They weren't regular anyway. After I had skipped several months, I finally told Mom, and the old bag went into hysterics. She took me to the doctor's and when we found out I was pregnant, she wanted me to get an abortion. I told her she wasn't going to screw with me anymore, and I would have this kid if I wanted to. That's when she kicked me out and I went to live with my grandmother. I haven't seen her since. My grandmother understands me better.

Lucy also shared the fact that her father had left home when she was four, and had never come back. She did not reveal the name of her expected infant's father and stated that she did not intend to do so. She expected to receive child support from Welfare and to continue living with her grandmother. She did not intend to return to school, saying, "I hate school."

Since Lucy was in the early latent phase of labor, an assessment was made of her knowledge of the labor and delivery process. Lucy said, "No, I don't know anything about what is happening, except Grandma says it will hurt like hell." Not only was Lucy unprepared, but she had some negative information about childbirth.

Lucy responded to basic instruction about labor and breathing patterns as if it were some sort of a game. Terms that Lucy could understand were used as the nurse explained how the cervix dilated and how discomfort could be alleviated with relaxation and concentrated breathing. Lucy practiced the slow, deep respirations for early labor and rapid, shallow respirations and panting for later labor quite willingly, however.

Lucy was also encouraged to get out of bed and walk around. She walked to the nursery with the nurse and there she became very excited upon seeing the babies. "Aren't they so cute," she exclaimed, and as she pointed to a large baby girl, she said, "I'm going to have a baby just like that one, all pink and cuddly."

When breakfast arrived, Lucy was upset that she received no solid food. The nurse explained to her that digestive processes are slowed during labor and that the stomach may not empty for hours; she then asked Lucy if she liked Popsicles. Lucy said, "I would rather have a hamburger, but I will settle for a Popsicle." A box of Popsicles was ordered from the main kitchen, and Lucy enjoyed them immensely during her early labor. Lucy was also encouraged to void regularly.

By 8:00 A.M., Lucy was 4 centimeters dilated and 95% effaced, and she told the doctor that she was now hurting more. He decided to do a paracervical block. He carefully explained what he intended to do, but when Lucy caught a glimpse of the needle, she began squirming and screaming. She continued to struggle and shriek throughout the procedure. Although one nurse quietly and calmly encouraged her, "You're doing well," she had to be restrained by a second nurse. Within five minutes after receiving the paracervical block, however, Lucy had relaxed and requested that the television be turned on.

Lucy's grandmother returned (she had gone home to rest because Lucy was given a mild barbiturate on admission), and Lucy said, "Everything is fine, Granny, you didn't have to come back yet." Her grandmother assured her that she came because she wanted to be with her. Lucy told her grandmother how well she had done with the injection to relieve the pain. The nurse's encouragement, "You're doing well," apparently was heard and was helpful to her amidst her screams of fear. Her grandmother praised her for this, and Lucy smiled with satisfaction. Her self-esteem was bolstered as she received recognition from her major support person.

Lucy remembered the instructions about slow, deep respirations. She did well with the contractions for an hour or so and relaxed well between them. As the frequency and intensity of Lucy's contractions increased, she began to moan and to breathe very rapidly. She asked, "Why does it hurt so much?" Her grandmother replied, "It will get a lot worse, honey." Lucy, pale and wan, complained of dizziness. The nurse turned her on her left side, lowered the head of the bed, and repeated the breathing instructions, encouraging her to breathe very slowly; she explained that she had hyperventilated from breathing too rapidly. Lucy, now in the active phase of labor, was weary and focusing more intensely on her pain. Lucy screamed, ''I've got to have some help. I need some painkiller.'' Her grandmother patted her hand and said, ''Now, Lucy, you try to be good. I told you how it would be.'' At this, Lucy, now distraught, screamed, ''Get out of here, you old bitch.''

The grandmother stepped back, her face registering a shocked expression. The nurse asked her to step outside the room into the hall. There the nurse interpreted to the grandmother the changes in behavior that occur during the active phase of labor, and Lucy's increasing feelings of panic and aggressiveness. The nurse explained that Lucy did not mean what she had said and that her outburst was her desperate way of coping, of trying to maintain control over what was happening to her body. The grandmother expressed appreciation for this explanation and went for a coffee break as suggested.

The doctor was notified that Lucy needed relief from pain; she screamed so loudly that he heard the screams over the phone. The nurse continually tried to calm and quiet Lucy by coaching her with her respirations during contractions, by frequent position changes, and by sacral massage. She screamed, ''Don't touch me,'' as she turned from side to side and pulled her hair. Her face was red and perspiring.

The doctor returned and gave her a second paracervical block, amid a struggle no less agitated than the one that accompanied the first paracervical block. He told her, ''You will have less pain soon. You will get through this fine!'' He also assured her that it would not be much longer for her. Lucy's aggressive, hostile behavior as the labor progressed was similar to that usually occurring with any woman. Her screams of ''don't touch me'' and ''get out of here,'' were panic responses indicating a need for emotional support. One of a laboring woman's greatest fears is that she will be left alone. It was very important for the nurse to accept Lucy's hostile and aggressive behavior without recrimination. Lucy, because of her immaturity and lack of external support resources, perhaps had a lower stress tolerance level than some mothers might have. Lucy had the ability to focus, with direction from the nurse and the doctor. The doctor's telling her at the time of the second paracervical block, ''I know you will get through just fine,'' gave her positive feedback that she badly needed for maintenance of her ego. Perhaps it assuaged her deepest fear, that she might die.

By noon, when the doctor examined Lucy, she had entered the transition phase of labor. He ruptured the membrane and ordered Demerol 50 mg and Vistaril 10 mg to be given intramuscularly. The medication helped Lucy to relax shortly. She had hyperventilated again and was screaming loudly. The medication enabled Lucy to breathe more slowly as she groaned slightly. At 2:00 P.M., however, she began screaming loudly, ''I have to push. Get this kid out of me!'' Lucy was nauseated and vomited a small amount. She began crying. She was bathed with a cool cloth and comforted by the information that the baby would soon be here. Since she was now completely dilated, she was encouraged to push, which she did very effectively.

Lucy was transferred to the delivery room unhurriedly, but it was difficult for her to grasp what was happening. She received a saddle block, which precipitated a fighting, screaming ordeal. As soon as she experienced pain relief, she quieted.

With constant coaching, encouragement, and praise for her pushing efforts, she soon pushed a big boy, weighing 4,140 grams (9 pounds, 2 ounces), over a midline episiotomy. Lucy said, "I had wanted a girl." The baby cried immediately, and Lucy said, "Well, he has a big mouth like me." Lucy fondled the baby and smiled at him when he was handed to her; she said, "Well, it's you and me against the world now, baby." Lucy stated that she planned to breast-feed her son. Later in the recovery room she told the nurse, "Now I have a real live baby doll to play with." Her grandmother smiled with pleasure. Lucy was in a gay and talkative mood the next day when several of her teenage girl friends were visiting her and admiring her baby.

The nurse caring for Lucy during labor was able to establish a trusting relationship during the labor process. Because of the nurse's simple, concrete descriptions of the labor process and respiration techniques for coping, Lucy was able to maintain control much of the time. Rather than become discouraged by Lucy's seemingly flippant and playful attitude during these explanations, the nurse realized that Lucy was responding as a 14-year-old child. Warm supportive care through touch and encouragement helped meet her dependency needs.

This 14-year-old girl had an unrealistic concept about caring for an infant: she perceived him as something to play with. Her lack of feeling of support from significant others, "It's you and me against the world now, baby," suggests that she is at risk for parenting. Lucy will need close follow-up by public health nurses and a social worker to ensure her growth and that of her infant.

DONNA

Donna, a 15-year-old black primigravida, gained only 4.6 kilograms (10 pounds) during her pregnancy; her hemoglobin was 11.7 grams and her hematocrit 34.4%. Her close support system included her mother, boyfriend, and sisters. The mother and boyfriend took turns staying with her during labor. Her sisters and several friends waited in the waiting room. Donna had attended the high school for pregnant students and had had classes on pregnancy, labor and delivery, and child care. Labor began exactly one month after her estimated date; however, since her periods had been irregular, establishing an exact EDC was difficult.

When Donna was admitted at 7:00 A.M., she was one fingertip dilated, with the fetal head at minus 1 station. A large sign on the labor room door read "No one under 16 allowed." Donna vomited shortly after admission and was tense and anxious during the day. At 10:00 A.M. her membranes ruptured spontaneously and were meconium-stained; she was 3 centimeters dilated and completely effaced. Since she was continuing to vomit, she was given Vistaril 50 mg and Nisentil 40 mg intramuscularly at 10:40 A.M. This helped Donna to relax and rest quietly. An ultrasonic transducer for monitoring the fetal heart was positioned on Donna's abdomen.

At 1:30 P.M. she became agitated, and a drop in the fetal heart rate was noted. Donna was placed on her left side. She was now 7 centimeters dilated, and the fetal head was at plus 1 station. Turning on her side was helpful; the fetal heart rate immediately returned to within normal limits. Donna's mother and her boyfriend gave her support by holding her hand and rubbing her forehead or her back.

The nurse who planned to stay with Donna throughout the remainder of her labor and her delivery entered her room around 2:00 P.M. and introduced herself. Donna looked at her, and then looked away. The nurse told her that she was doing a good job and that she would sit with her and be there if she needed her. Donna did not respond to this. As the nurse checked Donna's vital signs, she asked her if she would like to hear the baby's heart. Donna nodded and the nurse turned the audio on so that Donna could hear. Donna listened, and the nurse commented that the baby's heart sounded good. Donna smiled momentarily, then cast her eyes downward. The nurse squeezed Donna's hand and wiped her brow with a damp cloth. The nurse realized that Donna at this stage of labor (nearing transition) would be serious, less communicative, and possibly using withdrawal as a coping mechanism.

Donna quietly sighed. As a contraction began, the nurse slowly and quietly coached, "Take a deep breath down to your tummy, slowly, good; now, let it out. Good. It's almost over now, another deep breath, good. All over." Donna looked up and established eye contact for the first time, but she still did not speak.

Donna did not answer when asked how she was feeling, but looked, wide-eyed, at the nurse. When asked if she would like medicine for pain, she shook her head no, and turned towards her boyfriend.

The nurse then told Donna that she would rub her back; she asked Donna to squeeze her hand when a contraction came and said she would breathe with her during the contraction. The nurse rubbed Donna's back for 15 minutes, then sat in a nearby chair. Donna spoke to the nurse for the first time: "Why did you stop rubbing my back? It feels good." The nurse now sensed the dependency in this young laboring woman, as well as withdrawal, and she resumed rubbing Donna's back. Donna smiled.

Around 3:15 P.M. Donna said, "I have to go to the bathroom—no—I want to push." The nurse had the boyfriend rub Donna's back as she went to get the doctor to check Donna. Donna was now 8 centimeters dilated and the fetal head was at plus 2 station. The doctor encouraged her, "You are doing a great job, keep it up." The nurse interpreted to Donna that the baby's head had moved lower and that that was why she had suddenly felt a need to push. Donna was encouraged to pant in order to avoid pushing. Donna became more restless, although she remained silent. She began to tremble and perspire. Her boyfriend left the room and her mother entered. "Oh, Mama, it hurts so bad," Donna said, then turned to the nurse and commanded, "Don't stop rubbing my back." It seemed that Donna could now express what she was feeling; she could act dependent yet be directive. Perhaps she had not felt free to do so when her boyfriend was in the room. Her stoic quietness may have been part of her playing an adult role to help support her frightened boyfriend's ego.

Donna's mother gently stroked her head and said, "It's all right, baby." Donna continued, "I want to push. It hurts so bad." Her mother said, "It won't be long. Mama knows, honey." This quiet assurance of her progress and of her mother's understanding seemed to help Donna gain control at this difficult point of labor. The nurse again showed Donna how to pant, and panted with her; Donna was able to do this.

The fetal heart rate dropped to below 100, and positioning Donna on her side did not help. Her bed was placed in Trendelenburg position and the oxygen mask was placed on her face. The fetal heart rate returned to the 120 to 140 range. The doctor examined Donna and told her that she was almost complete, and that with a few more contractions she could push. Donna said, ''I don't want this thing on my face, I can't breathe.'' The rationale for the mask was explained—that both she and her baby needed it—but Donna was frightened and her anxiety had reached a panic level as she said, ''Please, I don't want this thing.'' The nurse held Donna's hand; she encouraged Donna to take slow deep breaths and talked slowly to her.

By 4:15 P.M. Donna was completely dilated and began pushing. She said, ''I feel like I have to go to the bathroom—or I'm going to rip.'' The nurse explained that the baby's head was right down on the perineum and that even though the pressure of the baby's head caused that sensation, Donna would not rip. Donna asked, ''Will I bleed? Will I tear?'' Her short, disjointed phrases all focused on herself and on her fear of mutilation. She was extremely vulnerable at this point.

Donna continued pushing, with much coaching, encouragement, and praise for her hard work. Her mother went with her into the delivery room. The physician did a pudendal block, an episiotomy, and a low forceps delivery. Her 3,345 gram (7 pound, 6 ounce) daughter had Apgar scores of 7 and 9. Donna asked, ''Is it out? It didn't hurt at all.'' The doctor held her baby up and said, ''Yes, a girl.'' The grandmother at this point expressed her disappointment that the infant was not a boy, saying that she had wanted a grandson. Donna was allowed to hold her daughter and said, ''She is beautiful.'' Donna's uterus would not contract, and bleeding was profuse. The pitocin that had been added to her intravenous fluids was not contracting the uterus and another 10 units of pitocin was given slowly by intravenous push. Following fundal massage and vaginal packing, the bleeding stopped.

Three hours later, when the nurse went by the recovery room, Donna was eating a sandwich. Donna said. ''That wasn't so bad. It didn't hurt.'' When told that she had done a beautiful job, she replied, ''That's what they all told me. I'm not tired. . . . You know what we named the baby? Tanya.'' Donna was happy and her self-esteem was high. She had lived through the experience, and could coolly say, ''That wasn't so bad.'' One can conjecture that it was not so bad as her expectations. How bad were they?

Donna illustrates the need for the nurse to be patient in establishing rapport with the youthful mother. It took time and touch on the nurse's part for Donna to accept her as a person who sincerely wished to help and who was committed to helping her. What was considered initially as withdrawal, during the late active phase of labor, was also increasing dependency and an inability to express this need. Donna expressed these needs when her frightened boyfriend left and her mother entered, however. The nurse can help promote and meet these dependency needs, as this nurse did by providing backrubs and wiping her face with a cool cloth. These comfort measures fulfilled many needs for Donna. They indicated that someone cared and would help her; they allowed her to be cared for in her increasing dependency state; and they helped her to relax and remain in control. It is important to recognize the teenage father's fears and concerns during labor. He also needs to be reassured that everything is progressing normally. Withdrawal from the labor room is important for him at times to regain his composure.

Did Donna's uterine atony following delivery reflect her immense fear for her safety, with its consequent jolt of epinephrine—i.e., "Will I bleed? Will I tear?" and her panic at having the oxygen mask on her face?

THE MIDDLE ADOLESCENT

The middle adolescent's fantasies of herself are highly glamorized; thus she tends to maintain a stoic front during stress. Her perceptions of an infant tend to be more realistic than the early adolescent's. Her motives are often altruistic.

LINDA

Linda, a 16-year-old Caucasian primigravida, had an uneventful prenatal course except for some slight nausea during early pregnancy and occasional headaches throughout pregnancy. Her hemoglobin was 13.6 grams and her hematocrit was 40.3%. Her mother and boyfriend were her major support system.

Linda had been enrolled in a special program for teenage mothers which enabled her to attend classes on prenatal care as well as high school academic subjects. An important part of this special program included stressing the mother's rights. Linda learned from the time that she began the program about her rights and her infant's rights, so that she was well informed about making decisions that affected the two of them.

Linda began labor some two and one half weeks after her estimated date for delivery. She was admitted at 4:00 A.M., in early labor; her cervix was 1 centimeter dilated and 50% effaced, and the fetal head was at minus 1 station. Linda's mother and the father of her baby were both present during the labor. The young father did not stay in the labor room for very long periods; he seemed very uneasy in the setting.

At 1:00 P.M., Linda was still only 1 to 2 centimeters dilated, and her mother called the doctor at his office and demanded that he do something. Linda had been moaning with each contraction for the past nine hours, and both Linda and her mother were exhausted. The doctor came and ruptured the membranes; since the amniotic fluid was meconium-stained, he inserted an internal electrode for fetal monitoring. Linda received Demerol 50 mg and Vistaril 50 mg intramuscularly. Her contractions became less intense and farther apart. At 3:15 P.M., intravenous pitocin was begun. Linda continued to leak greenish amniotic fluid all afternoon. At 7:30 P.M., Linda was 5 to 6 centimeters dilated and the fetal head was at 0 station. At this time she received a paracervical block. Fetal bradycardia as low as 90 occurred for 14 minutes; it was thought this was due to the paracervical block. The fetal heart rate improved after Linda was turned on her left side and received oxygen by mask.

Linda smiled but did not comment when the nurse entered and introduced herself. Both Linda and her mother appeared very tired and were not at all talkative. Linda's labor was advancing rapidly, however, and withdrawal was expected at this point. By 7:40 P.M., Linda had only a rim of cervix left and the fetal head was down to plus 1 station. Linda remained quiet during this period, dozing and even watching television occasionally. She continued to doze as her mother and her boyfriend came into the room. The paracervical block was effective in diminishing her pain. Shortly, she was completely dilated, and she grimaced when she said, "It's starting to hurt again.'' Linda was reminded how to push effectively, and she was coached as she pushed with each contraction: ''Take a deep breath in, let it out. Take another deep breath, hold it and push, push. Take another breath and push, push; good, Linda. Now relax.'' Directions were kept concise because of her narrowed field of perception, and the atmosphere was kept quiet so that Linda was not overloaded with stimuli. She maintained ego control well.

Linda was offered some nitrous oxide but responded, ''I don't know.'' She was unable to make decisions at this point. She continued to respond to pushing directions and coaching. She was placed in lithotomy position for the delivery and prepped. An explanation of the pudendal block was given, ''You'll feel him probing around so he can find the proper site for the injection. Now you'll feel a stick, followed by a little burning as he injects the medicine. Are you OK?'' Linda responded, ''Yes, but I'm starting to have pain again.'' She became excited and began to lose control, and the anesthesiologist gave her some nitrous oxide at that time. ''Linda, this will relax you. The mask is the worst part because it's like a big old rubber bowl. Now just breathe slowly, close your eyes, and relax. You'll feel the doctor probing again; he needs to numb the other side. Now a stick and the burning. That'll help a lot.''

Linda was encouraged to push, and low forceps were used to deliver the infant girl, amid a gush of meconium-stained amniotic fluid. The baby was flaccid and cyanotic. She was suctioned and intubated. Her respirations were soon well established and her color became pink. Linda, who was very concerned, asked, ''Is she OK?'' The nurse showed her the baby at that time so that Linda could see her before she was taken to the intensive care nursery.

In the recovery room Linda fell asleep and slept through explanations about the infant's condition to the mother and to the boyfriend: ''She had to go to the nursery right away because she had a little trouble at first. She had had a bowel movement while inside her mother's uterus. When she was born she seemed to aspirate some of this fluid into her lungs and it caused her to be depressed at birth. After she was suctioned out well, she began to do better. But she has to be watched closely to see if her lungs will be irritated. The pediatrician has examined her and ordered an X ray. He will talk to you as soon as he reads the X ray.'' Though both Linda's mother and boyfriend were relieved, neither asked questions or was talkative.

The nurse who was with Linda described how threatened she felt because of her inability to ''break through'' to communicate better or to establish a rapport with Linda. She felt awkward, although she realized that Linda was nearing transition when she first met her and was withdrawn because of the advanced stage of labor. These frustrating feelings extended throughout Linda's postpartum stage, however. Linda never communicated in more than monosyllabic answers. She had no questions about child care, and gave no feedback to the nurse for any kind of help received during her stay. The nurse gave instruction in the presence of Linda's mother and boyfriend after she saw that Linda would not communicate. In addition she wrote down the kinds of information related to formula, feeding, and infant care that she felt were especially important for Linda to remember. As they went to the car on the day of discharge, the mother and the boyfriend thanked the nurse. Linda made no response.

This clinical case is very important in that it illustrates how much of our satisfaction is derived from positive feedback from patients. The nurse in this case was dissatisfied with the entire experience, although she was aware that she had followed through and had tried to establish an effective relationship with Linda.

Any number of factors may have influenced Linda's response, but the feedback of apathy and no response affects any nurse's enthusiasm. Perhaps Linda had learned rather well at the special school and would be learning more there about infant care; she was returning with her infant to the school. On the other hand, she may have intended to rely on her mother to care for the infant and to teach her infant care. Linda may have grown up in a very uncommunicative family. Linda may have hesitated to expose any lack of knowledge and therefore did not "blow her cool" by appearing as if she did not know. Linda's mother may not have encouraged Linda to become independent, in order to maintain full control. It was her mother who called the doctor and demanded that he do something.

Close attention to the youthful mother, supportive help through touch during labor, and continued close instructional help, however, are not unrecognized by her even if they appear to be ignored. Including the teenager's mother and major support persons in counseling and teaching is a valuable learning experience for them and helps ensure that the young mother and her infant will receive better care.

Sandra

Sandra, a 17-year-old Caucasian unmarried adolescent, had decided to relinquish her infant for adoption. She had moved from a rural area to the city in which she delivered and had stayed at a residential home in the city during this pregnancy. She received prenatal care and psychosocial counseling through an adjacent hospital clinic. Her prenatal course had gone smoothly, without complications. Her parents came to the hospital when she went into labor, but two girlfriends stayed with her as support.

Sandra arrived at the hospital at 7:00 P.M., very apprehensive and tense, with two girlfriends. Her cervix was 1 centimeter dilated and she received Seconal grs. iii at 9:00 P.M. She requested that she be allowed to spend as much time with her infant as possible, even though she planned to relinquish the infant for adoption.

When the nurse entered the room and introduced herself at 10:00 P.M., Sandra said, as she grimaced with a contraction, "How long will this go on? The other nurse gave me a pill and told me to go to sleep, but I can't. The pain keeps me awake. See." She rolled to her side, and literally gulped air. The nurse began rubbing her sacral area and said, "Try not to hold your breath. Does this help at all?" Sandra replied, "Oh yes, rub harder."

Realizing that it is hard for an adolescent to admit that she does not know, the nurse asked her, "Has anyone explained to you what these contractions are for, or what they're doing?" She phrased the questions deliberately so that Sandra would not feel that it was her fault if she did not understand what was going on. Sandra answered, "No, I guess they're to help have the baby." The nurse was careful to avoid overly detailed explanations of labor, for Sandra's anxiety level was such that she could not have assimilated details and her anxiety could have been increased. The nurse began, "Each contraction is important, because it helps to dilate your cervix, the opening to your uterus. You're getting closer to delivering your baby with each contraction." Sandra asked, "The pain gets worse, right?" The nurse continued, "The contractions will get stronger. I'm going to help you try to stay as relaxed and as comfortable as you can. But the stronger the contractions get, the closer you are. Sometimes that is hard to remember, so I'll remind you once in a while, OK?" Sandra asked if the nurse would stay with her all of the time, and the nurse reassured her that, except for very brief periods when she had to leave, she would. The nurse explained that when she had to leave, she would let her know exactly when she would be back. Sandra then asked, "I wonder why they don't have a TV here. My friends are out watching TV." When asked if she wanted her friends to come in, she said, "No, not now." The nurse realized that time was passing slowly for Sandra and said, "It can get sort of boring with nothing to do. If I could find a radio, do you think you'd like to listen to it?"

Sandra immediately perked up. "Yeah. Hey, what time is it?" When told the time, she noted that one station was playing comedy albums. Sandra then asked that her friend, Judy, be asked to come in.

When the nurse returned with a radio, Judy immediately confronted her, "She's taking so long. She's been having pains about a week, and she's hardly been sleeping. She walks around all night. It took me four hours to have my baby. Why is it taking her so long?" Sandra joined in with her angry friend, "Yes, why is it taking so long?" The nurse took this opportunity to explain more about the labor process to Sandra:

> Your labor was exceptionally short, Judy. Sandra is doing very well, and her labor seems about average. I was going to go over what labor is about with Sandra. Maybe that can answer some of your questions, too. The cervix is the opening of the uterus, or womb, as some call it; it is sort of like the neck on a jug, and when you aren't pregnant it feels firm, like the tip of your nose. [Sandra reached up and touched her nose at this point.] During pregnancy the hormones make the cervix softer, and when contractions begin, the cervix gradually shortens and flattens. Then it begins to open. The contractions all last week probably were softening your cervix, and may have been making it shorter— what we call "effacement."

The nurse used her hands and fingers to illustrate the uterus and cervix in effacement and dilatation. Judy was very interested, and so was Sandra, at this point; the information seemed new even though Judy had had a baby. The nurse said, "I know it's hard to visualize all of this. I can look for a picture." Sandra said, "Yes, I want to see a picture. Do you have pictures of how the baby looks inside, too?"

The nurse showed Judy how to rub Sandra's back, in order to involve her in her care, and went to find a picture. She found a cervical dilatation card and a text that had pictures from the *Birth Atlas*. While she was being examined, Sandra crooked her fingers to illustrate how her cervix was effacing and was quite pleased with herself in doing so.

Sandra's contractions began to get stronger within an hour or so, and she began to lose control. The nurse told her: "You're doing really well, Sandra. Your contractions are stronger, which means you're closer. The next time you have one, I'm going to remind you not to hold your breath. Let's try taking some even breaths.'' The nurse began demonstrating the breathing and put her hands on her chest to demonstrate, ''In and out.'' Sandra did the same.

Sandra responded well to coaching. She dozed between contractions until about 3:00 A.M., when she complained of nausea and gagged but did not vomit. She began to shake and to complain of leg cramps.

At 3:30 A.M. the doctor examined her and ruptured her membranes artificially. She was 3 to 4 centimeters dilated and completely effaced. When asked if she wanted medicine for relief, she answered softly, ''It won't help . . . other pills didn't.'' The nurse explained that this was a different medicine that would relieve the pain somewhat, and Sandra asked if it would be OK for the baby. Her doctor assured her it was OK, and Sandra agreed. Following an injection of Demerol, Sandra slept between contractions but had difficulty controlling her respirations during them. Her lips were dry and she was diaphoretic. She experienced nausea again. Sandra was soon at transition, then completely dilated. She began to yell, grasp, and grimace with each contraction. She propped her legs against the nurse's and doctor's shoulders and raised her head and pushed. She was taken to the delivery room, and following saddle block anesthesia she fell asleep. As the baby's head emerged from the vagina, the nurse awakened her and directed her attention to the overhead mirror. She drowsily looked up and saw the baby as she was born.

Shortly the nurse took her daughter to her, and as Sandra smiled and stared at her she said, ''She has my lips.'' After the baby was placed in the warmer, Sandra looked all around the room and called the anesthesiologist's attention to the fact that her glucose bottle was almost empty. Sandra asked to hold her baby and was told that she could hold her baby when she got to her room.

When Sandra was transferred to the recovery room, as she went past her family and friends, they congratulated her and hugged her. She made little response. According to Deutsch and Rubin a woman has a need to feel that she is giving her baby to another person as a ''gift.''[47,48] Perhaps Sandra felt that none of the people congratulating her wanted her baby, that part of herself that she had just worked so hard to deliver.

When the nurse visited Sandra the next day, some 16 hours later, Sandra's primary concern was that she had not seen her baby since the delivery. The nursery nurses would not bring the baby out while Sandra was still receiving intravenous therapy. The nurse went and convinced them that they should let her take the baby to Sandra. Sandra was both surprised and pleased and immediately reached out for her baby. She took her and held her close to her breast, and looked alternately at the baby's face and at the nurse's. Sandra was silent for a time, then began to unwrap her baby saying, ''She's uglier than I remembered.'' Sandra counted each toe and finger, and said, ''Oh, wow,'' when the infant closed her hand around her finger. Sandra remained completely absorbed in her baby until the nursery nurse came for her.

Sandra then began sharing about how it would feel to give her baby up. She presented arguments both for keeping the baby and for giving her up for adoption. The nurse agreed that this was a difficult decision, which only she could make. Sandra concluded that she would give the baby up, but added that she knew she would have six months in which to make her final decision ''before she signed the papers.'' The nurse suggested that, if she did decide to have the baby adopted, Sandra might ask her social worker if a small description of herself and some of the things she enjoyed could be given to the baby's adoptive parents, so that the child would eventually have an idea of the kind of person Sandra is. Sandra commented, ''If she wants to be involved in art, then she'll know she inherited it from me.'' Sandra talked of her long relationship with the baby's father, and of how he wanted her to marry him and wanted her and the baby to go and live with him. Sandra dismissed his idea with the statement that she really wanted to be an artist and did not think it was a good idea to give up her dreams and settle for that kind of life now. After verbalizing the pros and cons of marriage, she finally said, ''I really can't tell him I love him. I really can't tell anybody I love him.''

Through the nurse's nonthreatening approach in labor, Sandra learned about the labor process and how she could maintain control in labor. The nurse was sensitive to the teenager's needs and found a radio for her during labor. Through this relationship of trust, established during labor and delivery, Sandra used the nurse most effectively postpartum.

Sandra worked hard at problem solving. She used the nurse to listen to her views—both positive and negative—about the situation and reaffirmed her earlier decision to relinquish her daughter as she talked with her.

THE LATE ADOLESCENT

Although the older adolescent is more mature, she is not necessarily better prepared for labor; the nurse may have to spend more time during early labor preparing the 19-year-old, than would be required for some much younger mothers who are well prepared. The clinical cases of the older adolescents reveal differences both in the levels of knowledge they possessed and in their approaches to labor and delivery.

MAE

Mae, a 19-year-old Filipino woman, had nine brothers and sisters; her husband had six. No one in either family had ever talked to her about childbirth, however. She had not attended any childbirth preparation classes. Mae thought that the ''waters would break and the baby would come out.'' Mae and her husband George had been out late celebrating Mae's birthday the night before, and Mae awakened with a ''stomachache.'' After she vomited, George convinced her she should go to the hospital. Mae was approximately 5 centimeters dilated when admitted to the labor unit at 1:30 P.M. Mae asked the nurse, ''Is this what I'm having—labor? I guess I don't understand what that means.'' One of Mae's sisters had told her that she would feel as if she had to push down before the baby was born, but other than that Mae's knowledge about childbirth was nonexistent.

The nurse explained as simply as possible the early latent, active, and transition phases in labor in terms of the kinds of feelings experienced at each phase and of approximately how much time a woman having her first child spends in each of the phases. Mae asked, ''Will I have the baby in an hour? In two hours?''

Mae was talkative and alert even though she was near the active phase of labor. The nurse explained that labors are very different for each individual, so that progress is difficult to forecast, but that first babies usually take longer than two hours. She used pictures of the uterus and cervix to illustrate effacement and dilatation and explained that dilatation was slower with the first baby.

The nurse tried to determine something about Mae's pain threshold and how she coped with pain. Mae explained that the only pain she had ever had was a headache and that when she had one she took aspirin or lay down and it went away. Mae asked, "Is this going to hurt?" The nurse explained that the contractions would get harder than the contractions she now had, which were about 2 plus quality and lasting 30 seconds. The nurse explained breathing techniques and coached Mae in trying them. Mae said, "That really helped." Mae said that George would go to the delivery room with her because she felt better when he was with her. George agreed that he wanted to help Mae as much as possible.

In an hour or so, Mae became diaphoretic and felt hot. She wanted water, and was given a wet cloth to suck on with the explanation that this was all that was permitted now, since anything taken by mouth might be vomited later. The nurse encouraged a change of position, but Mae said that she felt better either sitting up or lying flat. The nurse encouraged her to sit up.

Mae looked worried, and the nurse asked, "Is something worrying you, Mae?" Mae responded, "I guess I am a little scared now. Will I have to have a cesarean birth? My sister had one, and I look a lot like her. I thought I will have to have one too." The nurse explained that the size of the pelvis and the size and position of the baby usually determined whether one had to have a cesarean birth, and that because her sister had to have one did not mean that she would have to.

As the nurse rubbed Mae's back, she showed George how to rub it and apply counter pressure to the sacral area. This felt good to Mae.

At 7:30 P.M., about six hours after admission, Mae had made little progress. She was encouraged to get up and to walk a bit and to go watch TV. The bed seemed to represent safety for her, and she was hesitant to get up. However, once in the TV room, Mae seemed to be in better control of her contractions, which were getting stronger.

By 8:30 P.M., Mae's labor had accelerated; she began shaking and complained of bearing-down sensations. She returned to her bed, where the nurse reminded her of the breathing techniques and breathed with her. Mae kept in rhythm with the contractions and maintained control; the nurse praised her each time for her good work and told her the baby would soon be born, since she had entered the transition phase of labor.

Mae now closed her eyes and refused any comfort measures from George. The nurse assured George that this was normal behavior at this phase of labor. Mae cried out, "I can't stand it any longer."

Mae was examined and she was completely dilated. Mae began to lose control, but the nurse placed her hands on her shoulders and told her she was doing a good job, and not to let go now. Mae flashed a defiant look at the nurse, and began to push as instructed. She had had no medication and pushed effectively.

At 9:30 P.M. a baby girl weighing 2,495 grams (5 pounds, 8 ounces) was born.

Mae cried, then laughed when she heard the baby cry. She held her daughter for a while. Later, in the recovery room, when Mae was asked how she thought the labor had gone, she said that she did not remember very well. The next day when the nurse went to visit Mae, about 20 family members and friends were in her room; according to reports, they had been there all day. Although Mae's family had not prepared her for the birth experience in our sense of preparation, they had not implanted any negative feelings and their full-force support following the birth said to her that she had accomplished a lot. They provided emotional support for her and met her dependency needs in the early postpartum period.

In other cases, the Filipino husband has been observed to take a less active role than George did. Often, if the woman's mother is with her, the mother may act as the major support, and the husband and wife seem to accept this. Louise, a 19-year-old Filipino woman, had her mother stay with her, and her husband came in the labor room only occasionally. The mother worked at providing comfort measures with the nurse, and the family accepted that "women" care for the laboring woman.

CAROLE

Carole, a 19-year-old Caucasian had had pregnancy-induced hypertension during the last trimester of her pregnancy. She and her husband Larry had attended Lamaze classes. At 1:00 P.M. Carole was admitted to the labor suite. At 5:30 P.M. her membranes ruptured spontaneously and meconium staining was observed. Her blood pressure was 150/92, and she received magnesium sulfate intravenously by slow drip. An external tocotransducer was placed on Carole's abdomen to monitor contractions and an internal monitor was placed on the infant's scalp. Carole was 3 centimeters dilated with the fetal head at 0 station.

Carole and Larry had practiced relaxation and respiration exercises and were a very good team; Larry carefully coached her respirations and she did well. When she was 5 centimeters dilated, she had the urge to push, and hence had to be encouraged to blow. If Larry did not remind her, she would forget and push, and her cervix was becoming edematous. The anesthesiologist, in consultation with Carole and Larry, decided to give Carole an epidural anesthetic to relieve her urge to push. Carole became hypotensive and felt faint and nauseated following the epidural block. Shortly after her bed was placed in Trendelenburg position and oxygen was begun by mask, her blood pressure was 150/100.

Carole's contractions continued every 3 to 4 minutes and were of good quality and duration, and her husband frequently told her that she was doing a good job. She smiled when her husband praised her.

Carole began shaking, and an examination revealed that she was 6 to 7 centimeters dilated. She was assured that it would not be much longer. She complained of pain in her hip, and finally said she could not refrain from pushing any longer. Larry told her to "blow." Carole told him to "shut up." Larry said, "No, damn it, blow." Carole blew instead of pushing, and said, "I almost lost it that time." Larry told her, "But you didn't, Babe. You were dynamite." Carole beamed with Larry's praise; it was evident that Larry's praise was far more important than anyone else's.

Since the external monitor was not recording the uterine contractions, the doctor came to insert the internal monitor catheter. There was only a rim of cervix at this point, so he suggested that Carole be moved to the delivery room. Carole asked, "How much longer?" and as she was moved said, "I can't hold it anymore, I feel like I need to go to the bathroom." Caput was visible. Larry joined her in the delivery room after having gone to put on a scrub suit, and Carole scolded, "Where have you been? I need you."

As Carole pushed, she asked, "How much longer is it going to be?" The nurse told her, "Not much longer, look in that mirror and you can watch the baby being born." Carole became excited, "Oh, I can see it. Is that hair?" When she had pushed the baby out, Carole cried, "Oh, Larry, we have a little girl," and continued to cry softly. Larry's eyes also filled with tears. Although the cry was not lusty, the infant was soon pink, after she was suctioned. Carole looked lovingly into the baby's eyes when she was allowed to hold her, and touched the baby's fingers, "Look, Larry, she has a dimple in her chin like yours. Isn't she beautiful?" Larry said, "She's terrific; when do I get to hold her?" Larry was allowed to hold her for a while before she was taken to the nursery. The 3,685 gram (8 pound 2 ounce) baby was transferred to the intensive care nursery, and Carole and Larry began phoning family and friends on the portable phone to share their news. Carole had no complications following delivery, and her blood pressure was within normal limits upon discharge from the hospital.

Carole and Larry had prepared for childbirth; consequently, when Carole reached a point in labor at which it was difficult to cope and expressed hostility and aggression to Larry, he was unfazed, coached her effectively, and praised her. Both Carole and Larry had achieved a more independent level of functioning than the other youthful parents described. The nurse's major role during labor was to be supportive to both Larry and Carole and to encourage his coaching.

SUMMARY OF CLINICAL DATA

The behavioral responses of the early, middle, and older adolescent in labor are difficult to differentiate by age. Lucy's flippant response to labor preparation instruction was about the only response that could really be viewed as different from any response that one would see in an older woman. The physiological risks for the infants were similar; Donna, Linda, and Carole all had meconium-stained amniotic fluid which necessitated intensive care for their newborn infants. Donna, a younger adolescent, had a postpartal hemorrhage due to uterine atony following the third stage of labor, and Carole, an older adolescent, had pregnancy-induced hypertension.

A long latent phase was experienced by all except Mae and Carole, the older adolescents. Mae, however, failed to progress beyond 5 centimeters dilatation for about six hours following her admission to the hospital, which suggests that this was an anxiety-inducing experience for her that perhaps slowed the progress of her labor. Mae, at 19, was probably the least prepared for childbirth. Her family seemed to have viewed childbirth as an accepted experience that one did not discuss a great deal. The older adolescents were also the only ones who were married.

The labor room nurse learns much about the teenager's support system, special needs, and concerns that is important to share with those caring for her postpartally. Lucy's comment in the delivery room to her son, whom she wished had been a girl, "It's you and me against the world now, baby," suggests a frightened child without the adequate support system necessary for both her own development and for her ability to mother.

Client Advocacy

It is important to consider the teenager's rights from the perspective that if she has no support person to act as her advocate, the nurse has a greater than usual commitment to serve as this advocate. Linda's mother acted as her advocate. When she felt that Linda had labored long enough without making progress, she demanded that the doctor leave his office and come "do something." Judy, Sandra's friend, demanded to know why something was not being done for Sandra, who had been having contractions for a week. Mae and Carole used their husbands as persons who could speak and act for them.

When the client has with her a person who is able to act as an advocate, that person should be supported and encouraged by the nurse. Often the opposite occurs. The nurse is not always able to establish a trust relationship with the teenager, as was the case with Linda. Linda's mother and boyfriend needed encouragement and additional explanations so that they could interpret and reinforce any information that Linda did not grasp.

The nurse's sensitive response to Lucy's grandmother—who was shocked when Lucy, during her active phase of labor, yelled, "Get out of here, you old bitch"—helped the older woman to understand the situation. This was crucial, for no one else was available as support to Lucy; if Lucy's relationship with her grandmother had deteriorated, both Lucy and her child would have suffered.

If the family or the woman in labor have special requests for labor and/or delivery, such as having dimmed lights in the delivery room or delivery without the woman's legs in stirrups, the nurse is the health professional who is consistently present to speak out for the teenager's wishes. The nurse who was with Sandra during labor served as her advocate in going to the nursery and getting Sandra's baby for her. If the adolescent wishes her boyfriend with her and the rules state, "Husbands only in the delivery room," it is the nurse who must take action to be sure that this young woman is not deprived of her major support system.

When signs such as "No one under 16 allowed" are posted, it is important that the nurse initiate action so that the youthful client's friends and major supports— boyfriends, etc., are not excluded. Donna, the 15-year-old, was highly anxious and frightened. One cannot help but wonder whether that sign on the labor room door made her also feel unwelcome. With the trend toward sibling visiting on postpartal units, and even in some alternate birth units, such signs will perhaps soon be removed.

Unless the young woman has specified that she does not want medication in labor, this option should be explored with her. Medication enabled many of the young mothers just described to cope with labor and to have a satisfying experience. The anesthesia—paracervical, pudendal, and epidural blocks in particular—helped to make the experience one in which the young women were pleased with their performance. Donna, for example, could not believe her baby had been born, because "it didn't hurt." Barbiturates and analgesics timely administered can help to relieve some of the youthful mothers' anxiety and tenseness by enabling them to relax and regain control of their behavior. Ill-timed analgesics and barbiturates interfere with the labor process, as was observed with Linda, whose labor then had to be stimulated by pitocin. The nurse has the responsibility to try all relaxing techniques at her disposal before relying on medication. Often the nurse can also influence the drug or the dosage given, with comments such as "50 mg of Demerol and 50 mg of Vistaril? Is it OK if I give it in divided doses? I think she may need only 25–25 to relax." Or, "What would you think about Nisentil instead of Demerol? I think she is progressing rather rapidly, and maybe the Demerol would still be at a level that would depress her baby when she delivers."

It is imperative that a woman of any age be informed about the possible effects of any and all medications given during labor on both her fetus and herself. This is not intended to deny her the right to medication when needed, but to help her understand the importance of breathing and relaxation as methods of decreasing the amount of medication needed. Providing this information is also a responsibility in informed consent. Preferably, effects of analgesics and anesthetics are discussed during the antepartal period or very early in labor.

As an advocate for the client, it is important for the nurse to assess whether a support system exists for her. In the case of Lucy, for example, the nurse is compelled to call a social worker to see the adolescent as soon as possible. Lucy needs to learn very early about the day-care centers and community resources available to her. Her aged grandmother cannot be depended upon for babysitting. The public health nurse would have to be contacted during Lucy's hospitalization so that she could plan a visit for very soon after Lucy was discharged. Lucy also needs vocational counseling. Contraceptive counseling and assistance to assure that her postpartal examination appointment is kept are her right and a valuable component of her health care.

In Elkins'[49] *The Rights of the Pregnant Parent,* basic human rights are outlined and include for every pregnant woman and her partner the right to a supportive doctor (or nurse-midwife), a healthy baby, childbirth education, a shared birth experience, childbirth with dignity, and a family-centered experience. Annas[50] speaks to the rights of minors and emancipated adolescents in *The Rights of Hospital Patients.* He offers a model for a "Patient's Bill of Rights." These recent publications—the former by a consumer and childbirth educator, the latter by a lawyer and a former fellow in medical ethics—represent efforts to protect the hospitalized parent and to guarantee her rights.

The teenager's rights to grant informed consent and to refuse treatments must be continually acknowledged, along with her right to be informed of her progress and of both her own and her infant's health status. According the youthful parents their rights fosters their self-esteem and personal development.

Early Postpartal Care

Postpartal care refers to the period following delivery through the first six weeks following delivery. Special health risks for the young mother during the postpartal period are identified and discussed. Special needs and implications for the care of the parents and the infant are viewed from developmental and cultural perspectives.

POSTPARTAL HEALTH RISKS OF MOTHERS

No specific health risk has been identified consistently in the published research. Two studies found a higher incidence of one-day fever in the younger mother; in Coates's[3] study the younger mothers were all unwed blacks 14 years old and under, and in Israel's and Woutersz's[51] study the younger mothers included all under 20 who had delivered in 10 hospitals from four states in a one-year period. In the latter study the incidence of anemia and prolonged labor was higher, and in both studies the incidence of preeclampsia was higher in the younger groups.

Other studies did not find significant differences between younger and older mothers in postpartal morbidity rates.[1,2,7,8] One study noted that the most frequently observed postpartal complications were urinary tract infection (3.1% of the subjects) and endometritis (2.9% of the subjects).[4] In assessing postpartal morbidity rates, other factors must be carefully weighed. If a group experiences longer labor, they also usually experience greater numbers of vaginal examinations and operative deliveries. Thus, in the Jovanovic study in which uterine dysfunction was common during labor, the most predictably common postpartal complication would be infection.

Hollingsworth and Kreutner[20] observed a 41% febrile morbidity (documented infections or fever of unknown origin higher than 37.7° [100°F] during postpartum hospital stay) in 394 consecutive deliveries of primiparous adolescents at the University of Kentucky. Active infections or fever were observed in 5.6% during labor. Causal factors of the postpartal morbidity were: fever of unknown origin, 13.2%; urinary tract infection, 11.2%; vaginitis with Trichomonas and/or Candida, 6.3%; endometritis, 6.1%; puerperal sepsis, 1.8%; postoperative wound infection, 1.3%. Acute mastitis, acute gonorrhea, abscess of the mouth, acute viral infection, staphylococcal infection, herpes simplex, pneumonia and bronchitis all accounted for less than 1% each. These adolescents, 46% white and 54% black, were from the lower socioeconomic class. A large number had had significant health problems prior to pregnancy; 120 of 525 identified health problems were iron deficiency anemia, 172 were urinary tract infection or asymptomatic bacteriuria, and 42 were venereal disease.

In one study in which little difference in postpartal morbidity was shown between younger and older mothers, the incidence of cystitis and pyelitis was much higher (6 : 1) among the younger mothers.[8] Based on data discussed in Chapter 12, Prenatal Care, which identified vaginal infections as one of the common antepartal complications observed in the teenager, on data reporting prolonged labors, and on Hollingsworth's and Kreutner's data, the youthful mother appears to be more vulnerable to urinary tract and other infections. Since the younger bladder is more sensitive to stimuli, any infection also has the potential of being more painful.

SPECIAL NEEDS OF YOUTHFUL PARENTS AND THEIR INFANTS

Special needs of young parents are dictated largely by their supportive resources, their level of development and by their cultural shaping. The mother from a different ethnic group, especially one who has difficulty with the language, presents additional challenges to the postpartal nurse. Assessment of both the mother's cultural background and psychological and cognitive development are crucial in planning care that is relevant. Some clinical situations are used to dramatize these points.

Eighteen-year-old Aisha had lived in this country for only a year when she delivered a son. She had moved with her husband from Lebanon. Although her pregnancy had been uneventful, she had to have a cesarean delivery because of a transverse arrest and severe fetal distress. Her infant had to remain on a respirator for six days, but he progressed to room air by eight days and was tolerating his bottle feedings well. Aisha did not fare as well. She remained febrile even though she was on triple antibiotic therapy. A week following delivery, a large wound abscess was found. Aisha had seen her son only twice at the end of the first week, the first time being the fifth postpartal day. She had not touched her baby and was concerned that his head had been shaved in one area.

Aisha was very upset about her labor, and told the nurse, "The belts that they put on me during labor to push the baby out, made the baby sick." Aisha, recalling that she had felt the pressure of the monitoring belts, and realizing that she had had to have a cesarean delivery shortly after having the "belts" attached, now reasoned that they had caused her difficulty. The nurse carefully interpreted the function of the monitor and compared it to a stethoscope that could be placed on the abdomen or chest to listen to heartbeats.

The day following the removal of the incisional abscess, Aisha spiked an even higher temperature and was continued on intravenous fluids and therapy. She explained to the nurse who found her crying that she was relieved that her son had been transferred from the intensive care nursery and that she could now walk down to see him. However, she was upset: "the hospital made me sick," and she believed that because she was sick, the baby was "sick." This youthful mother, in a strange country, and very ill with her postpartal infection, was depressed and frightened, and did not understand the sequence of events that had occurred.

Twelve days following her delivery, Aisha had to go to surgery because her incision eviscerated. Postoperatively, she was transferred to a surgical unit, and was unable to see her son for several days. Finally, by Aisha's twentieth postpartal day, she had been afebrile long enough to visit her son and was allowed to hold him. Aisha touched her son cautiously for the first time, moving her finger lightly over his face. She made hissing sounds to him, and he maintained eye contact with her. The hissing sound was a sound that this mother used regularly with her infant instead of cooing. When told that her son was looking at her, Aisha said, "He can't see yet."

Aisha and her son were discharged from the hospital at three weeks postpartum.

When the nurse went to visit her at her apartment, Aisha again asked the nurse why her baby had gotten sick and if "the belts made him sick." The nurse explained the purpose of the monitors again, noting that the monitor could not tell why the baby was sick, but only that he was having difficulty. The nurse described how the uterine contractions squeezed the baby's placenta and thereby decreased his circulation and oxygen supply. Aisha thought about this as she said, "I had a long labor," but she asked, "Did all of the examinations [vaginal] make him sick?" The examinations, which were intrusive and perceived as pressure on her, made her wonder if they, in addition to uterine contractions, exerted pressure on the baby.

Aisha, although she had been separated from her son for the first several days, had become very attached to him. Her mother was helping her. She told the nurse, "He likes me. He quiets when I pick him up, but he doesn't always quiet when my husband picks him up." Aisha said that the next day she would begin breast-feeding because she had so much milk.

Aisha then asked the nurse if she would have to have the operation every time she had a baby. The nurse carefully explained that many doctors preferred to do cesareans once the mother had had one, because the uterine muscle tended to separate at the scar tissue when distended and under the strain of labor contractions. Aisha maintained that she would wait three years before getting pregnant again so that her muscles would get strong and this would not happen to her again. She said she was fearful that she would "come apart" again. Aisha then asked if another doctor would know that she had had an operation. The nurse explained that he would, because of the scar; Aisha did not know what a scar was. The nurse showed her a scar that she had on her hand. Aisha then asked how big her scar would be, and if the doctor would cut in the same place if she had surgery again. When told that he would, Aisha said, "The doctor told me that, too." Aisha was seeking confirmation from several persons. Aisha said that in her country, they did one operation in the middle and one on each side, and that women were allowed to have only three children by surgery. Aisha then asked if she would get another infection. The nurse explained that there was no reason why she should. Aisha then said, "It was the doctor's mistake, not my mistake." It seemed very important to Aisha to determine that she had not made her baby sick or had not caused her own illness. This youthful mother seemed to have been dealing with guilt; she needed verification that she had not done something wrong.

When asked if she thought her son could see yet, she said "No. In our culture, we do not believe they see or hear until they are 40 days old. The woman's body is also open to everything for 40 days and must be protected from stimulation. For 40 days, the woman stays indoors, mostly in bed. The first place she goes after the 40 days is to church to have the baby baptized." Although Aisha said her baby could not see or hear, she continued to maintain eye contact when she held him, and continued to hiss to him and to talk to him.

During the first two or three days following birth, the woman has a period of taking-in in which she receives from others and enjoys food and gifts.[52] Then as she gradually takes hold of her own bodily functioning and of her new mothering role she moves from a passive, receiving individual to an aggressive, mothering person.[52] The mother who has had a cesarean birth has a longer delay in moving to mothering activities because of the physiological and psychological stress of surgery. In Aisha's case, her postpartal infection added to her feelings of malaise and her complications made it difficult for her to expand her view to include events beyond herself. Her body was literally bursting open, and this was most frightening to her. In searching for a cause for the strange complication that she was experiencing, she intellectualized that it was something with which she was unfamiliar, "the belts." She moved from the belts to the examinations, and finally to the doctor, as the cause of her difficulties. Although Aisha's taking-in phase was prolonged and she experienced a lengthy separation from her son, she dealt with the incongruities surrounding her labor and delivery experience, and was able to attach to her son, who "liked her." She followed the cultural custom of staying indoors for 40 days, and comfortably shared her beliefs with the nurse. The nurse did not argue that infants could see and hear. However, Aisha's interaction with her infant spontaneously included eye contact and affectionate noise-making, despite the fact that she maintained he could neither see nor hear.

Aisha illustrates the misunderstanding that can occur about some of the interventions, diagnostic methods, and monitoring devices that are commonly used. Her acceptance of the mutilation that her body had undergone required time and much careful review. Much had happened to her body image during a nine-month period; the evisceration had been far worse than anything she had anticipated. That she seemed to have resolved some of her feelings about what had happened was indicated by an increase in her cognitive grasp of the events that occurred during her labor and delivery. That these events had been so different from her expectations was a threat to this young woman, and as she carefully worked through the incongruity between the events and her earlier expectations for them in her own mind, she absolved herself of blame. In a sense, she experienced a grief process in terms of losing an expected experience for childbirth and in losing body intactness. The cognitive aspect of Aisha's reasoning process was also hampered by the necessity of translating a language with which she still had difficulty. The concrete kinds of deductions she made, however, suggest the kind of reasoning that might be expected of a younger adolescent mother.

Lynn, a 16-year-old who had no complications, either during labor and delivery or postpartally, illustrated some of the adolescent's work in dealing with the trauma of labor and delivery and with its impact on her body image. On the third postpartal day, Lynn complained that her sutures were pulling: "I can hardly get out of bed." When her sister, who was visiting her, commented that a friend who had delivered yesterday was walking without difficulty, Lynn said, "Yeah, but her baby was no bigger than that bottle of lotion, and she didn't have stitches." Lynn was suffering more; she had had a bigger baby, and she had been cut.

Lynn went on to say, "I looked at my rear end and it looked like a zebra's stripes." Her sister and girlfriend who were visiting giggled at this description, but her shocked boyfriend said, "You got up in front of this mirror and looked at your rear end?" Lynn said, "No, silly, I looked with this" (she opened her billfold and showed a small mirror). When asked whether her stitches were to the side or the middle, Lynn commented, "I don't know, I didn't see them," and as she laughed, "Oh, it hurts my stitches to laugh."

On the sixth postpartal day, when the nurse visited Lynn in her home, Lynn had on a pair of beige slacks that fit well. The nurse commented, "You really went down to your usual size fast." Lynn gave a large "hummphh," and said, "That's a girdle." She again complained that her stitches were hurting, and said, "There are five underneath, and five on top." When the nurse commented, "On top?" Lynn said, "Yeah, I saw him put them in. They let me wake up. I felt him putting them in. I told him about it, too, and he said he couldn't believe it." Since Lynn could not see her stitches in the hospital, the description of five underneath and five above reflects some fantasy occurring during the delivery process. She had felt the suturing; her assigning numbers to the stitches seemed to help her to deal with them. When asked what she felt about her hospitalization experience, Lynn said:

It wasn't anything to brag about. I hate hospitals. They gave me a paracervical or some kind of shot as soon as I got there. It didn't help at all. The shot in my arm is the one that helped. After it I don't remember anything. That hospital was all right, but it wasn't nothing to brag about. . . . I've got to lose a lot more weight. I'm too big. I want to get back down to what I was.

Lynn then mentioned that her boyfriend was leaving that night, going back to the Army base where he was stationed, "I'm tired of him already. He's getting on my nerves. I'll be glad to see him leave. He tries to get me up off the sofa, and he knows my stitches hurt me to move." Lynn was sitting on several cushions as she talked.

Lynn, a middle adolescent, was very concerned about the pain resulting from her cut perineum and about not achieving her prepregnancy size in one week. She projected an aura of knowledge in order to assimilate the experience of the sutures and one of braggadocio as she assessed her hospital experience. She had got through the experience. To deal with her boyfriend's returning to his army assignment out of state, she rationalized that she was tired of him. In actuality, she seemed to enjoy his attention and giving him orders.

It is important for the nurse who works with a mother who responds as Lynn did to respect the stoic (and perhaps frightened) front she maintains in striving for her independence. Lynn's mother praised her for her performance in labor and provided Lynn with help for her infant and for herself, thus fostering her self-esteem and nurturing her in her movement toward independence.

Bibring[53] described three psychological tasks of pregnancy and motherhood that are a part of a woman's development. The tasks include (1) being able to love the child while permitting him to grow up as a separate, unique individual, although emotionally he will always be a part of herself; (2) maintaining her sexual attachment to her husband as she grows in her mothering role; and (3) moving from being a child to her mother to becoming her mother's peer. The young adolescent who has a baby "to have someone to love" may have difficulty when she sees the child developing as an independent person and beginning to move out from her during the last quarter of his first year—the time when the infant usually begins to separate from his mother. Lynn, at 16, did not seem ready to maintain her sexual attachment to her partner. Until she has achieved the independence she longs for, she may not be capable of an intimate relationship with another.

Erikson states, "It is only when identity formation is well on its way that true intimacy—which is really a counterpointing as well as fusing of identities—is possible."[54] To become close to another who would see through her braggadocio or who would know her too well may have been too threatening to her at that time. With her mother's help, she was beginning to assume a peer role with her mother. Her mother encouraged and complimented her on her performance of womanly tasks, i.e., childbirth.

Premature birth poses additional concerns for the youthful mother. Special concerns of the adolescent mother whose infant is in the intensive care nursery are illustrated by Anne, a 16-year-old primigravida, who began having contractions following an amniocentesis at 29 weeks gestation. A diagnosis of hydramnios had been confirmed. Shortly after admission to the hospital her membranes ruptured spontaneously. She began labor and delivered a female weighing 1,200 grams (2 pounds, 10½ ounces) who had to be intubated and placed on a respirator. The infant had respiratory distress syndrome and the physician had discussed this with Anne. The next day when Anne went to the nursery, she was reluctant to touch her daughter, saying, "She is too tiny, I don't want to hurt her." When the nurse asked Anne if the doctors had explained the baby's condition to her, Anne replied, "She's doing just fine. I guess she'll be here awhile." She did not seem to comprehend the seriousness of her daughter's condition, yet she recognized that the infant would have to remain in the hospital for a long while. Anne added, "My mother was with me all the time in labor. She told me the baby was fine after it was born. I was worried that it would die right away or not be all right." The diagnosis of hydramnios had increased Anne's fear for her baby's welfare. Anne's confidence in her mother's opinion that the baby was fine and that no anomalies were found may have contributed to her optimism.

Although Anne did not seem to grasp the seriousness of her infant's condition, she noted improvement and change in her infant's behavior immediately upon entering the nursery a couple of days later. She carefully took in all that she saw. She noted the infant's feet, hands, and hair, and said that she looked like her father, but she still declined the encouragement to touch the infant. The nurse touched the infant gently as Anne watched intensely. The nurse used simple terms to explain the equipment. The doctor was also present and told her that the infant was still quite sick. Anne remained quiet and looked worried for a while. She appeared to understand that her infant was still seriously ill. By the time she returned to her room, she voiced the desire to get a bed for her infant before she took her home, however. She wanted this infant very much. She told the nurse that her parents were upset when they learned of her pregnancy and "wanted her to get rid of the baby," but she could never do that. Her mother later apologized to her for suggesting this.

Anne went home the next day, and when she returned to see her daughter she said that she had cried and cried when she got home, "Because it was like I had never even had her. I was all alone." Anne commented when she saw her, "Look at those big feet, have you ever seen such big feet?"

In three weeks Anne's daughter had been extubated and Anne was busy taking pictures of her to take home to show to her friends and family. Anne also confided that she had wanted pictures of herself as she became larger during pregnancy but the baby came so early that she had been able to have only one taken. When Anne was asked how she felt about getting larger, she said, "It was exciting. At first I didn't show very much, but then by the fifth month I did, and it was neat. All of the girls at school, we used to compare how big we were and how far along. . . . She was real active. I could feel her thumping around. That was neat, too."

Anne's infant was now under an oxygen hood in the Isolette. She observed, "She's tired today. I can tell. Yesterday she moved around more." Anne noted that the baby looked a little like her sister, and that her skin texture and color were changing. She asked, "Do you think that babies itch like we do?"

Anne's interest in her infant and her regular visits to the nursery indicated her growing attachment to her daughter. Her earlier pleasure in her advancing pregnancy suggests that she enjoyed this positive feminine identification. Although Anne was not continuing her relationship with the boyfriend who had impregnated her, she was working on her feminine and mothering roles.

Cindy, in contrast, offered little positive feedback or satisfaction of success to the nurse clinical specialist who worked with her. Cindy is the 17-year-old whose antepartal convulsions are described on page 250. Because of Cindy's eclamptic condition, she was delivered by cesarean section very soon after admission. Once Cindy was discharged from the hospital, she did not come to visit her daughter. She talked to the nurse on the telephone about herself and her feelings, but when she was encouraged to come to see her daughter she gave evasive reasons for not coming to visit. Cindy seemed to be having difficulty resolving the frightening experience of the convulsions that had occurred suddenly and the consequent cesarean birth. Cindy told the nurse during a telephone conversation:

> I really wish I had seen her being born. My mom was so happy at seeing her. [She had been allowed to go to the operating room with Cindy.] She told me how tiny she was when she first saw her. . . . I had to be in the hospital eight days after she was born. I hate hospitals, oh, I hate them so much. All those *shots* and *needles* and pills they give you. I hate them all. I never had to be in one before—just always going to get shots in my rear for being anemic. I guess they were giving me iron. I'm not sure.

Cindy had no desire to go to the hospital to see her daughter. The hospital setting, particularly the intensive care nursery, was too overwhelming. Her daughter was alive; therefore, Cindy could do without further exposure to the frightening milieu of the hospital. Because the nurse wanted to promote the attachment process between Cindy and her daughter, she continued to call Cindy and give her reports about the baby. Cindy told the nurse that her mother would take care of the infant and that she did not have to learn how. She said that she had been helping with her smaller brothers and sisters, "It's no big deal taking care of a kid."

Anne, in contrast to Cindy, enjoyed her pregnancy experience, and although it was marred by the complications of hydramnios, premature rupture of the membranes, and spontaneous premature delivery, she dealt with these events and slowly moved toward a beginning mothering role. Cindy, the middle-adolescent described above, remained deeply frightened by her antepartal eclamptic state and her subsequent cesarean birth. This added to her fear of hospitals, which made it difficult for her to visit her daughter.

Anne was working at the four tasks of mothers who deliver prematurely described by Kaplan and Mason.[55] The first task is to prepare for the possible loss of the infant who may die. Anne slowly began to realize the seriousness of her daughter's condition, but her strong hope for her survival was evidenced in her future plans. Cindy's withdrawal from her infant by refusal to visit may have reflected anticipatory grief. Anne seemed to face the second task, which is acknowledging a failure to deliver a term infant.[55] For Anne this task was made easier by the sequence of events. She could link the premature labor and rupture of the membranes to the amniocentesis. Since her daughter did not have an anomaly, she was relieved that the hydramnios had not been due to fetal pathology. This different kind of situation helped Anne in rationalizing that the premature birth was not her fault. Recall Aisha's detailed study and her resolution that the complications were not her fault. Guilt is a common emotion of parents who deliver prematurely or who experience complications.[56]

The third task of the mother who delivers prematurely is to resume the process of relating to her baby.[55] Anne did this in many ways; she pumped breast milk and brought it to the nursery. She made frequent visits to the nursery, where she talked to her daughter and eventually stroked and fondled her. Cindy was too overwhelmed to resume a relationship with her daughter in the early weeks. Whether because of guilt feelings about her frightening serious illness and the subsequent cesarean birth or because of her fear of the hospital, she was not able or willing to come to visit her daughter. The trauma to her ego may have been too overwhelming. A body that was so much out of control and that acted so strangely as hers had during the convulsions may have also lowered her self-esteem.

The fourth task facing a mother who has a premature infant is to learn how a premature infant differs from a term infant with respect to needs and care and to realize that these differences are temporary.[55] Anne began learning very studiously. She carefully noted respiratory changes, the infant's movements, and maturational changes in her infant's skin texture. Cindy, who had not achieved the first or second tasks, did not appear to be working on subsequent tasks.

Anne and Cindy illustrate that age is not a predictor either of readiness for interaction with a tiny premature infant or of psychological ability to integrate the labor and delivery experience and to resolve conflicting feelings.

Implications for Nursing Care

The nurse who cared for Cindy experienced far more distress than the nurse who worked with Anne. There was no opportunity to see the results of her teaching and counseling, of her attempts to help Cindy integrate her labor and delivery experiences, or of her attempts at facilitating mothering activities.

Continued contact by telephone, with reports about her daughter and encouragement to visit were appropriate for Cindy. Referral to the public health nurse was important. The nursery nurse or postpartal nurse could have telephoned the referral prior to Cindy's discharge from the hospital. A home visit by the public health nurse would have ascertained whether needed equipment—such as a bed and clothing—was available for the infant and whether Cindy's mother was available, willing, and able to provide nurturing care for both Cindy and her infant. Visiting with Cindy and discussing her experience might have facilitated her resolving some of her feelings about childbirth and the hospital so that she could have visited her infant. Cindy's awareness that persons were both interested in helping her and available to help her might have increased her trust in "the system." If Cindy's home setting was not conducive to her welfare, the public health nurse could have presented alternative options to Cindy, such as placement in a foster home or in a residential home for unwed mothers where she would receive needed support.

Although Anne was attaching to her infant and visited her regularly, a home visit by the public health nurse would also have bolstered her support system and would have helped assure Anne and her family that adequate care and support were available, especially after Anne took her daughter home from the hospital.

For all young mothers, special instructions about postpartal hygiene are important. The higher rate of infection sometimes observed suggests that this should be a priority health teaching item. The teaching should be given in nonthreatening, consistent, concrete terms. The material dealing with special cleanliness of the perineal area may be presented as applying to "all women who have babies," so that the adolescent does not feel offended because she is being told something as basic as how to clean her "bottom" or the direction in which to wipe. Since youthful mothers are very interested in their bodies, a review of postpartal physiology can help to allay their anxieties. For example, early postpartal diaphoresis may be especially bothersome because she may have been embarrassed earlier by the profuse underarm perspiring that young girls experience in normal adolescence. A brief description showing that the increased circulatory volume that occurred during pregnancy is no longer needed, and that perspiring is one way of reducing extra fluid volume, may relieve some anxiety.

The importance of good nutrition for both the young parents and their infant cannot be emphasized too strongly. The young parents need to know that a good diet can usually prevent anemia and thus help avoid excessive fatigue. Young parents need to know that an infant must have protein and other nutrients for the optimal growth and development of his brain. This knowledge adds to their motivation for healthy food habits.

Teaching usual, helpful comfort measures is especially important. Warm showers make congested breasts feel better, and hot sitz baths may relieve a painful swollen perineum. Learning to contract the buttocks before sitting may ease discomfort on the episiotomy.

Reminders to drink fluids and to empty the bladder regularly are helpful instructions, along with the interpretation that the bladder may not give the young mother the usual signals of fullness or filling for a week or so, because of bruising due to some of the pressures of childbirth.

Contraceptive counseling is an important part of regular care during the hospitalization period. The young parents may have heard and may believe that pregnancy cannot occur while breast-feeding. Although a few women do not ovulate during the time when their infants are totally fed by breast-feeding, many women do. This needs to be carefully interpreted. Ideally, contraceptive counseling is done with both the young mother and father. If there are no contraindications for intercourse, such as infection or extensive lacerations, the young couple should have foam and condoms to take home upon discharge. These may be ordered from the hospital pharmacy. If the couple choose an intrauterine device, this may be inserted before the mother's discharge from the hospital. Some physicians, however, prefer to wait until one month postpartum to insert the IUD.

The couple can be instructed to test for vaginal soreness by the female's or her partner's introducing two clean, lubricated fingers gently into the vagina. Many couples resume sexual intercourse after two weeks. If intercourse is contraindicated until the postpartal examination at one month, methods of mutual stimulation and achieving orgasm without vaginal penetration can be discussed. If a teenage mother states that she is not interested in a contraceptive, because she will not be having intercourse, this intention must be respected. Printed pamphlets about various contraceptive methods and places to receive contraceptives can be offered for her future information, however. Such information should not be "forced" upon a young woman, because to do so would indicate to her that you lack confidence in her ability to follow through with her intentions. It is important for the young person to feel that an adult has confidence in her. Because repeat pregnancies in the teen years are such a hazard to her and her infant's health, and because she may lack the cognitive ability to plan ahead, the young teenage mother needs close follow-up and health care supervision with contraceptive counseling readily available.

Promoting the quality and quantity of parent-infant contact is an important part of facilitating the parent-infant acquaintance and attachment process. Schweitzer and Youngs[57] suggest that the pediatric nurse practitioner examine the newborn at the mother's bedside. Mothers may be stimulated to ask more questions and express more interest when the infant is present. The mother, for example, can be encouraged to feel the fontanel as the nurse demonstrates how to shampoo the infant's hair. This affords the nurse an opportunity to determine the young mother's beliefs and attitudes about child-rearing and to encourage the mother in her child care activities.[57]

In teaching aspects of infant care, a *careful* assessment of the mother's knowledge and previous experience is important. The 16-year-old mother may be bored with bath demonstrations that she has observed many times at school. Or she may have actively participated in changing and bathing her brothers and sisters. What may be important for this mother to learn are some of the unique characteristics of her infant's temperament and personality. Giving a demonstration of her infant's reflexes and pointing out what her infant seems to like and dislike can help the young mother to recognize and begin to read her infant's cues, so that she learns to *respond* to her infant rather than act upon her own whims. If the young parents understand that an infant's cry is his only mode of communication, they may be less likely to classify him as "mean" when he cries. Young parents get excited about their infant's capabilities. Both young parents should be involved in these getting-acquainted sessions. The young father often enjoys the unfolding and maturation of his infant as much as the young mother.

In interpreting the purpose of well-baby visits to the doctor or clinic, stress that the infant's growth and development are carefully followed. Young parents feel highly rewarded for their efforts, just as older parents do, as they note their infant's progress. Concrete explanations about the importance of immunizations help to motivate the young parents to follow through with them.

Interdisciplinary Collaboration

If the older adolescent has a supportive system—her husband, her family—and if her cognitive level of understanding is such that she understands care for herself and her infant and the importance of follow-up care, she will usually follow through responsibly. The early and middle adolescent, however, usually need a more carefully planned follow-up program of care. A primary nurse, usually the one who is most familiar with the young family, may be assigned to assume responsibility for coordinating and planning their care. Health professionals who will be playing an active role in the family's welfare should work in a collaborative effort—the pediatrician, pediatric nurse practitioner or midwife, the public health nurse, the obstetrician, and the social worker. Observations concerning the young family and any particular problems or concerns identified in the hospital should be shared with and communicated to others on the health care team. Follow-up by the social worker is very important for the very young mother for at least a year. The teenager needs to be in communication with an informed professional who is a "friend," one who listens empathetically and reminds her of her options. As the infant develops and circumstances change, the youthful mother may decide that she is not ready to continue in the mothering role and that she needs someone who can give her alternate options for her consideration.

The nurse practitioner or the public health nurse often has information about the young girl's home situation and family interactions that other health professionals may not have observed; it is very important that a system for communication and collaboration be established. The young parents, who are a vital part of this team, need to know which persons may be consulted and for what. The unmarried father, for example, may find that the burden of continuing to contribute to the infant's support will keep him from pursuing his college career. He may need help in ascertaining whether other support or help is available to him and the infant that would make sacrificing his future unnecessary.

The physician who delivers the young woman's child and who sees her for subsequent checkups may have the least information about some of the problems troubling her. He may be perceived as a father image, and the young woman, hesitating to appear immature to him, may say and do only what she considers to be "adult." Because communicating relevant information to the physician is important, the nurse might say, "It really is important for your doctor to have this information. He is very interested in you and this information would be helpful for his prescribing for you. Do you mind if I tell him?"

Because the adolescent's infant has a higher morbidity and mortality rate during the neonatal period and the first year of life, the involvement of public health nurses who are able to plan visits throughout the year is important. Continued, careful assessment of the young mother's progress in the mothering role and of environmental factors that facilitate or impede her progress is vital.

The period occurring toward the end of the first month seems to be a crucial one for the mother and her infant emotionally. It has been observed that not only does the mother have difficulty meshing her responses with the infant's cues, but her level of hostility is particularly high at this time.[58] During this period when increased hostility is felt by the mother, from about two to four weeks, a home visit by a nurse is crucial. The nurse can help the youthful mother identify and verbalize her concerns and can help her explore what can be done about them. The transition to the mothering role is gradual; maternal feelings and emotions do not follow birth immediately or automatically. The disruption that an infant causes in a household can be exhausting. The mother may need a break or a couple of evenings out. The young mother needs to know that "all" mothers become exhausted in caring for a tiny, helpless infant who keeps them up at all hours during the night. Interruption of sleep and disruption of routine present two of the biggest problems for young mothers.

If the young mother realizes that all mothers experience similar frustration and exhaustion, she may feel it is safe to express her own feelings; otherwise, she may feel that her age is the cause, rather than lack of sleep and rest. If a young mother can say, "I really feel like sending her back sometimes," she is recognizing and dealing with her feelings. The young mother who denies that the baby poses any hardship in her life needs more careful and subtle help. The absence of maternal anxiety usually connotes a lack of emotional commitment to the baby.

In summary, the postpartal nurse, or a primary nurse in the hospital setting, bears a responsibility for setting in motion a team network of persons who are informed about the young woman's childbirth experience and her approach to early mothering. If the teenage mother is enrolled in a special school program, she continues to receive help through classes on child care. Social workers often have been involved with her during her pregnancy. Ongoing relationships with social workers, teachers, and nurses that worked with her antepartally are ideal because trusting relationships have probably been established, and the adolescent will be able to express her emotions more freely. If, however, the adolescent is not enrolled in a special program, the nurse has the responsibility to align individuals that are necessary to provide an individual special program. This team includes the pediatrician, well-child clinic or pediatric nurse practitioner, public health nurse, obstetrician or midwife, social worker, and, when available, vocational counselor.

The Mother Who Relinquishes Her Infant For Adoption

The adolescent who makes the decision to release her infant for adoption experiences a grief process similar to that of a woman who has a stillbirth or an infant with a defect. For the adolescent, however, the grief work may be hampered or intensified by vacillation in her decision making and because she willfully makes the decision to separate from her infant. She cannot rationalize that it was something "beyond her control." This grief process, as well as some implications for the care of such an adolescent both during her hospitalization and following her discharge, will be discussed in the section which follows.

GRIEF PROCESS

Hallett[59] evolved a concept of burden to interpret both the psychological changes that occur during pregnancy and the grief work that follows the birth of a stillborn infant or an infant with an anomaly. The growing burden is illustrated in Figure 13–1, by the process of psychological and physical development and bonding that occur during pregnancy. The diminishing burden is illustrated by a process of separation through a grief process when the newborn is dead or deformed.

The pregnant woman, during the growing burden of pregnancy, also prepares for the bodily separation of her baby through birth and the severing of the umbilical cord. The pregnant adolescent who makes the decision to release her infant prepares

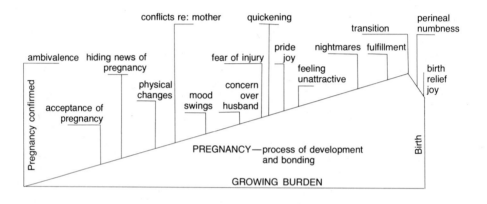

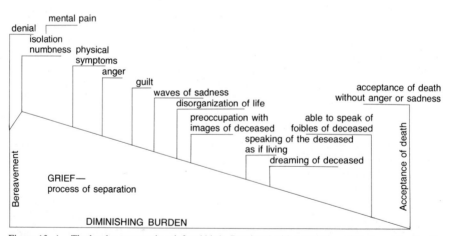

Figure 13–1. The burden concept in grief and birth. Reprinted with permission of *Birth and the Family Journal,* copyright, 1(4):21, 1974, and with permission of and adaptations requested by the author, Elizabeth R. Hallett.

for this physical separation of her infant from her body and for permanent emotional and physical separation from her infant. Therefore, during the usual time of growing burden, because of the projected imminent separation from her infant, the adolescent may not achieve a similar level of bonding to the infant growing within her. However, at birth, there may be an increase in bonding as the young mother becomes acquainted with the child she has produced and experiences continued ambivalence about her choice. Separation is her choice, and the grief work which ensues is a consequence of her choice. Some differences in the concepts of growing and diminishing burdens for the pregnant adolescent are illustrated in Figure 13–2.

Although she recognized that there is much individuality in grieving and that permanent changes evolve as a result of that grief, Hallett[59] projected time spans in the grief process of two to three years for widows, nine to ten months for a stillbirth, and four months for an abnormality. We do not know the temporal impact of releasing a child for adoption; research is needed to suggest the length of time during which follow-up is needed for these mothers.

The young woman who feels pleasure in her performance in giving birth and in seeing a healthy, normal baby, has increased self-esteem immediately postpartum. As she becomes acquainted with the infant whom she carried for nine months, she very likely becomes increasingly attached to him or to her. She may see in the infant some of the characteristics that she is able to see in her boyfriend or in a family member. She establishes a firm reality image from which she must separate, rather than an obscure fantasy. She experiences ambivalence each time she interacts with her infant. Recall Sandra's experience, which was described on page 321. It was necessary for Sandra to review all of the reasons why she wanted to keep her daughter and the consequences if she did. She then carefully reviewed all of the reasons why she did not wish to rear her daughter and the consequences if she made that choice. This careful mental work promoted the young woman's comfort with her decision. Once Sandra had reaffirmed that she was not capable of a close relationship with anyone and that she did not wish to give up her goal of an art career, she began planning for her future. Even the younger adolescent is often able to reason, with articulate wisdom, that at her age she is incapable of parenting a child. Further, the young adolescent can visualize the disruption to her parents' household and to her siblings' routines that an infant could cause.

It takes great strength and courage to love enough to give one's child to someone else who is ready to parent. Young, sensitive mothers are often concerned about the long interval between the time when they are caring for and feeding their infants and the time when the adoptive parents receive the infant. This delay is even more worrisome when the infant has to be released to a foster home before adoptive parents can have the infant. The young mother seems to be particularly sensitive to feelings of isolation and alienation at this time; they are feelings she may have experienced often during her pregnant state.

When she returns to school without an infant, the teenage mother may no longer receive the special attention that she enjoyed in her pregnant state. She may become disappointed and angry. Thus, not only does she feel emptiness without her infant, but she feels the loss of peer attention. This loss and other losses are so extensive for some adolescents that they do not relinquish their infants for adoption. Giving up the

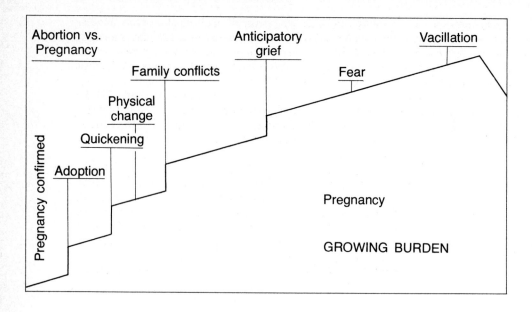

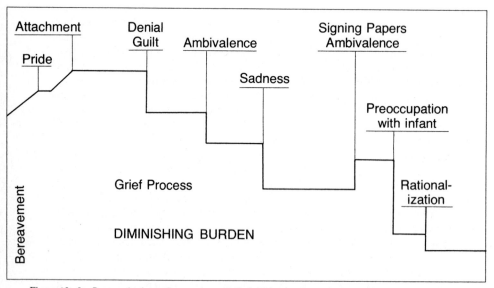

Figure 13–2. Proposed schema for growing and diminishing burden around adoption of infant. Adapted from Hallett's schema of The Burden Concept in Grief and Birth, with permission of Elizabeth R. Hallett and *Birth and the Family Journal*.

infant may mean loss of free health care, financial aid, social worker or other support, and nice living quarters in a residential home. Severely disadvantaged adolescents have confessed that their sole reason for maintaining custody of their infant was to retain these advantages and avoid returning to a parental home of deprivation.

Depending upon the state laws and the arrangements that are made for the adoption, the time leading up to the young woman's signing of the final release papers is another period of extreme sadness for her. She rethinks her decision and has to carefully weigh the implications. Sixteen-year-old Nancy verbalized some of her feelings about this at two weeks postpartum:

> I'm a little uptight because the lawyer has contacted me for an appointment for us to sign the final papers. It is scary. It has really made me think. You know if I met up with her [the baby] in 16 years, of course I'll be looking to see if I can recognize me in her. She might really be a pretty girl, but she won't be mine because she'll have grown up with other folks and will have become what their love and care has made her. Other than carrying her and having delivered her, I won't really have influenced her growth. . . . But I'm not ready to settle down yet. No way am I able to mother her.

At three weeks postpartum this young woman expressed much sadness about not being pregnant. She expressed sadness about her flabby abdomen and not having anything to show for it. She was angry at not receiving as much attention in school. She was able to express her feelings to the maternity nurse practitioner and her boyfriend. They were the only persons who she felt understood. After she verbalized her sadness and anger, she began rationalizing and intellectualizing by saying that she was glad that she had given the baby up while she was in the hospital and that during the short time she had had with her daughter, she had felt close to her. Nancy added that she thought she had done the right thing and again said that she was not ready to settle down. The nurse told her that her feelings were expected and that it took courage for her to make her decision. This reinforcement of her self-esteem seemed to help her.

At six weeks Nancy described occasions when, while she was absorbed in what she was doing, something would suddenly remind her of the pregnancy and adoption. She described these as very sobering experiences, but they seemed to help her express her feelings. She always cried when this happened. Mother's Day was difficult for her. She broke into tears and cried uncontrollably for some time because it was difficult ''to be a mother without a child.'' Indications of Nancy's progress in the grief process were reflected in her expressed anger at her flabby abdomen and at the meager attention she now received at school, in contrast to the large amount she had enjoyed during her pregnancy state. On occasional moments when she would remember her daughter, the reality of the separation jolted her into crying and expressing her sadness. She fantasized ahead 16 years when, she projected, she would search for resemblances of herself in 16-year-old girls. Her grief process was intensified when she had to sign the papers. Denial that she was losing her daughter could no longer be used once she signed the papers. All of her feelings of ambivalence and guilt were exacerbated at that time.

IMPLICATIONS FOR CARE AND FOLLOW-UP

Nancy illustrates the importance of the young mother's becoming acquainted with her infant following delivery. Not only does she have a mental picture of her daughter, but she also has an image about which to grieve more completely.

The young woman needs to have access to someone who can skillfully listen without making judgments or recommendations. This most serious decision has to be made by the young woman herself after carefully weighing all of the pros and cons for retaining and releasing custody of her child.

Follow-up counseling for the young woman by the social worker, nurse practitioner or clinical specialist, and physician, is helpful and is necessary to assure her continued progress. If she has a good rapport with the health team, when she is sad and depressed she will be more likely to call them. She will be sad, and she will grieve; this will be painful. But with help, she can grow because of the experience and become a stronger person, so that, in time, she will be able to talk about her infant without experiencing undue sadness or anger. However, adults who have relinquished infants during their earlier years have said that all pangs of sadness are never totally erased. The memory of the normal, pretty infant whom she held and kissed offers some solace to the mother, however.

Summary

The adolescent's increased anxiety and fear around the time of labor may lead either to the prolonged duration of her labor process or to hypertonic contractions that are ineffectual. The nearer she is to the age of puberty, the more likely her chances of physiological, psychological, and emotional immaturity.

The adolescent's age is not necessarily a predictor of the kinds of help that she needs during the childbirth experience. The young woman's cultural background, previous life experiences, level of understanding, and support systems are all important factors as well. The young adolescent who receives basic, consistent instruction and warm, nurturing support may do as well as her older sister. The 19-year-old, who would be expected to have a more sophisticated knowledge and to have a higher level of cognitive functioning, may be more naive and do less well. Care for adolescent parents during the childbirth experience is most effective when it is individualized. Including young parents in the decision-making processes and recognizing their special developmental needs will increase their interest and involvement.

There is a lack of agreement among research reports about the increased health risks for the adolescent childbearing mother. Pregnancy-induced hypertension with its concomitant complication of abruptio placentae and premature birth remains a threat to both the mother and the infant. Anemia is a threat along with the increased rates of infection. When labor is prolonged due to dysfunctional uterine activity, this adds to the risk of infection.

Comprehensive care of youthful parents during hospitalization includes careful counseling in hygiene, sexual activity, child care, parent-infant bonding, infant stimulation, and careful planning for follow-up care.

The adolescent's infant suffers greater health risks. This seems due in large part to the lower socioeconomic level of the youthful mother, rather than to her age factor alone.

Because the youthful parent may be less sophisticated in dealing with the health care system, the health care professional has a deeper commitment to serve in the advocate role and to support any advocates the client may already have. The nursing professional who has a better understanding of the special needs and concerns of the adolescent is the one most responsible for communicating these special needs to her colleagues. When her individuality and basic human rights are recognized, the youthful parent's potential for growth from the experience is increased.

REFERENCES

1. Hassan, H. M., and Falls, F. H. "The Young Primipara." *Am. J. Obstet. & Gyn.* 88(2):256–269, 1964.
2. Dwyer, J. F. "Teenage Pregnancy. *Am. J. Obstet. & Gyn.* 118(3):373–376, 1974.
3. Coates, J. B., III. "Obstetrics in the Very Young Adolescent." *Am. J. Obstet. & Gyn.* 108(1):68–72, 1970.
4. Jovanovic, D. "Pathology of Pregnancy and Labor in Adolescent Patients." *J. Reproductive Med.* 9(2):61–66, 1972.
5. Mussio, T. J. "Primigravidas Under Age 14." *Am. J. Obstet. & Gyn.* 84(4):442–444, 1962.
6. Aznar, R., and Bennett, A. E. "Pregnancy in the Adolescent Girl." *Am. J. Obstet. & Gyn.* 81(5):934–940, 1961.
7. Bochner, K. "Pregnancies in Juveniles." *Am. J. Obstet. & Gyn.* 83(2):269–271, 1972.
8. Briggs, R. M., et al. "Pregnancy in the Young Adolescent." *Am. J. Obstet. & Gyn.* 84(4):436–441, 1962.
9. Semmens, J. P. "Implications of Teen-Age Pregnancy." *Obstet. & Gyn.* 26(1):77–85, 1965.
10. Semmens, J. P., and Lamers, W. M., Jr. *Teen-Age Pregnancy.* Springfield, Ill.: Charles C Thomas, Pubs., 1968.
11. Friedman, D. "Parturiphobia." *Am. J. Obstet. & Gyn.* 118(1):130–135, 1974.
12. Deunhoelter, J. H., et al. "Pregnancy Performance of Patients Under Fifteen Years of Age." *Obstet. & Gyn.* 46(1):49–52, 1975.
13. Aiman, J. "X-Ray Pelvimetry of the Pregnant Adolescent." *Obstet. & Gyn.* 48(3):281–286, 1976.
14. Efiong, E. I., and Banjoko, M. O. "The Obstetric Performance of Nigerian Primigravidae Aged 16 and Under." *Brit. J. Obstet. & Gyn.* 82:228–233, 1975.
15. Scher, J., and Utian, W. H. "Teenage Pregnancy—An Inter-Racial Study." *J. Obstet. & Gyn. Brit Commonwealth* 77:259–262, 1970.
16. Gabbard, G. O., and Wolff, J. R. "The Unwed Pregnant Teenager and Her Male Relationship." *J. Reproductive Med.* 19(3):137–140, 1977.
17. Smith, P. B., et al. "The Medical Impact of an Antepartum Program for Pregnant Adolescents: A Statistical Analysis." *Am. J. Pub. Health* 68(2):169–172, 1978.
18. Clark, J. F. J. "Adolescent Obstetrics—Obstetric and Sociologic Implications." *Clin. Obstet. & Gyn.* 14(4):1026–1036, 1971.
19. Donnelly, J. F., et al. "Fetal, Parental, and Environmental Factors Associated with Perinatal Mortality in Mothers Under 20 Years of Age." *Am. J. Obstet. & Gyn.* 80(4):663–669, 1960.

20. Kreutner, A. K. K., and Hollingsworth, D. R. *Adolescent Obstetrics and Gynecology*. Chicago: Year Book Medical Pubs., Inc., 1978, pp. 140, 233, 258–259.
21. Baldwin, W. H. "Adolescent Pregnancy and Childbearing–Growing Concerns for Americans." *Population Bull.* 31(2), 1976.
22. Gill, D. G., et al. "Pregnancy in Teenage Girls." *Soc. Sci. & Med.* 3:549–574, 1970.
23. Menken, J. "The Health and Social Consequences of Teenage Child-bearing." *Fam. Plann. Perspectives* 4(3):45–53, 1972.
24. Erkan, K. A., et al. "Juvenile Pregnancy Role of Physiologic Maturity." *Maryland State Med. J.* 20:50–52, 1971.
25. Dott, A. B., and Fort, A. T. "Medical and Social Factors Affecting Early Teenage Pregnancy." *Am. J. Obstet. & Gyn.* 125(4):532–536, 1976.
26. Rich, O. J. "Temporal and Spatial Experience as Reflected in the Verbalizations of Multiparous Women During Labor." *Mat. Child Nurs. J.* 2(4):239–325, 1973.
27. Watson, Sister J. M. "Four Behavioral Patterns of the Ego in Multigravidae During Labor." Doctoral dissertation, University of Pittsburgh, 1971.
28. Affonso, D. "Crisis of Labor and Birth. In Clark, A., ed. *Maturational Crisis of Childbearing*. Honolulu: University of Hawaii, 1971, 23–39.
29. White, R. W. 'Strategies of Adaptation: An Attempt at Systematic Description." In Coelho, G. V., et al., eds. *Coping and Adaptation*. New York: Basic Books, Inc., 1974, 47–68.
30. Stroup, P. E. "The Influence of Epinephrine on Uterine Contractility." *Am. J. Obstet. & Gyn.* 84(5):595–601, 1962.
31. Zuspan, F. P., et al. "Myometrial and Cardiovascular Responses to Alterations in Plasma Epinephrine and Norepinephrine." *Am. J. Obstet. & Gyn.* 84(7):841–851, 1962.
32. Morishima, H. O., et al. "The Influence of Maternal Psychological Stress on the Fetus." *Am. J. Obstet. & Gyn.* 131(3):286–290, 1978.
33. Newton, N., et al. "Experimental Inhibition of Labor through Environmental Disturbance." *Obstet. & Gyn.* 27(3):371–377, 1966.
34. Newton, N., et al. "Effect of Disturbance on Labor." *Am. J. Obstet. & Gyn.* 101(8):1096–1102, 1968.
35. Newton, N. "The Effect of Psychological Environment on Childbirth: Combined Cross-Cultural and Experimental Approach." *J. Cross-Cultural Psychol.* 1(1):85–90, 1970.
36. Matthews, A. E. B. "Reflections on the Pain of Labour." *Nurs. Mirror* 118:550–554, 1964.
37. Woodrow, K. M., et al. "Pain Tolerance: Differences According to Age, Sex and Race." *Psychosomat. Med.* 34(6):548–556, 1972.
38. Mead, M., and Newton, N. "Cultural Patterning of Perinatal Behavior." In Richardson, S. A., and Guttmacher, A. F., eds. *Childbearing—Its Social and Psychological Aspects*. Baltimore, Md.: Williams & Wilkins Co., 1967, pp. 142–244.
39. Atwood, R. J. "Parturitional Posture and Related Birth Behavior." *Acta Obstet. & Gyn. Scandinav.* Supplement 57, 1976.
40. Liu, Y. C. "Effects of an Upright Position in Labor." *Am. J. Nurs.* 74(12):2202–2205, 1974.
41. Engelmann, G. J. *Labor Among Primitive Peoples*. St. Louis: J. H. Chambers & Co., 1882.
42. Austin, S. H. "Coping and Psychological Stress in Pregnancy, Labor and Delivery with 'Natural Childbirth' and 'Medicated' Patients." Doctoral dissertation, University of California, Berkeley, 1974.
43. Cogan, R. "Use of Relaxation and Breathing after Labor Contractions Begin." *Birth & Fam. J.* 1(3):16–18, 1974.
44. Willmuth, L. R. "Prepared Childbirth and the Concept of Control." *JOGN Nurs.* 4(5):38–41, 1975.
45. Chertok, L. *Motherhood and Personality: Psychosomatic Aspects of Childbirth*. Great Britain: Tavistock Publications, 1966.
46. Clark, A. L. "Labor and Birth: Expectations and Outcomes." *Nurs. Forum* 14(4):413–428, 1975.
47. Deutsch, H. *Psychology of Women, Vol. 2, Motherhood*. New York: Grune & Stratton, 1945.
48. Rubin, R. "Maternal Tasks in Pregnancy." *Mat.-Child Nurs. J.* 4(3):143–153, 1975.
49. Elkins, V. H. "The Rights of the Pregnant Parent." New York: Two Continents Pub. Group, Inc., 1976.
50. Annas, G. J. *The Rights of Hospital Patients*. New York: Avon Books, 1975.
51. Israel, S. L., and Woutersz, T. B. "Teen-Age Obstetrics." *Am. J. Obstet. & Gyn.* 85(5):659–668, 1963.

52. Rubin, R. "Puerperal Change." *Nurs. Outlook* 9(12):753–756, 1961.
53. Bibring, G. L. "Some Specific Psychological Tasks in Pregnancy and Motherhood." In *1st International Congress of Psychosomatic Medicine and Childbirth, Paris, 8–12 July, 1962.* Paris: Gauthier-Villars, 1965, pp. 21–26.
54. Erikson, E. H. *Identity: Youth and Crisis.* New York: W. W. Norton & Co., Inc., 1968, p. 135.
55. Kaplan, D. M., and Mason, E. A. "Maternal Reactions to Premature Birth Viewed as an Acute Emotional Disorder." In Parad, H. J., ed. *Crisis Intervention: Selected Readings.* New York: Family Service Association of America, 1965, pp. 118–128.
56. Mercer, R. T. *Nursing Care for Parents at Risk.* Thorofare, N.J.: C. B. Slack, Inc., 1977.
57. Schweitzer, B., and Youngs, D. D. "A New Professional Role in the Care of the Pregnant Adolescent." *Birth & Fam. J.* 3(1):27–30, 1976.
58. Mercer, R. T. "Research Project: Attainment of the Maternal Role by Teenage Mothers." 1976.
59. Hallett, E. R. "Birth and Grief." *Birth & Fam. J.* 1(4):18–22, 1974.

14

The Adolescent Parent

RAMONA T. MERCER, R.N., PH.D.

Parenting is an adult role requiring adult skills and maturity for its successful negotiation. The adolescent who opts to assume the parenting role, either by choice or by default, relinquishes the usual social moratorium[1] of experimentation and role play in safe settings that permits vacillation between dependence and independence. The abrupt break in the continuity of her development which the adolescent mother faces when she must move from a child's dependent role in which she *receives* care, to the independent parent role in which she *gives* care, is profound and often traumatic. If she chooses to marry, she assumes an additional adult role that also requires much facility in role adjustment.

The early or middle adolescent whose cognitive abilities have not reached the stage of conceptualizing and abstract problem solving is handicapped in assuming adult roles. Further, she may be very egocentric—unable to view situations from another person's perspective—and her social skills in role attainment may be quite undeveloped. Whether the adolescent can provide nurturant, empathic, and growth-inducing physical care for an infant depends upon her level of cognitive, emotional, and social maturity.

Additionally, the intrapsychic disequilibrium that occurs concomitantly with a woman's psychological adjustment to pregnancy and impending motherhood[2,3,4,5] may intensify the disequilibrium the adolescent is already experiencing in evolving her adult identity.

During adolescence the resolution of reemerging childhood conflicts fosters ego maturation.[6] Motherhood provides another opportunity for further development via "emotional symbiosis," which is described by Benedek[7] as a spiral of reciprocal mother-child interactions that create developmental changes in both. At each "critical period" of the child's development the parent's unresolved conflicts of that period reemerge; if the parent resolves the conflict, a higher level of personality integration is achieved.[7] Has the early or middle adolescent reached a level of maturation that is capable of this higher level of integration? Does her child's mirroring of her conflicts threaten her to the extent that her defenses do not permit her continued growth?

Deutsch[8] suggested that pregnancy in early adolescence may be crippling to an

348

immature personality, whereas motherhood in late adolescence has the potential either to consolidate maturity or to be traumatic.[9] Pregnancy has the potential of acting as a catalyst for the maturational process of the older teenager, whereas it may be a disorganizer for the young teenager.

In this chapter the challenge of adolescent parenthood is viewed from the perspective of the risk for young parents and their infants. Vignettes of early, middle, and late adolescents highlight both the developmental problems and the achievements of these young mothers during their first year of motherhood. The teenagers' responses to mothering are compared to the older mothers' responses. The process of achieving a maternal role is discussed along with ways of facilitating the adolescent's parenting role and some of the resources for promoting quality parenting.

Scope of the Challenge

There are approximately 608,000 teenage births annually in this country, and nine out of ten of the teenage mothers keep their babies.[10] Figure 14–1 illustrates the choices teenagers 15 to 19 years of age made about the disposition of their babies in the early 1970s. Approximately 547,200 infants per year are born to adolescent mothers who retain custody of them. What is the outcome for these infants and their parents? How can health professionals and community leaders best meet the health and social needs of these youthful parents?

REPORTED RESEARCH

Physical, sociological, and psychological risks for teenage parents are discussed in some detail in Chapters 11 and 13. The risks for the adolescent's infant, as reported in research, receive greater attention here.

The adolescent mother's infant receives a disproportionate burden of the hazards of youthful pregnancy because the high morbidity and death rates for the infant place him at greater medical risk than the mother.[11] Menken[12] reported additional hazards for the teenager's infant; negative environmental influences add to high postneonatal death rates, especially for infants whose mothers are under 15 years of age.

A comparative, controlled study over a ten-year period of mothers under 18 years of age and mothers 18 years old or older found significant deficits or impairments in children of the younger mothers.[13] Children of younger mothers had been reared by someone other than their parents more often, and were less often reared in families that were described as healthy by social workers. The group of younger mothers had more children within a six to eight year period than the older mothers. The younger mother exhibited less anxiety and wanted her child to have freedom to behave independently more often than did the older mothers. The children of the younger mothers were characterized as dependent, distractible, outgoing, and having more infantile behavioral and acting-out problems more often than the older mothers' children, however. The younger mothers' children were underweight, shorter, and had poorer reading skills and a lower IQ more often than children of the older

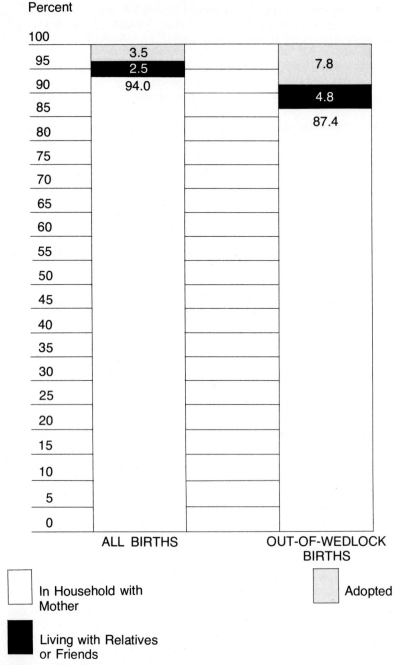

Figure 14–1. Disposition of babies born to females aged 15–19, United States, 1971. Reprinted with permission from *11 Million Teenagers: What Can Be Done About the Epidemic of Adolescent Pregnancies in the United States,* published by the Alan Guttmacher Institute, New York, 1976.

mothers. Since the subjects were matched for socioeconomic status, child's birth weight, race, and numbers of previous live births, researchers believed differences to be attributable specifically to youthful age.

A follow-up study of a program for low-income pregnant teenagers assessed infant's development and behavioral style, and mother-infant interaction of 60 mothers and infants during the first year of life.[14] Infants' average birth weight was 312 grams (11 ounces) below the national average. At 1 month, 74% of the infants were below the 50th percentile in weight, although at 6 months the infants' weight resembled that of the population at large. There was an overall weight decrease at 9 months when 55.9% were below the 50th percentile, and at 12 months, with 61.6% below the 50th percentile. Both strengths and weaknesses were observed in mother-infant interactions. The mothers were high in warmth and physical interaction and low in verbal interaction with their infants. High measures of activity and lower ratings of affectivity and responsivity were observed in these infants.

Child-rearing attitudes of 80 black mothers, aged 15 to 19 years, were tested prenatally by questionnaire.[15] The teenagers indicated a preference for physical punishment or coercive persuasion for aggression against parents. Their responses to the questionnaire suggested that there had been inconsistency in their own childhood disciplining. They had little knowledge of the value of praise and sensory stimulation in promoting the child's early development. The teenagers, however, expressed a basically warm and motherly attitude toward children, especially newborn infants, and some sensitivity to a child's needs.

Williams[16] reported that fewer young mothers breast-fed their infants. He also observed that young mothers talked less to their children, were less sensitive to the children's cues than other caretakers, and seemed to decide on options from their point of view rather than the child's.

Singer[17] described child-rearing practices of young 11- to 22-year-old non-addicted mothers in a special program for adolescents from a heavy drug use area as socializing the children into the drug culture. The young mothers, intent upon "showing the baby who is boss," fed babies according to their preference rather than when the infant indicated hunger. An infant or toddler was not expected or permitted to explore or to request attention, and was expected to go to sleep when told to do so. The baby was dressed so that his appearance was pleasing to the mother rather than appropriate for the climate. The young mothers began toilet training before the infant was a year old, and all used physical punishment. Because age-specific exploratory behaviors reflected poor mothering to the young mothers, they were viewed as bad. Strict enforcement of compliant behavior kept their children dependent, so that when the child was sent to school or to the street at age six or seven, he did not know how to function.

DeLissovoy[18] studied 48 teenage couples during their first three years of parenthood. He found the young parents as a whole to be rather intolerant. They were impatient, insensitive, irritable, and likely to use physical punishment with their children. The severe frustrations experienced by the young parents were attributed to their inexperience, unrealistic expectations of child development, lack of economic resources, and a general disappointment in their lives.

Crumidy and Jacobziner[19] studied 100 unmarried primigravidas under 21 years of age for 18 months to determine whether intensified social work would be of benefit to the group. All of the mothers kept their infants. Many of the subjects were hostile and ambivalent about their babies; the majority were unhappy in their roles as unwed mothers. Although the young woman's attitude toward child care was similar to that of her parents, the young mothers were very interested in receiving help with emotional problems, education, and employment. The young mother under 16 played with her infant as if he were a live doll and was content to have her mother assume responsibility for his care. With individual, highly intense, sympathetic, and understanding care, the young mothers were helped in job finding, work perform-ance, and personality development, all of which increased their self-confidence.

LaBarre[20] studied 71 pregnant school-age girls during pregnancy and at a one-year follow-up interview. An assertion of independence by the young mothers as they began to voice their dissatisfactions was observed. They experienced problems in returning to school when plans for baby care were disrupted by illness or other family crises. The married mothers experienced more problems than single mothers in their living situations because of the multiple tasks of school work, housework, and feeding and caring for their infant and husband. In an earlier pilot study of 10 white, married teenage mothers, LaBarre[21] observed that the mothers grew during the experience of pregnancy and possessed much optimism and courage in the face of crises.

Those working with teenage mothers have reported that their youth and its resiliency, energy, and capacity to have fun are their major assets.[16,22] The teenage mothers' willingness and capacity to learn about child development and parenting have been demonstrated in an interdisciplinary program in which after one year they were observed to have gained confidence and competence in their new role.[23]

One residential program for the "child-mother" and her infant provides care for the dyad until the mother achieves her educational or occupational goals.[24] The mother and child are equal as clients in this program that utilizes an extended family concept in which staff members care for both the infant and the mother. Mothers learn how to care for their children in a sharing kind of atmosphere. Benas[24] noted that often a mother needs only two years, from 16 to 18, to learn the necessary parenting skills.

Teenage parents indeed present unique problems and challenges for health care professionals. As they learn to parent, they need nurturing guidance to achieve their own developmental milestones.

Clinical Cases

Eight vignettes are presented which describe the first year of motherhood for two early adolescent mothers, three middle adolescent mothers, and three late adolescent mothers. Outcomes at the end of the first year are discussed in relation to the developmental level of the mothers and the impact of motherhood on the adolescent's growth.

Data for the eight vignettes are from a study of teenage mothers during their first year of motherhood. A naturalistic field approach was used for the purpose of describing the transition of the young women to the maternal role and evolving hypotheses for continued study. During the year, 12 interviews were held with each young mother in which the teenager expressed her feelings and perceptions about her experiences and the impact of the mothering role on these experiences.

THE EARLY ADOLESCENT PARENT

PAM AND HER DAUGHTER, AMY

Pam, a 14-year-old single black girl delivered a term but small for gestational age (2,183 grams, or 4 pounds 13 ounces) infant girl spontaneously following a 6-hour labor. She described her labor on her first postpartal day: "It wasn't bad at all, except the last 15 minutes of it. Then I liked to [have] died the pain was so bad." Pam's daughter, Amy, remained in the hospital for two days following Pam's discharge to her mother's nicely furnished modern apartment. Amy weighed 2,240 grams (4 pounds 15 ounces) upon discharge and gained about 454 grams (1 pound) a week in the next two weeks. Amy weighed 8,618 grams (19 pounds) when she was 10 months old. Pam's mother remained home from work for a week to be with Pam during her first week home from the hospital. Pam breast-fed Amy for about six weeks.

Pam had many girlfriends who had had babies. When asked if she felt lonely or left out of things since she had had a baby, she replied, "No, all of my friends have babies."

Pam demonstrated that she was comfortable with the physical care-taking skills of holding, changing, and feeding her infant. She said that she had learned these skills by taking care of her cousins' babies, rather than in classes "over at the school."

Pam went back to school when Amy was two weeks old. Amy stayed at her great-aunt's while Pam was in school. Pam did not like the special school following her delivery, however. She commented, "All those big stomachs over there. Everyone either has had a baby or is going to have one." When Pam went to a regular high school, she liked it better. Amy stayed at the family development center when Pam changed schools. During the summer months Pam worked part-time as a file clerk but found it hard to get up and get both herself and Amy dressed.

Pam never volunteered information about Amy's father. When asked, she noted that he came to see Amy, but Amy cried when he came. Pam commented that he never held her. He moved out of the city during the year and never provided any financial assistance for Amy. Pam dated occasionally during her first year of motherhood and was on contraceptive pills.

Pam was frank when answering questions about what it was like for her, being a mother. At one month, she related, "It's pretty bad. I get so mad I want to hit her. . . . She takes up all of my time." Yet, when asked how motherhood had affected her personally, Pam said, "You are the same person you were before."

At three months, Pam reported that she was getting Amy over her "spoiled" behavior. When asked how this was being done she replied, "When she cries, I don't pick her up."

At the monthly interviews Pam always handed Amy to the interviewer to hold in a very sharing way. On one visit, Pam had forgotten that the interviewer was coming, and she apologized because Amy was at her aunt's. Pam often watched television during interviews. There were many silences while she remained absorbed in the television performance.

Pam consistently referred to diapers as the hardest thing about being a mother. Amy was allergic to disposable diapers and this worked a hardship on Pam, who had to wash the diapers by hand, soak them, then take them to the laundromat.

Pam found that the nicest things about being a mother included Amy's quiet periods, her playing, and her mimicking of Pam's faces. From all observations, Amy indeed seemed like a younger sister, and Pam was a developing teenager who found it difficult to place or consider Amy's needs before her own. She commented about Amy's cruising and crawling, "She is so bad, she is into everything."

Pam's mother helped her with feeding and caring for Amy, and Pam said that she liked this help. Pam's older sister, who was 16, also helped care for Amy at times convenient to her. Pam related that both her sister and her mother "spoiled the baby." Amy reportedly had also "taken over everything in the house" by one month of age.

During interviews Pam teased Amy until she cried. Once when Amy was eight months old, Pam's mother heard Amy cry and intervened by slapping Pam's thighs; after a struggle she retrieved Amy from between Pam's legs and took the baby to another room.

Pam made derogatory remarks about Amy throughout the year. In referring to how ugly Amy was at birth Pam shuddered, saying that Amy had been hairy, flaky, and scrawny, with legs like a frog. Later she referred to Amy as having "fat old legs and triple chins." Amy in reality was an exceptionally pretty infant with delicate features.

Pam seemed to be compulsive about cleanliness; when Amy burped, Pam ran her finger in the baby's mouth with a diaper to clean her mouth. When Amy was eight months old, Pam maintained that she had 30 dirty diapers daily. At one year of age, Amy was being toilet trained.

Amy had measles when she was five months old and had a cold at every visit afterward during the year. At eight months of age, her ears had been infected and "running" and she received ampicillin. At one year, Pam was unconcerned about Amy's cough and chest congestion and the fever that she had had earlier.

Amy laughed and responded eagerly to Pam, just as she cried readily when Pam teased her by holding objects out of her reach. When Pam held her at the one-year interview, Amy sucked her thumb and twisted her hair as she dozed against her mother's breasts. Pam maintained that motherhood had not affected her life at all: "I'd be living here with my mother, going to school, and going skating on weekends. It wouldn't be any different. . . . I never will feel like a mother. She is more like a sister."

VIOLET AND HER SON, TOMMY:

Violet, a black 14-year-old, was delivered by cesarean section following a six-hour labor with the baby in a frank breech position. She had a 3,572 gram (7 pound 14 ounce) son, who was diagnosed at four weeks as having a ventricular septal defect. This was treated with medication, and when her son, Tommy, was eight months old, Violet was assured that the medication had corrected his heart defect and that surgery would not be necessary.

During her postpartal hospitalization Violet asked the nurse to bring her a coloring book because she was bored. Violet handled her son with ease and seeming confidence from the first initial contact and referred to him as "Beautiful. It's hard to believe that I birthed anything so beautiful." However, during the first week after her discharge from the hospital she said to Tommy, "I'm sick and tired of you."

Violet lived with her mother who had a chronic heart disease and also drank rather heavily. Their home was in a run-down section of town.

Violet returned to high school at approximately six weeks postpartum after much encouragement and after special arrangements had been made by the nurse, who was visiting her frequently. Violet told the nurse, "I have to finish school or it's always going to be like this, nothing to do. . . . I won't be able to do anything but have babies and clean house, I can't stand it anymore." Social workers and teachers were pleased with the Violet who now smiled and seemed so happy; she was very different from the sullen, withdrawn Violet who missed many days of school during pregnancy. This new optimism about Violet was short-lived, however. When Violet became ill and missed some days at school, the teachers speculated that she was cutting school "just as she did before." Violet soon met their expectations and dropped out of school again.

Tommy's father, Frank, lived with Violet at Violet's home much of the year. Around the third month following Tommy's birth, Violet's mother was hospitalized and there was much moving back and forth of the young couple and infant from Violet's to Frank's home. During this period of instability Tommy became ill with an upper respiratory infection and Violet did not keep appointments for him at the cardiac clinic or give him medications that were ordered. Tommy became wan and thin and was hospitalized for failure to thrive syndrome and the upper respiratory infection. Violet was heard to say to Tommy during a clinic visit before his hospitalization, "I hate you, I hate you." Although placement in a foster home was encouraged by the public health nurse for both Violet and Tommy, both Violet and her mother resisted. When Violet's mother became well again, she went with Violet to all clinic visits for Tommy. With the grandmother's emotional support, Tommy did well.

Frank worked at his fathering role early by holding and caring for his son. Frank was also warm and playful with Violet, yet he used physical violence in anger. Violet related, "He slapped my face." Violet pouted when Frank chided her about not helping her mother with household chores.

Violet became pregnant when Tommy was seven and a half months old. Violet had been taking a contraceptive pill, but when the heavy bleeding that she was experiencing did not subside, she stopped taking the medication. Violet had met the expectation of her mother, who had told her that she would be pregnant again before Tommy was a year old.

When Tommy was nearly a year old the public health nurse arranged for Violet to live at a residential home so that she could return to school and have adequate care for herself and Tommy. Her mother was physically unable to care for the infant while

Violet attended school. Both Violet and her mother were ambivalent about the residential home. Violet's mother felt that she had not been adequately involved or consulted in this planning, and both felt it a disadvantage that "there were no colored there. There was one black baby-sitter, but she acted white." Both Violet and her mother expressed the opinion that blacks were "warmer and more affectionate with their babies than whites," and they did not want Tommy to grow up "thinking he is white." Violet was, however, also seeing positive aspects about the move: "It's a real pretty place. They're gonna give me a room alone. I have to get up at 8:00 A.M. and dress the baby before breakfast and take him to the nursery next door." Violet, well into her fourth month of pregnancy, was relieved to be over her morning sickness. She was experiencing conflict between the opportunity to go to school and to live in a better environment and the necessity to move from her mother's home in order to do so. Still a child needing her mother's approval, she was unable to mother her son independently. Although Violet moved to the residential home, she stayed only two weeks. She preferred living with her mother.

Discussion: The first year of parenthood had a decidedly disorganizing impact on Violet, whereas Pam, because of her immature cognitive reasoning faculty, maintained that "nothing had changed." Violet's motherhood indeed seemed to have trapped her in the cycle of "being able to do nothing but have babies and clean house," as she had feared during earlier months of motherhood. Violet's inability to resume her schooling has made it difficult for her to continue to develop her potential. Her immature judgment and behavior were demonstrated when Tommy became ill and had to be hospitalized during the grandmother's illness. Because of illness, Violet did not have the physical support from her mother that Pam had had. Apparently, the physical and emotional help that Pam received from her mother made it possible both for her and for Amy to grow and develop.

Both Violet's and Pam's emotional maturity were such that they were not able to place the needs and demands of an infant before their own. Their cognitive immaturity was reflected in their insensitivity to normal cues and responses from a developing infant.

The case studies of Violet and Pam suggest the importance of a continuing mother figure for the young child-mother, one who is able to provide nurturing care for both the mother and infant. It seems that without a strong mother, or surrogate mother, the young teenage mother cannot continue her own growth and development.

Both Pam and Violet expressed hostility to their infants that reflected some of the anger they felt in their premature mothering roles. Though anger and conflict play important roles in motivating mothering behavior, when teenagers are faced with the emotion of anger and with conflicting emotions, they need help in channeling these feelings into constructive mothering or other appropriate role responses.

Although neither Pam nor Violet attained a mothering role in the sense that their infants were central to their lives and they were able to assume responsibility for their infants' welfare, they were not particularly aware of this. The immaturity of their cognitive reasoning seemed to preclude their recognizing their shortcomings. They did not express anxiety or worry about their infants' welfare, suggesting detachment. Both seemed to enjoy, and need, their dependence on their mothers.

Violet dramatizes so vividly the danger involved when parents, health care workers, or educators have preconceived notions or stereotypes about adolescent behavior. Violet seemed to give up and meet the expectations of her teachers that she was not actively interested in her education and would drop out of school. Likewise she met her mother's expectations that she would be pregnant before her infant was one year old. Pam's mother treated her as if she were a sister to Amy, and Pam "felt like a sister" to Amy.

The self-concept is socially defined. Significant other persons' responses to us in our day-to-day interactions with them convey our characteristics and our worth, which we ultimately introject and later project.

THE MIDDLE ADOLESCENT PARENT

Dottie and Jim, and their daughter, Joan

Dottie, a vivacious 16-year-old Filipino, had to have a cesarean delivery because of cephalopelvic disproportion and fetal distress. She reacted to the spinal anesthesia and had two seizures on the operating table. She had an infection postpartum and was not allowed to hold or touch her daughter for three days. Her daughter, Joan, weighed 3,459 grams (7 pounds 10 ounces) at birth.

Jim, a 19-year-old Caucasian, had lived across the street from Dottie. They dated for two years before she became pregnant. Their daughter was born about five months following their marriage. Dottie related that they were lonely and had had intercourse to achieve closeness and a feeling of security. Dottie and Jim lived in a large, roomy apartment across the street from Dottie's parents' home.

Dottie was deeply concerned about social approval. She worried about whether the doctor or nurse would judge that her daughter was gaining "too much or not enough" weight. She hated to leave Joan with sitters for fear that she might be fussy and that the sitters might think that Dottie was not a good mother or might not want to put up with fussiness.

Dottie's parents had marital problems during her first year of motherhood. They separated, then went back together. The separation posed a hardship for Dottie since her father baby-sat for her while she worked, and when her parents separated the father had to move. Dottie judged that her father was better with Joan than her mother was.

Dottie experienced much fatigue during the first postpartal weeks. By three months, boredom and isolation were overwhelming. Dottie had completed high school requirements during her pregnancy. She felt that her husband did not understand what it was like to be home all day "doing the same thing over and over." When she began working during her fifth month of motherhood, her feelings about herself improved, and the money she earned helped with expenses.

Both Dottie and Jim enrolled in college when Joan was six months old. This seemed to be an exciting outlet for Dottie; she planned a career in a helping profession (she was not sure what she would choose ultimately).

An invitation to speak at a national conference on school age parents when Joan

was six months old also boosted Dottie's self-esteem. Both Jim and Dottie participated in a state conference on school age parents a couple of months later. Dottie felt
that the latter experience was helpful to their relationship since Jim had an opportunity to express his feelings to professionals and to other teenage parents. Dottie was
then able to understand some of the feelings that Jim had had during early parenthood.

Dottie was concerned about her relationship with Jim from the beginning of their
parenthood, and worried lest Jim should feel left out when she breast-fed Joan. On
the other hand, she was irked when Jim came home and did not want to care for Joan
while she prepared dinner. Her continued concern about her marriage was rewarded,
because the couple experienced much growth in their relationship over the first year
of parenthood. She stated, "We have worked together in so many things and have
grown together so much. Our relationship is so much richer. I enjoy so much the
feeling of our own family and being a part of it. It really is just great to see Jim and
Joan romping and squealing."

Although Dottie experienced conflict about her mothering role, she became surer
in the role and enjoyed it increasingly over the year. In her ninth month of
motherhood she felt competent in the role and sure of herself, so that she "did not
feel a need to ask anyone what to do or what to expect." Although she had felt
motherly before that time, she had not felt competent.

Joan's growing up was exciting for Dottie to experience. Dottie remarked that
Joan looked so precious falling asleep that it brought tears to her eyes. Dottie had
tears in her eyes as she shared the poignant moment.

Dottie had much insight into Joan's impact on both herself and Jim. When Joan
was six months old, she commented, "We have had a baby right when we were
developing our own identities, and we have to consider this dependent baby before
ourselves. Our growth gets stunted. Jim and I have to really work at our own growth
and our marriage."

Dottie also described herself as a "misfit." "I don't look like a mother or
anything when I go out. I can't talk to my girlfriends who are getting ready for the
senior prom. They would not understand what I'm talking about." Jim described
himself as a "boy-man" following an incident which emphasized the asynchrony of
the social system. He was denied the privilege of purchasing a bottle of wine. Dottie
very frustratedly commented, "Here he is a father and could be drafted to serve his
country, and he can't even buy a cheap bottle of wine."

At the end of her first year of motherhood, Dottie said, "When I come in from
work and she runs to me and hugs me, it is wonderful. She laughs with me and is
glad to see me. I know that I am doing a good job and she trusts me."

MARIE AND HER SON, MIKE

Marie, a black 16-year-old, was preeclamptic during labor (B.P. 200/110) and
had a third degree laceration when her son, Mike, was delivered by low forceps. He
weighed 3,203 grams (7 pounds 1 ounce). She described her labor as "a two-day
labor." Marie was hospitalized for acute endometritis at two weeks postpartum and
had a uterine infection at five months. She was hospitalized again at 11 months for
uterine and urinary tract infections.

Mike's health fared no better than Marie's. During his third week following birth, he was hospitalized for a gastrointestinal series, barium enema, and proctoscopy to determine the cause of his rectal bleeding and diarrhea. Following these procedures he had no further bleeding. He had an upper respiratory infection at two and one half months and ear infections at five and nine months of age which required ampicillin to treat the infection with a fever of 40°C. (104°F.). Marie noted that all of Mike's colds seemed to end in ear infections.

Marie moved from her parents' comfortable, old, well-furnished home to an apartment of her own at three months postpartum. She moved to another apartment with a boyfriend when Mike was nine months old. After a couple of months with her boyfriend she moved in with her sister for a short while before moving back to her parents' home. Marie talked warmly with the interviewer, although she was not home on four occasions to keep appointments. At all visits with Marie, either the television, radio, or stereo was on.

Mike's father, Ray, was in the hospital with Marie for her labor and delivery, and again when she was hospitalized two weeks postpartally. Ray continually pressured Marie to marry him. He held Mike, fed him, and reacted warmly with him. When Marie was in the hospital at two weeks postpartum, Ray wanted to take Mike to his mother's so that she could care for him. Marie spurned Ray's offer of help and his offers of marriage. She observed that Ray was too dependent on his mother to get out on his own; he wanted her to move in with his mother. He reportedly was also jealous and possessive. Marie's mother reaffirmed these statements.

Marie began dating Don when Mike was one month old. At five months after Mike's birth, Ray confronted Don while all of them were at Marie's sister's wedding and said, "Give me my baby." Ray threatened to take legal action to gain custody of his son at that time and periodically during Mike's first year. Marie retaliated that she would move out of the state if he did so and would not appear in court. Ray never followed through on his threats.

Marie wished to return to school; she had been in the eleventh grade when she dropped out after becoming pregnant. She noted that Ray had talked her into cutting classes before she became pregnant. Marie felt that now she could appreciate school; she even spoke of going to college. Marie did return to school when Mike was two months old, but had to drop out when he became ill and there was no one to care for him. After she was in her own apartment she could not find a baby-sitter and she talked of studying to pass the GED test to get her high school diploma and going on to nurses' aid school or to clerical school. Marie went back to school a second time when Mike was seven months old but dropped out when she moved to another part of town with her boyfriend Don. Marie had a job offer to work in a convalescent home at the end of Mike's first year, but was unable to find a baby-sitter or funds to pay for one.

Marie had a large support system: her mother, two younger brothers, two older sisters, girlfriends who were pregnant, her boyfriend, and Ray's mother and sisters. There was a perceivable warmth within the family unit; the young males enjoyed interacting with Mike, and a 12-year-old brother later went across the town to spend the night with Marie in order to baby-sit. Before she moved, her brothers got up at night to feed Mike.

Marie maintained that Mike knew his father, Ray, but added, "You know I have been going with Don since he was born and Mike loves Don too, and Don plays with him."

Marie described herself as "very independent, basically." Marie felt that motherhood contributed to her independence. She noted that her relationship with her mother had changed and that her son had given her something to live for. Before she became pregnant she became depressed when she and her mother argued, and felt that she had nothing to live for. "Now, we get along better. She talks to me like I'm grown up, and if she fusses I look at Mike and know that I have something to live for."

Marie's mother was an important role model and authority figure. Her two older sisters also served as role models. Her mother supported Marie by her statements and by praising her capabilities and behaviors to the interviewer.

Mike was an active boy; he walked when he was one year old. Marie commented, "He is a bad boy. When I spank him, he spanks me back." Marie enjoyed watching Mike grow and was thrilled when he called her "Me-Me." Marie had grown up around small children and helped her older sisters with their small children before Mike was born so that she always felt competent in caretaking skills.

At the end of the first year of motherhood Marie reflected, "When he was sick with the bleeding bowels I knew then what it was like to worry about him being sick. It shook me up a lot. I worried and I was scared. Like he was just over two weeks old. And I knew what it was like being a mother."

HELEN AND HER DAUGHTER, THERESA

Helen, a 17-year-old Latino, delivered a 3,856 gram (8½ pound) daughter spontaneously. She suffered a fourth degree laceration and a postpartal urinary tract infection that necessitated her being in the hospital for nine days. She was not allowed to hold her daughter, Theresa, for five days.

Helen lived with her parents in an older home. Although it was not luxurious, it was comfortably furnished. With the birth of Theresa it became a four generational household, since Helen's maternal grandmother lived in the home. Helen related that her mother had always preferred her older sister to her and that her father called her "dirty" for having had a baby out of wedlock. "He worries about what people say," she said. Although her father would not let her boyfriend, John, come to the house to see her following Theresa's birth, John wanted to marry Helen. Helen said that she had never had close girlfriends because her father had embarrassed her older sister when her girlfriends came to their home. Helen described her father as "weird and moody."

Helen returned to high school at one month postpartum. She had been accelerated during the year of her pregnancy so that she managed to graduate the same year. Helen also began attending beauty school, although she stated that that was not what she wished to do for a life's occupation. She saw preparation as a cosmetologist as a form of security until she was better prepared at college. Helen passed her cosmetology test and received her license when Theresa was eight months old. Helen also passed her driving test and received her driver's license at about the same time. She manifested typical teenage pride in passing her driver's test and noted that her mother let her drive her car.

Mothering was a lot of hard work throughout the year for Helen. She had to get up at 5:30 A.M. to get Theresa and herself ready for the day so that she could get to school on time. Theresa was ill several times during her first year—diarrhea at five and eight months, an ear infection and rash at nine months, and stomach flu at ten months. Throughout the year, Helen worried about Theresa's illnesses and whether she should move into an apartment. She said, "There is so much to think about that it takes up *all* of your mind."

To Helen, the nicest thing about being a mother was expressed in the words "I have her, and she is all mine. That's something, the only thing that I have that is all mine." Helen was warm and sensitive with Theresa and Theresa clearly chose her mother for solace and comfort.

Helen's feelings for Theresa's father, John, seemed to vacillate. Shortly following Theresa's birth, she said she loved him very much and wanted to get married when they could afford it. Later, when he lost his job and was ineffective in obtaining another one, she stopped seeing him. Helen observed, "Men think they are superior, and if you marry them they treat you as if they are superior." She declared that it was much easier to live with just a baby than to live with a man. "A baby can't complain or argue with you, and you always have control." Undoubtedly, much of Helen's judgment about men was based on her observations of her father.

John helped Helen pay for her cosmetology license, and when she started college, he paid $15.00 weekly for a baby-sitter. Helen lacked complete trust in him, though, and said that she would go to summer school rather than let John get used to the extra $15.00 he paid the sitter during the summer. Helen had decided, when Theresa was a year old, that if her father would allow them to rent the upstairs apartment in the parents' home she would marry John. She was not fully convinced about the security in this and observed that she did not wish to get married in the church since she didn't know "if it would last." If her father did not agree to their living in an upstairs apartment she planned to move out to an apartment with John but to remain single. The welfare money she received would be essential to their livelihood and her continuing in college if they had to pay high rent for an outside apartment.

Helen denied a changed relationship with her mother during Theresa's first year. She viewed her mother as the person who had been the most helpful to her and added that her mother did not get mad if she did not follow her advice. Helen attributed her success in remaining in school to her mother. She felt that if she had lived in a residential home (which she had gone to visit and had considered moving into before the birth of her baby) she would not have had the encouragement to continue her schooling.

Helen observed that having a baby "forces you to grow up in a hurry." Otherwise, she felt that things in her life had not really changed all that much. She had finished beauty school, was enrolled in college, and, as she remarked, "I couldn't have gone out any more than I do anyway." Helen confided that she did not have money or a car to enable her to "take off" even if she had not had Theresa.

At the end of her first year of motherhood, Helen reflected that it was most difficult to see "Theresa in a setting without a home or a family of her own, and with few material things." Helen's desire for a traditional nuclear family setting of her own mirrored her need to become completely independent and on her own.

Discussion: The three case studies of the middle adolescent reflect a more mature perception of capabilities, greater sensitivity to the feelings of others, and much more growth during the first year of motherhood than was observed in the early adolescent. Motherhood appeared to have accelerated the middle adolescents' growth and to have helped consolidate their maturity.

The educational accomplishments of Dottie and Helen were remarkable. Marie, faced with illness and with moving a number of times, was unable to remain in school despite two efforts to continue.

Motherhood served to increase the self-esteem of all three young mothers. They all received social feedback of approval regarding their mothering roles. Their infants gave them a sense of purpose and responsibility in life.

Dottie, Marie, and Helen possessed the emotional maturity to consider their infants' needs before their own, although they experienced the usual conflict in doing so. They exhibited anxiety in caring for their infants during illness and in health. They enjoyed their infants' responses to them, and Marie and Helen, who did not have husbands, noted that their infants were especially important in the sense of having someone to love.

The young fathers and boyfriend were all emotionally and physically involved with their children. They enjoyed father-child interactions and, except for Ray, assumed financial responsibility in the child's care. The extent of the father's involvement with the child seemed to be largely limited and controlled by the youthful mother. The involvement of the younger brothers in helping to care for the infants also suggests that males are just as interested as females in caring for tiny, developing infants. Their interest and eagerness seem unaffected by old social stereotypes that view the woman as largely responsible for parenting. This masculine enthusiasm must be cultivated and expanded to foster the development of greater richness and humanness for us all!

All three of the middle adolescents seemed mature beyond their years in assessing their situations realistically. Marie and Helen astutely weighed the pros and cons of marriage. Helen continued to see the father of her infant; Marie had a meaningful relationship with another boyfriend. Although Helen had a biased view of masculinity because of her father, all three of the middle adolescents seemed comfortable with their femininity and in their self-concepts in relating with men.

Dottie's great concern about her new marriage may have been increased because of her own parents' dissolving marriage. However, her healthy anxiety and concern about including her husband in their daughter's care and about sharing communication seemed to have contributed to a stronger marital relationship.

Although Helen felt that her mother had always preferred her older sister, she also felt that her mother was supportive and recognized her capability in the mothering role. Dottie's and Marie's mothers recognized their capabilities as mothers also. Marie experienced the greatest change in relationship with her mother.

Marie and Dottie became more secure in their feelings of competency as mothers than Helen. Helen remained a little unsure about what she should be teaching her daughter.

Marie's situation points to the need for an active relationship with a counselor or social worker the first year following the birth of a child. If Marie had had help in finding infant day care or in transferring to different schools when she moved, she might have continued her education. That she was motivated was indicated by her two attempts. Persons in Marie's social system apparently did not value education to the same exent as did those in Dottie's and Helen's.

The middle adolescents in these vignettes possessed the maturity to grow through the experience of motherhood, and to further their educational and professional goals with proper supportive help from the social system.

THE LATE ADOLESCENT PARENT

ANN AND HER DAUGHTER, THELMA

Ann, an 18-year-old black high school graduate, had a daughter delivered by low forceps over a third degree laceration. Her postpartal course was uneventful. Ann's personal appearance throughout the first year of motherhood was always attractive and well-groomed, and she was eager to get her "waistline back." Ann, a very slender young woman who soon attained her prepregnancy size, breast-fed her daughter, Thelma, her entire first year.

Ann had moved with her mother, stepfather, two sisters, and one brother from the Midwest when she was seven months pregnant. Ann wore a wedding band and stated that her husband was in the army. During the first days after delivery, Ann spoke of joining her husband; however, she never initiated any conversation about him later, nor did she ever call him by name. He reportedly telephoned her from time to time, but Ann dated others and was active in a local church. Ann also received welfare and medical aid.

Ann and her family lived in a new four-bedroom apartment. Her parents valued education and upward mobility very highly. They encouraged Ann to go to college.

The grandmother, an attractive woman in her thirties, said that all Ann had to do in the house was to take care of Thelma. The grandmother was an authority figure and role model for Ann, who never argued with her. Ann often related how her mother had done things for her as a child, and compared and fantasized about how things would be similar for her daughter. The grandmother played a lot with Thelma and acknowledged that Ann did things differently than she had: "They cling to each other, and I put my kids down in a playpen. I toilet trained my children right away and didn't hold them all of the time."

Ann reacted warmly with her daughter. She verbalized that she had wanted a son because daughters require "so much more in the way of clothes and in being spoiled." Ann attributed cognitive functioning to her daughter early; at one month Thelma reportedly became bored and yawned during television commercials. Ann kept Thelma up to watch television with her until 1:00 or 2:00 A.M.

The television seemed central to their lives. It was always on during interviews throughout the year, and Ann frequently watched television as she talked with the interviewer.

When Thelma was at the clinic for a checkup at the end of her sixth month, it was noted that she had not gained weight for the last two months. Ann reported that Thelma had lost over 454 grams (1 pound) at her five-month checkup, but the nurse had told her to bring Thelma for weighing later, since the scales were working improperly. A physical examination revealed no cause for failure to gain or to grow. Conferences were held with social workers, physicians, and nurses who were caring for her. Ann had started attending secretarial school for four hours daily when Thelma was four months old, the apparent time of Thelma's cessation of growth and gaining. Ann was advised to quit school, but this did not alleviate the problem. Thelma did not gain or grow until her ninth month. While health care workers worked at ruling out maternal depression, maternal deprivation, and possible physical factors in Thelma—sickle-cell anemia, kidney dysfunction, etc.—Ann worried.

The pediatric nurse practitioner diagnosed the etiology of Thelma's failure-to-thrive syndrome as overstimulation and sleep deprivation. When Ann began putting Thelma to bed earlier in the evening, around 8:00 P.M. or so, Thelma began gaining weight. At the end of her first year, Thelma weighed 7,456 grams (16 pounds 7 ounces); she had weighed 3,232 grams (7 pounds 2 ounces) at birth.

Ann, without responsibility for household chores, had kept Thelma up late for company. Since, in addition, all members of the household had been playing with Thelma during the day she had not been getting sufficient rest for her growth.

Ann was bored and somewhat depressed after she dropped out of secretarial school. She returned to school when Thelma was nine months old, and, although the commuting was tiring, she was excited about preparing for a career so that she could move into her own apartment.

Although Ann reacted warmly with Thelma and the mother-infant pair had much body contact, Thelma had a somber expression after one month of age. Thelma smiled in response to her uncle and aunts, but she lacked the spontaneity of an infant soliciting responses. She manifested stranger anxiety at five months. She developed neuromuscular skills early; she was drinking from a cup she held herself at five months and walking alone at ten and a half months.

Ann, early in motherhood, described being a mother as "great" or "marvelous." At the end of her first year of motherhood, Ann said, "I wonder if it is really worth it to have kids." In addition to Ann's worry about Thelma's failure to gain or grow, there was some indication of Ann's loss of pleasure in an infant who had begun to individuate. Ann said, "It is so hard keeping her from hurting herself. She crawls, walks, and is into everything. It's hard to keep up with her."

JANE AND HER DAUGHTER, KATHY

Jane, an 18-year-old Caucasian, delivered her daughter two weeks postmaturely on the date on which she had had a spontaneous abortion one year earlier. The 3,416 gram (7 pound 8½ ounce) girl was delivered spontaneously and Jane had a vaginal hematoma postpartally. Both pregnancies were unplanned; Jane had been on the contraceptive pill both times. Jane and her husband had been married when she was 15 and he was 20. Her husband had wanted a baby, but Jane had not. Jane related, "I just knew it would be a girl. I just couldn't picture myself with a boy."

Jane described her husband as a slob who expected her to pick up after him, and who did not cook or help around the house. During the latter part of her pregnancy, Jane moved in with her parents because she did not feel like taking care of him any longer and because she needed emotional support which he was unable to give. Jane's husband was with her during labor and delivery, but Jane went back to her parents' nice, well-furnished home when she left the hospital.

Her daughter, Kathy, was in the intensive care nursery for two weeks following birth; she had hypoglycemia and anorexia and was on intravenous feedings. The first postpartal week, Jane related, "I don't really feel like a mother yet. I've only seen her three times, and I haven't held her at all."

Jane remarked at two weeks postpartum that it was good to be a mother, but that it was "scarey, too. I'm on welfare and medical aid. When you have children, you want something better for them, you know."

At six weeks postpartum Jane stated that her mother could not wait to get rid of her; Jane planned to move to a place of her own. Jane observed that her mother just did not like children and said, "If I hadn't been her own kid, she would have hated my guts."

Jane's father seemed to feel differently about babies, however. He enjoyed playing with Kathy and got up during the night to feed her while Jane slept. Jane breast-fed Kathy for about one month but never in her father's presence. "He's very conservative and would be shocked if I did." Jane viewed her Dad as "great. He thinks I'm wonderful because I did the greatest thing — give him a grandchild." Jane also commented, "Mother and I are the only ones who don't pick her up when she cries. As long as she's dry and fed and nothing's wrong, I'll just let her cry herself to sleep."

At three months postpartum, Jane admitted that she didn't like being a mother, but added, "I know it doesn't sound good." She said that she had wished Kathy back inside her so that she could eat and go as she wished. Jane enjoyed playing with Kathy and hearing her laugh and watching her when she fell asleep, however.

When Kathy was about four months old, Jane gave her baby to the young father to rear. Jane said at that time that he was better with Kathy than she: "He is a better mother than I am." Jane said that she had never felt like a mother, that she had feelings of being trapped, and that she was much happier now that Kathy was with her father.

At six and eight months postpartum, Jane said, "I hate babies. When they get about four years, I can relate to them. I can't stand little babies because they use and manipulate grown-ups. I've always felt that way."

Jane moved to her own apartment when Kathy was in her second month, but she could not swing it financially. After she gave Kathy to her father, she moved in with a man who was "in the same boat as me. He gets his two children on the weekend." Jane saw her daughter over the weekend at her parents' home where she "did not have complete responsibility." She maintained that she was relieved when Kathy's father came to pick her up.

Jane was repulsed by Kathy's drooling at three months. "I can't stand that. I'll wipe it off and then it's on my pants, and I look at all that spit, and I don't like it at all." Eight months after Kathy's birth, Jane said, "Changing a diaper is just horrible. It still nauseates me. People told me that I'd get used to it. But I never did. I still throw up. I can't stand the sight of it or the smell of it." Jane had conflicts about relinquishing Kathy, however, for she said that sometimes it was hard to see her go, and that when she saw a woman hug a small child she thought about her own daughter.

Ambivalence or conflict about Kathy was not the only ambivalence for Jane, however. Jane mentioned that she did not want a divorce because by remaining married she could not get married again. She reasoned that it would take six months to get a divorce and by that time she would be sure whether it would be a mistake to marry or not. Jane was also ambivalent about her feminine role. She seemed to identify strongly with her mother, and her feelings about babies were very much like those she had perceived in her mother. Jane also identified with a male role, commenting several times that she had taken over the "male role" in seeing Kathy on weekends only. She reiterated later that she "had all of the privileges of a man without any responsibility."

Jane planned to enroll in modeling school to learn poise, charm, and aggression, which she considered necessary "to get ahead." She emphasized what she regarded as Kathy's beautiful features—her eyes, eyebrows, complexion, etc. Eight months following delivery, Jane was working on her feminine identity; there seemed to be no energy for working at a maternal identity.

Jane was always neat and well-groomed and she liked her apartment and activities orderly. She complained about her inability to get caught up during the early months when she had Kathy with her. Jane also needed to feel that she was in control. "I used to hate having my reflexes tested. I still do. I guess I just have to be in control. I don't like to have my leg move without my controlling it." With Kathy, there were many uncontrollable factors, and an infant's schedule created chaos in her household.

At the end of the year following Kathy's birth, Jane's mother told her that she would never be independent. Her mother had earlier said that Jane was not capable of taking care of herself or her infant.

Jane, one year after giving birth to Kathy, moved out of the state to show her mother that she could be independent. Jane planned to keep the fact that she had had a daughter from friends that she might meet. Jane reported that one man lost interest in her when he found out that she had given her daughter up. Jane said, "It is no one's business, unless we get really serious or something."

SALLY, LARRY, AND THEIR SON, PAUL

Sally, a 19-year-old Filipino, delivered a 3,175 gram (7 pound) son by low forceps without complications. Sally had wanted a girl "for my mother," but her husband, Larry, had wanted a boy. Sally's father named their son.

Sally began considering whether she would let her mother and dad take her son back to the Philippines during her first postpartum week. Sally felt that if she permitted this it would make up for her elopement. She added that this was an Oriental custom. Sally vacillated about this decision until after her son, Paul, was over three months old, before deciding against it.

Sally and Larry, who was ten years her senior, had dated for three months before they eloped. Her parents had consented to their marriage, but had requested that Sally go back to the Philippines to discuss her decision with her grandmother. However, both Sally and Larry feared that if she did this, she would be unable to return to the

United States and to get married. They felt her grandmother would keep her in the Philippines.

Sally talked about her father's attachment to his grandson Paul a lot. The grandfather sat near the crib and watched Paul for long periods of time. He also baby-sat for her when Sally went to work. Sally also recalled having read letters that her father had written to her mother when she was pregnant with Sally about wanting a son.

Paul maintained eye contact with his mother when he was two weeks old; he also smiled early and often. Sally derived much pleasure from the eye contact, even when she was unsure whether she would permit her parents to take Paul to the Philippines.

When Paul was one month old, Sally let her parents keep him overnight so that she could get some rest. He had been colicky and awake every two hours for several nights. Sally commented, ''Boy, did I miss him.'' Sally also told about awakening to find Paul on the floor. She had apparently fallen asleep with him on her chest and he had rolled off onto the floor. She said that he had just a small bump on his head which soon disappeared. Paul was not taken to a doctor following the incident.

Sally enrolled in key-punch school at one month postpartum and began work as a key puncher a couple of months after finishing the course. When Paul was ten months old, Sally began to have migraine headaches and ''passed out'' at work, apparently from exhaustion and the headache medication. She was also disturbed by her obesity. She had been rather stocky and overweight following Paul's birth. She had continued to gain, never losing the weight gained during pregnancy. Her sister-in-law also moved into their apartment around this time. Larry worked the midnight to 8:00 A.M. shift and Sally worked from 2:00 P.M. to midnight. They saw little of each other and had little privacy.

After Sally obtained a day job she no longer experienced headaches. Sally also observed that her parents were less demanding of her: ''They let me have more time to myself.'' Paul had done well over the year. He was underweight when he was five months old, after just recovering from the flu, but by one year weighed 12.5 kilograms (27 pounds).

Sally initially found it hard to believe she was a mother but stated that she now knew what her ''mommy'' had gone through and could appreciate all that she had done for her. Partly because of her working so late in the evenings, getting up during the night was one of the most difficult aspects of mothering for Sally during her first few months in the role. She felt exhausted all of the time. Mothering was hard for Sally, and she felt that the responsibility was very great.

Sally enjoyed Paul most when he was asleep; she ''touched him and really thought about what it meant to be a mommy.'' She enjoyed picking out clothes for Paul.

Sally said that the first time she really felt like a mother was when Paul recognized her and went to her rather than to anyone else in the room. She noted, ''I wouldn't feel the way I do now if I had let Paul go to the Philippines to live.''

Although Sally denied having had any difficulty in her relationship with Larry as they incorporated Paul into the family unit, she had felt that Larry was not understanding of her fatigue. He had not helped her with the household chores. Sally added that Larry had wanted a child whereas she had not, so he had been better prepared for it. She felt that Larry's maturity had made it less difficult for them to adjust to an infant.

At the end of the year, Sally noted that mothering gets "harder and harder," the most difficult aspect being that she had no time for herself. Sally felt she had matured in the role, however, more than if she had not had Paul. Sally said that now she "thought more of others, particularly my family." If she hadn't got married, Sally observed, she would just think of herself, whereas now, "the first thing that comes into my mind is my son, my family."

Discussion: The vignettes of the late adolescent indicate that generalizations cannot be made that the late adolescent will have less difficulty with the mothering role than the early adolescent. Sensitivity to an infant's needs and the emotional ability to respond to these needs seem to be cultivated and learned behaviors. Although Ann was emotionally involved with Thelma, she had no cognitive awareness of or sensitivity to Thelma's physical need for rest. Rather, Ann met her own needs for companionship by keeping Thelma up with her. This was not intentional inconsideration on Ann's part. Ann experienced much guilt, anxiety, and worry when doctors were unable to find a reason for Thelma's failure to gain. Her guilty feelings were accented because she was queried often about how much she fed Thelma and how much attention she gave her. Ann's mothering was questioned, but perhaps in Ann's perception her keeping Thelma up and close to her reflected good mothering.

Jane's emotional immaturity was such that she was unable to incorporate the disorder and household disruptions of a growing infant into her life. Neither Ann nor Jane were accurate in their perceptions of an infant's cognitive capabilities at very young ages. Both saw their infants as planning and making judgments. Jane's lack of emotional involvement with Kathy led to her rejecting the maternal role, and even though Ann achieved the mothering role she wondered "if it was worth it."

Sally, the 19-year-old, did not have an easy first year of motherhood. Sally felt guilt about eloping, and this probably contributed to her vacillation about whether she would relinquish Paul to her parents. However, she became attached to Paul and could not relinquish him, despite her physical fatigue and heavy work schedule. She was mature enough to give to a dependent infant, but she also received positive feedback from Paul. Paul's early eye contact, smiling, and later recognition of Sally and his running to her were rewards for her mothering. She gained empathy toward her own mother and appreciated her earlier sacrifices in the mothering role. Sally felt that she and Larry had had no untoward difficulty in their relationship, although she experienced somatic symptoms and depression late in her first year of motherhood that perhaps reflected a lack of empathy on Larry's part.

Lynch[26] observed that depression in older adolescents may evolve from the resolution of the tasks of late adolescence, which necessitates finally relinquishing or modifying longtime idealized images of self, parents, and the world. Sally's getting married and becoming a mother forced her to acknowledge that her parents were neither all-powerful nor all-knowing. Her refusal to allow Paul to go to the Philippines to live presented Sally with the reality that her judgment could be superior to that of her parents, and she perhaps felt a sense of loss in recognizing that her parents were not omnipotent. Likewise, Jane no doubt experienced a similar feeling of loss when she finally realized that she could not depend on her parents for continued emotional and financial support as she had during her pregnancy and the months following it. Sally's reference to her mother as "mommy" suggests that vestiges of the little girl remained.

GENERAL DISCUSSION

These vignettes suggest developmental differences in the early, middle, and late adolescent; i.e., the early adolescent needs an adult role model in order to function in the maternal role, and she does not appear to achieve or internalize the role in a one-year period. However, the case of Jane illustrates that an older adolescent may be less advanced in her psychological and emotional development than the middle adolescent or early adolescent.

Cognitive development is quite variable according to age, as was noted earlier. Blasi and Hoeffel[27] point out that formal operations, or the ability to subordinate reality to possibility and to reflect on one's thoughts, are logical explanations for the universal characteristics of adolescence but may not hold true in all cases. They suggest that in considering the concept of possibility, the major difference between the youth's cognitive structures of formal operations and concrete operations may be the style in which a problem is approached. For example, formal operations cannot automatically be assumed to be better than concrete operations. Whereas formal operations involve making deductions for specific instances from general and implicit causal structures, a concrete operational approach involves responding to a specific problem on the basis of earlier relevant experiences. Concrete thinking may be adaptive to the extent that an individual has had rich and varied earlier experiences.[27]

One example which illustrates Blasi and Hoeffel's point is that of an adolescent living in very deprived social conditions. Because of the adolescent's extended experience of this situation, she may achieve, based on informally learned rules within her culture, a more cogent solution in dealing with a problem than the nurse who is postulating several alternatives from a nonexperiential or noninteractive base.

Blasi and Hoeffel[27] note that the ability to reflect on one's actions exists long before adolescence and long before the stage of formal operations occurs. They maintain that at adolescence what is new is the adolescent's attempt to capture the common source of action and to get at meaning and consistency within the self.

Blasi and Hoeffel's theoretical propositions are both especially intriguing and helpful in dealing with the question which often confronts the health care worker: "What do you do when the teenager does not have a cognitive level of understanding sufficient to learn infant care or sufficient to make decisions about her future?" These theorists offer one explanation for the wisdom sometimes observed in the very young, as well as some encouragement for the health care worker who is dealing with young people. Rather than her age per se or her facility with language or symbols, we must assess the young woman's earlier experiences in depth. What kinds of experiences has she had? In what kinds of situations? Was she able to respond flexibly, or does she have only rigid responses? Has she grown up helping to care for children or has she never held a small baby?

The vignettes dramatized that the adolescent's support system has the greatest impact, more, even, than age. Whom does the young woman have that she can depend on in emergencies? Does she have a loving and helpful mate? Does she get positive feedback from others in her setting?

Likewise, the development of a feminine identity occurs at different rates, dependent again upon the individual's mother (response to daughter, role model), background experiences, and opportunities to practice the feminine role.

Intervention for adolescent parents must focus on many more parameters than the age of the parent. A review of early problems in parenting for any parent yields a perspective that is useful in counseling adolescent parents. Following this review, a discussion of stages in assuming new roles in general is followed by postulation of phases in the process of attaining the maternal role for adolescent parents.

How Different is the Teenager's Response?

The adolescent mothers in the vignettes found that their mothering roles included a lot of hard and frustrating work. They expressed positive, negative, and ambivalent feelings about the role. These responses to the mothering role are not uniquely different from those observed in older mothers.[28,29,30] Barber and Skaggs[28] found that women who were first-time mothers in their late twenties and thirties tolerated their frustrations with an infant more easily than the younger mothers. They deduced that the more mature mother had a stronger desire for a child and a more mature view of life.

Robson and Moss[31] observed, in their sample of 54 primiparas aged 18 to 34 years, that 59% had positive feelings, 34% had no feelings, and 7% had negative feelings at the time of their first contact with their infants. These mothers found the first three to four weeks at home very demanding, and noted that they were fatigued and insecure. They expressed fears about harming their infants and frustrations at being unable to stop their crying or to communicate with them. During the fourth to sixth week the mothers experienced a transition period during which they were more confident in caring for their infants, who seemed more personable and had somewhat predictable eating and sleeping schedules. These findings do not sound terribly different from the adolescent mothers' responses.

Enjoyment of the infant's social response seems universal. Robson and Moss[31] also reported that mothers found their infants' smiles and recognition highly gratifying. Paul (Sally's son) might have ended up in the Philippines if it had not been for his winsome smile!

The exasperated feelings expressed by the teenage mothers about losing order in their lives also seems universal among mothers. Difficulty in adjusting to the baby's needs made up almost half of the responses among 33 primiparas describing their greatest stress at three months.[29] Worry about their ability to cope was also frequently mentioned. In another study, almost all of the 62 18-to-28-year-old first-time mothers indicated that they had not been prepared for the extent of the fatigue, disorganization, postpartum physical complications, and terrible feelings of inadequacy that they experienced in addition to the demands of both the infants and their husbands.[30]

Cohler and associates[32] noted that all mothers express ambivalence about the caretaking role which must be recognized and expressed if the mother takes a realistic approach to child care. They observed a greater denial of child-rearing concerns among 35 mothers admitted to a mental health hospital than existed among 35 nonhospitalized women who had never sought psychiatric care. The teenage mother's expression of ambivalence about the maternal role suggests a healthy expression of concerns.

Support and recognition from her mother seems to be an important factor in the teenage mother's growth during the year. When the mother was not supportive or did not recognize the daughter's capabilities, the teenager had difficulties in dealing with the mothering role. This may result from the strong identification a teenager has with her mother. If her mother does not judge her capable and competent, she cannot feel capable or competent. Achieving independence from the mother and becoming a peer in doing so did not appear to be a viable option for the younger adolescent. Bibring[33] observed that a woman's unresolved relationship with her mother, whether it reflects excessive submissiveness or defiance, can create disturbances in the early mother-child relationship. To be a healthy, happy mother, the woman must evolve from her earlier childlike relationship to her own mother and become coequal with her mother as a mother.

A positive relationship with her mate appears to enhance a teenager's self-esteem and to contribute to her sense of feminine identity in the mothering role. Russell[34] found that the transition to parenthood was less of a crisis when the level of marital adjustment was high; for the woman, the longer she had been married, the less severe was the crisis. A favorable relationship with the father of the child was a significant factor in the successful adaptation of 18- to 28-year-old mothers to the maternal role in another study.[30]

The postpartal morbidity observed in the teenage mothers during the postpartal period raises questions about their physical risks. In my study,[25] from which the vignettes are taken, eight of the 12 mothers (66%) experienced postpartal morbidity. Three had fever and infection following cesarean section; two had urinary tract infections; one had preeclampsia and endometritis; one had a vaginal hematoma; and one had influenza at four weeks. This compares unfavorably with a 20% morbidity rate found in a sample of 18- to 28-year-old subjects.[30] Fatigue and malaise due to illness deplete a mother's energy supply—energy that is needed for mothering.

A serendipitous finding from my study of teenagers has implications for the health care worker. Once the young women agreed to participate in the study, difficulties arose in making appointments for interviews, and on 12 occasions no one was home at the prearranged appointment time. The seeming lack of commitment to keeping appointments for interviews reflected a difference between this teenage population and a 20- to 25-year-old population.[35] Out of 80 interviews for the 20- to 25-year-old population no appointment was missed, and only 6 were changed for reasons such as the inadvertent scheduling of the doctor's appointment at the same time.

The 12 teenage mothers also made a total of 19 residential moves, which made it difficult to maintain contact with them. Further, their penchant for watching television during interviews suggests that a one-to-one interview may have been too intense for them.

Highley[35] observed three phases occurring in the 20- to 25-year-old mothers over a year: biological-physical restructuring, psychosexual and psychosocial moratorium, and identity restructuring. During the first short phase of biological-physical restructuring, mothers voiced concern about the immediate past. The teenage mothers' comments suggested that the experience of the labor and delivery and their fears about bodily damage were too overwhelming to discuss. Violet told the nurse who had been with her during her labor, "Don't tell me about it (cesarean section). I don't want to hear about getting cut up." Pam maintained that she had almost died during the last 15 minutes of labor, the pain was so bad. At the one-year interview, Pam shuddered when she described seeing the doctor holding her baby up immediately following delivery. Rubin[36] observed that 25% of the primiparas' (ages not stated) role-taking responses in the postpartal period related to body image. Only 6% of the teenage mothers' total responses referred to body image.[25] The question is raised whether feared and actual trauma to their bodies during labor and delivery are too overwhelming for some young mothers to discuss in the early postpartal period.

The second phase observed in older mothers,[35] declaration of a temporary psychosexual and psychosocial moratorium in which mothers looked to a more distant past, e.g., courtship days before marriage, was not observed in the teenage mothers. Only one of the young women, Jane, had been married longer than nine months before the child's birth (two years). The young women simply did not have the romantic and historical past that the older women had. This may be a handicap. A successful historical past provides ego strengths and a positive attitude when approaching challenging new roles.

The third phase of identity restructuring observed by Highley,[35] internalization of the role with adaptation to changes in her style of life, was observed in three fourths of the teenage mothers. The timing of internalization of the maternal role occurred later, within approximately six to eight months for the teenage mothers, whereas it occurred within approximately three months for the older mothers. The 20- to 25-year-old women had probably resolved the earlier task of establishing an identity apart from the maternal role, a task the younger mothers were working on at three months. Even though the young woman is projected into the maternal role prematurely, Erikson's[1] epigenetic principle of development seems applicable; perhaps the young woman must work at tasks of achieving her identity in relation to other roles during the optimal time of ascendancy before she resolves the tasks that usually come later, in the period of generativity.

The four mothers in Highley's study all achieved the maternal role. Three of the teenage mothers rejected or did not achieve the maternal role. Two other mothers had difficulty in the role; this was manifested by the physical symptoms of their children. Robson and Moss[31] found that 3 of 54 mothers (18%) remained detached and unreactive to their infants through three months postpartum.

One half of the teenagers' infants in my study experienced neonatal morbidity; five of the six infants required special hospitalization care beyond the usual newborn period. Two who were born postmaturely were in an intensive-care nursery during their first two weeks of life; one infant was small for gestational age; one had hyperbilirubinemia following birth and a fractured skull at one month; one was diagnosed as having a ventricular septal defect at one month; and another had rectal bleeding at two weeks. Of the two infants who experienced failure to thrive syndrome at four months one had a ventricular septic defect; the second infant had experienced no illnesses other than upper respiratory infection. What impact did the early illness and separation from their infants have on the mother's attachment process?

Although one infant's failure to thrive seemed to be a result of emotional deprivation and lack of physical care, the other failure was a result of sleep deprivation and overstimulation. In both cases, the young mothers had not perceived and assessed the environment or the needs of their children accurately. These perceptual deficiencies are part of a psychological constellation conducive to inadequate mothering.[31] Although generalizations cannot be made from the small study of teenage mothers, a recent study of referrals for child abuse supports these findings. Lynch and Roberts[38] compared 50 children who were referred to the hospital for actual or threatened abuse with 50 controls. Each control child was the next child born after the abused subject, at the same hospital. They found that the mother who was under the age of 20 when she had her first child was more likely to abuse her child than the mother who was over the age of 20; 25 of the 50 mothers in the child-abusing group were under 20 when their first child was born, in contrast to 8 of the 50 in the control group. More than twice as many abused children, in comparison with nonabused children, had been in a special care nursery.[39] They found that other factors prominent in the group of abused children included the existence of diffuse social problems rather than defined problems in the family and concern about mothering, which had been recorded in the hospital maternity records almost five times more frequently in the abused group.

Process in Attaining a Maternal Role

The incorporation of a new role involves the learning of behaviors required for acting the role and the reordering of the life-space to include a new social position of the role. The young woman giving birth to a child must learn the tasks inherent in a mothering role as she simultaneously assumes the position or status of "mother" within her social structure. Her sociocultural structure specifies some of the role behaviors and the status of mother, but she is not a passive learner. The individual brings a unique self to the situation that interacts with the role. The self both adjusts and adapts to the role and alters the role during the process.

Role taking is both a behavioral and an affective cognitive process involving active interaction with another person or partner. Gestures, vocalizations, and other behaviors are directed to a partner in the role-taking process; the role taker then reflects on how the partner perceives the behavior and modifies or adapts the behavior accordingly.[40]

The ease with which role transitions are made depends upon many factors. Anticipatory socialization for the role, role clarity, role conflict, role strain, the extent to which the role permits the achievement of other desired goals, length of time to be spent in a role, availability of substitute gratifications in frustrating roles, importance of the role, and the amount of change a role causes in the person's life, all affect the individual's transition to a new role.[41]

Thornton and Nardi[42] described role acquisition as a dynamic process progressing through four stages—anticipatory, formal, informal, and personal. In each of the stages, the individual interacts with external expectations in the environment as each attempts to influence the other. The anticipatory stage is the period that precedes moving into the social position of the role; during this time the individual learns generalized and stereotyped expectations of the role. The formal stage of role acquisition occurs as the individual begins viewing the role from the actual social position, rather than as an outsider. There is general agreement within the social system about expectations of the required behaviors in the role and the role taker usually conforms to these expectations. The third stage (informal) involves learning informal attitudinal and cognitive behaviors in the role, or the permissive latitude of a role. At this point the role taker shapes the role to fit himself in view of past experiences and future goals. In the final, or personal, stage, a mutual transformation of self and role occur so that harmony of self and role is achieved. In the process of modifying the role to make it congruent with self, a sense of balance is achieved. The anticipatory stage of the maternal role begins during the woman's pregnancy. She moves into formal, informal, and personal stages following the birth of her child.

Rubin[36] described five operations of maternal role attainment—mimicry, role play, fantasy, introjection-projection-rejection, and grief work—which begin during pregnancy. Mimicry and role play involve learning about expectations and performance in a role. Fantasy and introjection-projection-rejection involve a beginning internalization of the role. The woman imagines herself in the role and searches for models to fit her fantasy of herself in the role. Based on whether the models are judged compatible to her style, the role taker either accepts or rejects the models. In the operation of grief work, a relinquishing of roles that are incompatible with the mothering role occurs. The maternal role is internalized as part of the mother's identity when there is a sense of comfort in the role. This sense of comfort described by Rubin appears to be congruent with the personal stage of balance in role acquisition described by Thornton and Nardi.

The maternal role may be considered to have been attained when the mother feels internal harmony with the role and its expectations. Her behavioral responses to the role's expectations are reflexive and are seen in her concern for and competency in caring for her infant, in her love and affection for and pleasure in her infant, and in her acceptance of the responsibilities posed by the role.

Phases in Adolescent Maternal Role Attainment

Based on data from my study[25] and subsequent observations, four phases that teenagers experience in assuming a maternal role are suggested: (1) a fairyland phase; (2) a reality shock phase; (3) a give-and-take phase; and (4) an internalization of the maternal role phase. The phases are described and are related to Thornton and Nardi's[42] and Rubin's[36] work. This discussion focuses on role taking after the infant's birth; therefore, the teenager's work in the anticipatory phase and the role-taking operations for that period are omitted.

THE FAIRYLAND PHASE

Writers have frequently used the word "honeymoon" to describe the early period in a role during which others overlook the role learner's inadequacies and promote a sense of well-being for the new incumbent. That term did not seem appropriate for the young mothers, especially since this phase did not extend beyond the hospitalization period. Though a hospital can hardly be considered a "fairyland," an aura of irreality surrounds this phase. The attention, praise, and gifts that the teenager receives give an initial impression that being a mother is really wonderful. This initial social response in the early formal stage of role taking is misleading to the young role taker. She may also be somewhat dazed from postpartal fever and/or discomforts and very relieved that labor and delivery are over.

The young mother may view her infant as "cute" and "precious." Except for their feeding their infants, there are usually no formal expectations by others of the women in their new role. Motherhood is a largely rewarding experience during the fairyland phase. One 18-year-old, Ann, at the end of her first year of motherhood, recalled the fairyland phase: "Like, I'm happy now. But *then* I was really happy and it was different."

REALITY SHOCK PHASE

The reality shock phase (a phenomenon observed by Kramer[43] among new nursing graduates) begins shortly after the young woman leaves the hospital. It may reach its acme during the second postpartal week. All of the good things (praise and gifts) about being a mother become harshly overshadowed by the realities of mothering; the "precious" infant becomes a "demanding" infant who wreaks havoc in her life. The discrepancy of the fairyland and reality shock phases may be met with much hostility and/or rejection. During this phase, deprivations in the role far outweigh any gratifications. The glowing, spontaneous remarks about being a mother during the "fairyland" phase are gradually tempered by feelings of ambivalence and rejection. Expressions of hostility may be higher during this phase than at any other period.

Formal role expectations become more reality oriented. Formal expectations are that the young mother will get up during the night and take care of her infant. Changing and washing diapers are part of the tasks in the role. This is a dramatic contrast to the occasional feeding of a clean, sweet-smelling infant that was experienced during the fairyland phase. The young mother's difficulties in dealing with the formal expectations of others may be reflected in her infant's physical difficulties, such as colic, skin rashes, feeding problems, etc. The fairyland phase and the reality shock phase make up Thornton and Nardi's formal stage of role acquisition. All of the operations of role taking described by Rubin may be occurring.

GIVE-AND-TAKE PHASE

A transition period seems to occur near the third month, so that by the fifth month the young woman reaches a balance between perceived gratifications and deprivations in the role; there is a stabilization or balance of "give-and-take." This phase also seems to herald a first stage of identity restructuring, in which some adaptation is made to the disrupting changes that have occurred in the young woman's life. In the "give-and-take" phase the young woman may make decisions about how much of her life she is willing to "give" and she seems to decide what she is going to "take" from life. The young mother may seek employment or additional schooling in response to feelings of boredom and financial need, and a restructuring of role identity apart from the motherhood role may result.

Changes also occur in the infant around the beginning of the "give-and-take" phase. The infant becomes a more active social interactor in his response to his mother. The infant's accomplishments and recognition of his mother at this phase enhance the young mother's feelings of warmth and enthusiasm.

The young mother begins to achieve comfort in learning some of the informal role behaviors and in adapting them to her unique situation. She becomes more comfortable in "giving" of herself because she sees that she may "take" options needed for her own development. The reader will recall that Jane judged the demands of motherhood to be more than she wished to give and she rejected her daughter during this phase. She had felt that "now" was the time for her own development, a time which could not be shared with other responsibilities. The give-and-take phase is congruent with Thornton and Nardi's informal stage of role taking and somewhat overlaps the personal stage. The operations of introjection-projection-rejection and grief work as described by Rubin are most active during this phase.

INTERNALIZATION OF THE ROLE PHASE

From the sixth to the eighth month another transition seems to occur. This transition period ushers in what appears to represent an "internalization of the maternal role" phase, a second part of the woman's identity restructuring. It seems that the teenage mother needs to work toward a role other than mothering before incorporating the maternal role.

Gratifications in the mothering role begin to outweigh the deprivations at this time. The infant's recognition of the mother and his physical approach are very rewarding experiences for the mother. The baby's rapidly changing behavior, increasing mobility, and developing autonomy account for both rewards and frustrations in mothering.

Feelings of competency emerge as mothers begin to feel secure about their decisions in their new role. One young mother's description of her experience summarizes these feelings:

> When she does something wrong in the kitchen I can slap her hands, because I know that what I am doing is right, that it is my job to discipline her, I feel really good. I really feel that I am competent and that I'm doing a really good job, and that she trusts me and loves me and I know it is good.

With internalization of the maternal role, the young mother usually perceives that her personal growth and development are accelerated. She may view herself as more sensitive to others and as having greater skills to care for another. Surprisingly, she may not view the premature state of motherhood as having been a handicap, although she will describe it as most difficult. Her pleasure and satisfaction in her role and achievements are evident once internalization of the maternal role has been achieved; this phase corresponds with Thornton and Nardi's[42] personal stage of balance and harmony—the end point or role attainment.

Facilitating and Promoting the Adolescent's Parenting Role

Many professionals are involved in helping young parents as they begin the parenting role. The public health nurse, maternity and pediatric nurse clinical specialists, social worker, physician, educational or vocational counselor, and teachers, all play vital roles as an interface between the young parents and society in providing a supportive climate. Initially, the nurse may have a more extended period of time with youthful parents, especially during the early postpartum period. Later, the teacher may be the person who observes the young mother feeding and interacting with her infant and may be more influential. The social worker or the public health nurse may be the person who has the lengthiest contact. The efforts of each are strengthened if communication and collaboration among all are effective. Careful collaboration also emphasizes to the young parents that all are interested in them and are working together.

The coordination of efforts of those working with young parents is particularly important in view of their mobility. When parents move to a different part of the city, the school teacher or the social worker may be the first to know. Whoever has knowledge of the intended move is the one to remind and encourage the parents to tell the local well-child clinic, public health nurse, and physician. Young parents sometimes simply do not think of doing this, and a concerned public health nurse may have to spend half a day in detective work tracing the whereabouts of a family.

The nurse working with adolescent parents is particularly concerned with their follow-up health care. The higher incidences of complications for both mother and infant make it very important that frequent physical examinations be maintained. The young parents' economic hardships and lack of experience in planning add to implications for continued nutritional counseling. Continued reinforcement and teaching about foods high in protein and iron are needed to ensure that the infant receives adequate nourishment for his rapid brain and general physical growth during his first year. The increased burdens of caring for an infant are also more easily borne by a mother and father who themselves are not anemic.

Since some adolescent mothers are hesitant about discussing their bodies following their labor and delivery experience, special opportunities should be provided for them to do so. The young woman who is afraid that she has no sex appeal because of a cesarean birth scar may have other questions about her body image or possible damage to her body. If the youthful parent does not have an opportunity to verify the intactness and normal functioning of her body, her fears about possible damage may grow. Providing an opportunity for the young mother to ask whether her clitoris might have been damaged during childbirth may elicit further questioning from the mother and the father. It is important to review carefully the hormonal changes during pregnancy that led to hypertrophy and softening of tissues so that they could expand to permit an infant's head to pass through, and it is helpful to note the postpartal change in these tissues to near-usual elasticity and pre-pregnancy state. The youthful husband may have difficulty believing that the vaginal canal will ever be small enough so that he can enjoy intercourse again.

Although it is assumed that many opportunities to discuss body change or damage would have occurred during the early postpartal period, the mother may not have been able to discuss some of her fears in the fairyland phase. Her physical response to medications or to labor and delivery may have been somewhat exaggerated, or this phase may have been too threateningly close to the event. Her fears may be enlarged because of the adolescent's increased vulnerability to body damage and because the bladder and other organs may have had a more generalized or systemic and sensitive response to pain. Further, in the reality shock phase, the young mother may be so preoccupied with learning formal expectations of the role that she does not have time to deal with concerns about possible body damage in labor and delivery. She may talk more freely about her concerns during the give-and-take phase, sometime after the third month. However, the sooner the young parents have the opportunity to have fears about bodily harm or bodily functioning dispelled, the sooner they have additional energy released to devote to their infant. Ultimately their feeling of well-being enables them to enhance the quality of all facets of their child's and their own lives.

Young parents may need help in realizing that their feelings of fatigue, anger, exhaustion, disorganization, and despair are really no different from those that *any* parents experience. Young mothers frequently ask about other young mothers and how they are doing, whether they are having difficulties with their infants, etc. There seems to be a *need* to know how one measures up as a parent.

Knowledge of local child-care centers, day camps, baby-sitters, and organizations that assist families is helpful; it is important to share it with young parents. Younger parents with their shorter background of experiences, need increased opportunities for learning and help in managing adult tasks. Societal supports seem particularly important since often grandparents are not in a position to help. Some parents may need encouragement to let the grandparents keep their baby overnight so that they can get some sleep. This kind of break is particularly important for the parents of an infant who is irritable or colicky.

In assessing the young parents' experiences, their earlier experiences that are contributory or parallel to parenting skills may be emphasized. A parent may confide that a younger sibling made unreasonable demands and continually messed up his school projects. The recollection of the incident enables the parent to remember how he handled the situation with his sibling (often with his mother's assistance) and to realize that putting important papers or valuables that may be damaged by exploring fingers out of reach is easier, until a child is older. Such recall also awakens in the young parent and brings to a conscious level the memory that he had to *tolerate* a certain amount of interference from the younger sibling and alter his behavior with his younger sibling. This helps the parent to realize that his own child will need a similar kind of understanding and patient interaction. In situations which were less than desirable (e.g., if the parents were abused when they were children), psychological counseling is needed so that the cyclical cultural patterning can be interrupted. The young parent needs suitable role models; the nurse, teacher, and social worker all serve as role models to parents in their interactions with themselves and their infant.

Needs vary at different phases in the role-taking process. During the irreality period of hospitalization, the fairyland phase, the young mother's perceptions of her infant and of her role are based on very different kinds of feedback from that which she will receive when she is with her infant 24 hours daily and all household routines are disrupted. She needs much supportive physical help from someone who is aware of the difficulties during this transition period.

Supportive counseling seems especially crucial during the ''reality shock'' phase and during the transition period to the ''give-and-take'' phase at the third month. If available options for care of the infant and for her own care and development are presented clearly, the new mother can usually make workable decisions with help from those persons who are significant to her.

The young parents need much encouragement in adapting the parenting role to their lives so that they do not focus exclusively on adapting their lives to the parenting role. During the informal stage of role taking, the give-and-take phase, specifics about child care, such as limit setting with a growing infant, providing needed stimulation by using kitchen utensils instead of expensive toys, all help young parents to become creative in doing their thing, their way. If they enjoy camping, their child can learn to enjoy camping.

The gratifications that teenage parents derive from interacting with their infant and watching him grow and develop can be encouraged. Through sharing knowledge of growth and development and appropriate sensory stimulation of the infant, youthful parents gain even greater pleasure and feelings of competency in their role.

Considering the important role of the young mother's mother, assessing the mother-daughter relationship and verifying with the young mother the kind of help she desires or needs from her mother seems important. Involving the grandmother with planning can provide reinforcement for her own mothering. With increased self-esteem, the grandmother can be more accepting of the daughter's less effective performance in the role.

If the young mother's mother is an unsuitable role model, perhaps her mate's mother will be used as a model. If the mate's mother is unavailable, an aunt or older relative may be selected by the young woman. Recognition by a revered, older mother that she is a capable, good mother seems to be very crucial for the adolescent mother. In the formal stage of role taking, if a revered expert acknowledges that one's behavior in the role is good, think of the joy. Any one of us experiences the need for this social acceptance in a new role. How much do we all seek approval from the boss in a new job? Until we are told by the boss that our performance in the role is acceptable, we are rather uneasy. Added attempts are made to prove ourselves; yet, if we have no role models in a particular job, we do not know what we may be omitting from the repertoire of behaviors usually required in the role.

As we assess the youthful parents' background experiences in relation to parenting, some of the feeling tone of their experiences emerges. When some experiences seem to have been particularly threatening, the nurse realizes that this type of experience will probably be difficult for the young woman to handle with her own child.

When young parents are troubled and unable to define their problems, special effort and help are warranted to help them do this. If parents view their infant as the cause of their deprivation, rather than their low-paying jobs, they will be more likely to display hostility to the child than to seek preparation for a better paying job. Sometimes the situation appears diffuse and confusing, but methodical, careful listening, with appropriate questioning, can help guide young parents to pinpoint some of the major problems. Once problems are identified, parents think about what they can do in the situation.

Health care workers must be especially sensitive to the financial difficulties facing young married parents, who in most states are denied welfare aid. These states deny any financial aid to mothers if they are living with their husbands or the fathers of the infants. Youthful parents who must pay high rent, buy groceries, clothes, and baby supplies often do not qualify for medical aid either. Their deprivations (and problems) may be far greater than those of the single mother who is living with her parents in a comfortable apartment and who has no responsibility for managing the household. If we value families and family life in our culture, we must direct more energy toward helping young, struggling families.

The youthful father cannot be overlooked. Like the mother, he needs constructive counseling about *how* he can improve his technical or professional skills so that he is not trapped for life in a low-salaried job. Societal support is crucial at this point in the young man's life so that he does not become disillusioned and discouraged about his future. Research findings all report that adaptation to parenthood is facilitated in a stable husband-wife relationship. To improve the quality of human life, human resources must be cultivated and nurtured.

Because of the intensity of the parenting role, younger, immature parents need more intensive follow-up efforts, especially for the first year or two. Phases that are postulated in assuming a mothering (or fathering) role pinpoint periods during which extra supportive professional assistance is needed. The progress parents make in their roles and their level of adaptation will indicate when intensive follow-up is no longer needed. Some young parents may be doing extremely well at nine months; others may still need extensive help from the social system at two years.

Resources for Young Parents and Health Professionals

Usually there are a variety of local organizations within a community that provide a number of varied services for young parents. There may be a senior citizens' group that provides "grandparenting" for young families isolated from their own families. Some of the grandparenting groups work in hospital clinics; they help by entertaining small children who must wait while their mothers are seen by the doctor. Others do baby-sitting, which is quite helpful and rewarding both to the young family and to the surrogate grandparent.

Sometimes churches have organizations that provide counseling and financial or physical help for new homemakers. If the churches do not sponsor the organization, they frequently permit the organization to use the church facilities.

Counties may contribute support to organizations that serve teenage parents. One example is the Friends to Teenage Parents organization, South San Francisco, California, which receives some support from the county, various local organizations, and the state. This organization's major thrust includes three areas: volunteer friends, who are available to teenage parents for visits or phone calls; an infant day-care center (sponsored by state funds) to serve young parents who are going to school or working; and a young parent advocates program which promotes public awareness of and responsiveness to the needs of adolescent parents.

The National Alliance Concerned with School-Age Parents (NACSAP) is a multidisciplinary membership organization that focuses on resolving problems of adolescent parenthood and sexuality. This organization offers such services as publications, in-service training, conferences, and program consultation and is an advocate for school-age parents. NACSAP has affiliate state organizations in California, Florida, Louisiana, Michigan, Ohio, Oregon, Washington, and Wisconsin. NACSAP is supported through membership dues, contributions, and government contracts. The organization headquarters is at 7315 Wisconsin Avenue, Suite 211–W, Washington, D.C. 20014.

NACSAP has developed a *National Directory of Services for School-Age Parents*[44] which is a valuable resource for health professionals. This directory includes names and addresses of directors of services available to adolescents in the United States. Examples of the kinds of services listed include: advocacy, abortion clinics, alternative school counseling/social-services, infant/day-care services, birth control, legal aid, medical services, maternity homes, entries from Planned Parenthood Directory, Child Welfare League of America Inc., Directory entries, transportation, and Women's and Infants' Supplemental Food Program. The directory is available from NACSAP headquarters.

Some high schools have classes in child development as part of their home economics or homemaking department curriculum. These departments sponsor nursery schools for preschool children in which high school students care for the nursery school students. High school students thus learn about child development and child care and gain a better understanding of themselves and their parents. Such experience enhances the high school student's ability to parent when he becomes a parent himself. The Department of Health, Education, and Welfare has published *Education for Parenthood: A Program, Curriculum, and Evaluation Guide* ''to assist school agencies and community-based organizations in developing effective preparation for parenthood programs for teenagers they serve'' (The Purpose).[45] The guide contains valuable resources for program planning and for teaching parenting concepts. Demonstration programs for Boy Scouts of America, Boys' Clubs of America, National 4–H Club Foundation of America, Girl Scouts of America, National Federation of Settlements and Neighborhood Centers, The Salvation Army, and Save the Children Federation, are described.

Summary

Teenage parents present a challenge to all who work with them. They are already overwhelmed by their work on their identities, independence, and other adolescent tasks as they take on the adult role of parenting. In order to become successful parents, they must become successful, self-confident persons.

Because of the variability in rates of development, generalizations cannot be made that 18- or 19-year-olds need less help. The very young adolescent parent always needs nurturing from an adult in order to continue his or her own maturational and growth processes. The wide range of cognitive, psychological, and social maturity in each phase of adolescence necessitates that we work with each parent in an *individualized* manner so that the young parent is not turned off by authoritative, oversimplified, and stereotyped language or attitude. Only through careful listening and interviewing can we learn of the richness of an individual's previous experiences and gain the information about his support system that may offer us the greatest clues we presently have about future directions in providing appropriate health care.

The needs of the youthful parent are so diverse that no one professional or group of professionals can meet these needs. Greater social consciousness and awareness are mandatory so that youthful parents have an opportunity to continue to grow themselves as they learn to care for and nurture their children.

REFERENCES

1. Erikson, E. H. "Identity and the Life Cycle." *Psychological Issues* 1(1), Monograph 1, 1959.
2. Bibring, G., et al. "A Study of the Psychological Processes in Pregnancy and of the Earliest Mother-Child Relationship, I. Some Propositions and Comments." *Psychoanal. Study of Child* 16:9–24, 1961.
3. Colman, A., and Colman, L. *Pregnancy: The Psychological Experience.* New York: Seabury Press, 1973.
4. Deutsch, H. *Psychology of Women,* vol. 2. New York: Grune & Stratton, 1945.
5. Winnicott, D. W. "Primary Maternal Preoccupation." In *Collected Papers: Through Paediatrics to Psychoanalysis.* New York: Basic Books, Inc., 1958, pp. 300–305.
6. Blos, P. *On Adolescence.* New York: Free Press, 1962.
7. Benedek, T. "Parenthood as a Developmental Phase: A Contribution to the Libido Theory." *J. Am. Psychoanal. Assn.* 7:389–417, 1959.
8. Deutsch, H. *Psychology of Women,* vol. 1. New York: Grune & Stratton, 1944.
9. Deutsch, H. *Selected Problems of Adolescence.* New York: International Universities Press, Inc., 1967.
10. The Alan Guttmacher Institute. *11 Million Teenagers: What Can Be Done About the Epidemic of Adolescent Pregnancies in the United States.* New York: Research and Development Division of Planned Parenthood Federation of America, 1976.
11. Dott, A. B., and Fort, A. T. "Medical and Social Factors Affecting Early Teenage Pregnancy." *Am. J. Obstet. & Gyn.* 125(4):532–536, 1976.
12. Menken, J. 'The Health and Social Consequences of Teenage Childbearing." *Fam. Plann. Perspectives* 4(3):45–53, 1972.
13. Oppel, W. C., and Royston, A. B. "Teen-Age Births: Some Social, Psychological, and Physical Sequelae." *Am. J. Pub. Health* 61(4):751–756, 1971.
14. Osofsky, H. J., and Osofsky, J. D. "Adolescents as Mothers: Results of a Program for Low-Income Pregnant Teenagers with Some Emphasis Upon Infants' Development." *Am. J. Orthopsychiat.* 40(5):825–834, 1970.
15. Gutelius, M. F. "Child-Rearing Attitudes of Teen-Age Negro Girls." *Am. J. Pub. Health* 60(1):93–104, 1970.
16. Williams, T. M. "Childrearing Practices of Young Mothers: What We Know, How It Matters, Why It's So Little." *Am. J. Orthopsychiat.* 44:70–75, 1974.
17. Singer, A. "Mothering Practices and Heroin Addiction." *Am. J. Nurs.* 74(1):77–82, 1974.

18. DeLissovoy, V. "Child Care by Adolescent Parents." *Children Today* 2(4):22–25, 1973.
19. Crumidy, P. M., and Jacobziner, H. "A Study of Young Unmarried Mothers Who Kept Their Babies." *Am. J. Pub. Health* 56(8):1242–1251, 1966.
20. LaBarre, M. "Emotional Crises of School-Age Girls During Pregnancy and Early Motherhood." *J. Am. Acad. Child Psychiat.* 11(2):537–557, 1972.
21. LaBarre, M. "Pregnancy Experiences Among Married Adolescents." *Am. J. Orthopsychiat.* 38:47–55, 1968.
22. Weigle, J. W. "Teaching Child Development to Teenage Mothers." *Children Today* 3(5):23–25, 1974.
23. Shaw, N. R. "Teaching Young Mothers Their Role." *Am. J. Nurs.* 74:77–82, 1974.
24. Benas, E. "Residential Care of the Child-Mother and Her Infant: An Extended Family Concept." *Child Welfare* 54(4):290–294, 1975.
25. Mercer, R. T. "Research Project: Attainment of the Maternal Role by Teenage Mothers," 1976.
26. Lynch, V. J. "Narcissistic Loss and Depression in Late Adolescence." *Perspectives in Psychiat. Care* 14(3):133–135, 1976.
27. Blasi, A., and Hoeffel, E. C. "Adolescence and Formal Operations." *Human Develop.* 17:344–363, 1974.
28. Barber, V., and Skaggs, M. M. *The Mother Person.* Indianapolis/New York: Bobbs-Merrill Co., Inc. 1975.
29. Larsen, V. L. "Stresses of the Childbearing Year." *Am. J. Pub. Health* 56:32–36, 1966.
30. Shereshefsky, P. M., and Yarrow, L. J. *Psychological Aspects of a First Pregnancy and Early Postnatal Adaptation.* New York: Raven Press, 1973.
31. Robson, K. S., and Moss, H. A. "Patterns and Determinants of Maternal Attachment." *J. Pediat.* 77(6):976–985, 1970.
32. Cohler, B. J., et al. "Childcare Attitudes and Emotional Disturbance Among Mothers of Young Children." *Genet. Psychol. Monographs* 82:3–47, 1970.
33. Bibring, G. "Some Specific Psychological Tasks in Pregnancy and Motherhood." In *1st International Congress of Psychosomatic Medicine and Childbirth, Paris, July 8–12, 1962.* Paris: Gauthier-Villars, 1965, pp. 21–26.
34. Russell, C. S. "Transition to Parenthood: Problems and Gratifications." *J. Marr. & Fam.* 36(2):294–301, 1974.
35. Highley, B. L. "Maternal Role Identity." In *Defining Clinical Content in Graduate Nursing Programs Maternal Child Health Nursing.* Boulder, Colorado: Western Interstate Commission for Higher Education, 1967, pp. 31–43.
36. Rubin, R. "Attainment of the Maternal Role, Part I, Processes." *Nurs. Research* 16(3):237–245, 1967.
37. Pollitt, E., et al. "Psychosocial Development and Behavior of Mothers of Failure-to-Thrive Children." *Am. J. Orthopsychiat.* 45(4):525–537, 1975.
38. Lynch, M. A., and Roberts, J. "Predicting Child Abuse: Signs of Bonding Failure in the Maternity Hospital." *Brit. Med. J.* 1:624–626, 1977.
39. Lynch, M. A., Roberts, J., and Gordon, M. "Child Abuse: Early Warning in the Maternity Hospital." *Develop. Med. Child Neurol.* 18:759–766, 1976.
40. Mead, G. H. *Mind, Self, and Society.* Chicago: University of Chicago Press, 1934.
41. Burr, W. R. "Role Transitions: A Reformulation of Theory." *J. Marr. & Fam.* 34(3):407–416, 1972.
42. Thornton, R., and Nardi, P. M. "The Dynamics of Role Acquisition." *Am. J. Soc.* 80(4):870–885, 1975.
43. Kramer, M. *Reality Shock: Why Nurses Leave Nursing.* St. Louis: C. V. Mosby Co., 1974.
44. National Alliance Concerned with School-Age Parents." *National Directory of Services for School-Age Parents.* Washington, D.C.: NACSAP, 1976.
45. Morris, L. A., ed. *Education for Parenthood: A Program, Curriculum, and Evaluation Guide.* Washington, D.C.: U.S. Dept. of H.E.W., Office of Human Development Services, Children's Bureau, DHEW Pub. No. (OHDS) 77-30125, 1977.

The Adolescent, The Health Professional, and the Health Care System

15

The Adolescent
and the Health Professional

Ramona T. Mercer, R.N., Ph.D.

The health professional's role and responsibility vis-à-vis the adolescent are as difficult as they are important. The adolescent usually assigns a low priority to the need for seeking health services; from his perspective he is functioning, perhaps performing athletic feats not previously accomplished, and preventive health is just not foremost in his mind. Yet, among the leading causes of death and morbidity for this age group, some are in large part preventable—accidents, suicide, and infections—and reflect the teenager's vulnerability. The interrelatedness of the adolescent developmental state, which involves rapid physical growth, mental turmoil, conflict, indecisiveness—all affecting the adolescent's health—suggests the need for subtle and sensitive observation of these factors so that the cycle may be interrupted when necessary to prevent accident and depression. This is an enormous responsibility, or, in the adolescent lingo, a "heavy trip" for the health professional. Giving a wrong or unthoughtful response to a frightened adolescent has the potential to cause far-reaching repercussions in the young person's life. A single, only chance for a health professional to influence a youth to adopt good, lifelong health habits may be wasted by hasty action or by lack of information, thought, and care.

Three universals that seem to lead to generational clashes include the real age differences, the slowing rate of socialization as one ages, and the basic physiological and psychosocial differences between the young person and the older person.[1] These basic human universals are affected by variations within specific cultures in the rate of social change, the complexity of the social structure, the extent of the individual's integration in the culture, and the individual's mobility within the social structure, or his ability to move from one class to another.[1] Social change, in the direction of increasing complexity, has been rapid since the 1940s. It is easy to see how a society with such complex problems as the possibility of nuclear warfare and destruction, space exploration, dwindling energy stores, polluted environment, and lack of employment, could potentially foster an increase in conflict between younger and older groups. The adolescent, rather than becoming more integrated into the society, is tending to remain closer to the periphery. Communes and various religious cults are attracting many adolescents who feel estranged, unnecessary, and unwanted in family groups.

Adults respond in frustration and anger. They feel helpless, resentful, afraid, and embarrassed. In what seems to be a situation in which they have lost all control, adolescents respond with similar feelings and emotions. The stereotypic responses to each other of adolescents and adults further heightens the conflict.

This chapter focuses on the responses of the health care professional and of the adolescent. Some special hazards inherent in counseling are reviewed and special problems in dealing with broken appointments and in communicating with the young person conclude the chapter.

The Professional's Responses to the Adolescent

STEREOTYPING

"I don't know why I bother; all of you are exactly alike. You don't intend to come to the clinic and you don't intend to follow the instructions because you think you know all the answers." Such thoughts and responses may be heard in the medical care setting, in the school setting, or wherever there are groups of adolescents. Some of the health professional's frustration because earlier instructions to the youth have not been followed is evident. But the stereotype "All of you are exactly alike," with the projection "you don't intend to follow the instructions because you think you know all of the answers," makes it psychologically impossible for a spunky youth to do so. He acts out the expectations of rebellion and rejection conveyed to him by authority figures or knowledgeable persons. If he were to "cooperate"—whatever that means—he would see himself as a traitor to all adolescents; therefore, he must meet expectations. Comments and expectations that stereotype another person do not permit any other response—because an adolescent, perhaps more than an individual of any other age, does not wish to be totally different from his peers!

Although the majority of adolescents respond and follow social indicators and customs smoothly and with little difficulty, it is the small percentage of adolescents who respond with extreme behavior that capture publicity, which in turn leads to stereotyping.[2] The one in ten high school students who has a baby is advertised; the nine in ten who do not, and who proceed through developmental tasks without difficulty or rancor, receive much less notice. The youth who steals a car for a lark receives much attention, whereas the youth who contributes his time to charitable organizations or to working with children or older citizens often escapes praise and recognition. Thus, even the conforming adolescent gets a distorted social view of his age group because of society's and the communications media's tendency to present the sensational or the unusual, often to the exclusion of all else.

Anthony,[2] summarizing adult stereotypic responses and reactions to the adolescent, states that the adolescent is seen: as one to be feared yet protected; as sexually potent and threatening; as maladjusted or vacillating; as enviable; and as one who will soon be independent and no longer need the adult's help. Society stereotypes the social adolescent as a big spender and a trend setter, and adolescence as a special age for extensive research.[2]

Does the health care professional, as an adult in today's society, harbor and perpetuate these stereotypes? If so, is it any wonder that the adolescent does not seek health care or does not seek out the school nurse to talk over sexual or health questions? Talk with a group of high school students and ask them whom they seek out to answer personal questions about their bodies or about reproduction. Very often the adolescent says he goes to the coach, physical education instructor, or science teacher. What is different about these persons? The coach and physical education teacher reinforce the youth's ability to perform, to play, to be a sport, to be a part of a team. His individuality, worth to the team, and individual uniqueness are valued. John is a top-notch passer or kicker to the football coach; he is not stereotyped as just a member of the team! The science teacher interprets knowledge accurately without embarrassment or subjectivity. The student is more comfortable learning about sexual behavior in mammals because the material is presented objectively and no personal questions are directed to the stereotype of the adolescent's masturbation or sexual habits. One group of high school students related that they did not go to the nurse because she always gave aspirins or an excuse from class. She had stereotyped the adolescents' somatic complaints rather than determined each individual's problem. Health care professionals could perhaps learn something from the kinds of interactions and relationships adolescents have with the persons they respect and seek out.

Important questions for all who work with adolescents are: How do I view adolescents? Am I able to relate to individual responses rather than how I think adolescents respond? Am I uncomfortable with this age group? Am I flexible enough to be tolerant with struggles and indecisiveness, or does my rigidity require that I work with completely dependent or completely independent persons? Am I flexible enough to tolerate difficult choice making without imposing my values or beliefs, even when the young person seems incapable of making a decision?

If individuals are not comfortable in those kinds of situations, and are not able to respect and relate to the adolescent as a unique individual, it is probably best that they choose another age group with whom to work. This is not meant to be uncomplimentary to the professional; not everyone is comfortable with all age groups.

"Teenagers today are just not like we were. I didn't do that when I was her age." Similar comments are frequently heard. They are true comments. But perhaps some reflection is merited as to why teenagers are different. If there is a 20-year age differential, the teenager has reached physiological maturity or puberty 8 months sooner than the older generation did; if there is a 30-year differential, puberty was reached an entire year sooner. But, because the teenager reached puberty one year sooner, this does not mean that she is better (or worse) prepared to cope with it psychologically. She is more apt, however, to be thrust sooner into adult roles for which she is quite unprepared. Even language changes as social conditions change. "Making out" was called "necking" 30 years ago. The adolescent also has difficulty perceiving life from the adult's perspective. One mother was bemoaning to her husband some of the difficulties of adhering to a very restricted dietary regime in order to lose 20 pounds. Her 14-year-old daughter commented, "Why worry so much about that? You're old!" To that 14-year-old, interest in one's appearance, the need to look attractive, all subsided by the forties. This mother remembered that period in her own life, however, and recalled that growing up seems to take forever at age 14. Her empathetic ability enabled her to respond in good humor, rather than with a hostile remark such as: "Young people only worry about being attractive and slim themselves, and they think they have a monopoly on the right to look good."

ANGER AND HOSTILITY

The emotional and behavioral problems of adolescents have been related to overt conflict with hostile adults.[3] Primitive cultures have institutionalized rites, such as removal of the clitoris or mutilation of the male genitals, which may reflect the adults' fear of and hostility to the budding sexuality of youth.

Hostility is often expressed through physical punishment of children by parents. Concomitant with corporal punishment are feelings of frustration, guilt, anger, and helplessness. Health care professionals also feel similar exasperated feelings in dealing with adolescents, especially the younger adolescent. "I wanted to shake her" (said of a 13-year-old mother of a premature baby in ICN who was arguing with her siblings about who would hold the infant) "and yell, 'Why don't you grow up!'" "I wanted to shake some sense into him" (said of a 13-year-old delinquent boy who refused to communicate and remained silent). These statements by health care professionals were not made callously but out of concern for the young persons; they reflect their frustrated feeling of helplessness and their inability to communicate verbally.

Anger at the adolescent is one of the primary emotional responses of health professionals when the behavior of the young person does not meet adult expectations. If the 17-year-old boy expresses his rebellion against years of surgery and constraining braces for treatment of scoliosis by refusing to follow through with his plan of care, the nurse gets angry because of her *concern* that he is damaging his health. The youth who was restrained from activity for so long and who had no control over movement is learning to exercise control, however detrimental. Both the nurse and the youth must recognize what is happening rather than continue in conflict. The adolescent boy who refuses to care for his body and to be involved with his peers also evokes anger. This behavior may indicate signs of depression, and such a youth cannot cope with the fear of an angry adult's response at the same time. The adult fears loss of control in the situation; the adolescent fears the responses of a hostile adult.

Recognizing one's anger is a first step in modifying one's behavioral response to anger. The adolescent may be told, "When you ignore instructions that endanger your health like that it upsets me and I get angry at you for not caring more about yourself.'' The sensitive adolescent *perceives* the adult's anger; therefore a frank acknowledgment of what caused the anger may relieve him or even motivate him to take better care of his body. It is important to convey the idea that the health professional cares and is truly concerned about the adolescent's welfare. Once the health professional expresses these feelings, the adolescent may clarify his behavior. Sometimes physical or economic constraints prevent the adolescent's following a regimen of care. By dealing with anger in an open manner, the health professional also provides a role model for an acceptable way of handling anger.

FRUSTRATION

Frustration, one of the most common emotional states of health professionals who work with adolescents, results from feelings of disappointment in the youth's response, and may often lead to feelings of defeat. There are feelings of helplessness or lack of control in the situation. These feelings lead to feelings of inadequacy and incompetency: What can I do? How do I cope with the situation? Where do I turn next? It is important for the health professional to recognize that the adolescent's parent must also experience these same feelings. Thus, an empathetic approach when communicating with parents is very helpful. It can also enable parents to be less defensive in their responses.

Josselyn[4] reflected that the adolescent needs to have persons over 30 to dialogue with and to test ideas. It is important for the professional person relating to the adolescent to differentiate between tolerance for the individual and permissiveness, between argument and agreement, between authoritative and authoritarian attitudes, and between the real meaning of a statement and the meaning assumed by the professional. In assisting the youth, it is important that no attempt be made to mold him into an image of what the professional thinks he should be.[4] The fact that we encourage the adolescent to express his divergent thoughts and views or are tolerant of his erratic behavior does not suggest that we must agree that he is correct or deny that our knowledge extends far beyond the young person's.

The health professional is obligated to present the knowledge and understanding at his command in the relevant situation. The young person is encouraged to think about choices; if the situation is too intense, he may be asked to imagine what a hypothetical individual in a similar situation would do and how he might feel. By projecting, the adolescent can express feelings and, by verbalizing them, can weigh the values involved and eventually arrive at choices that are meaningful to his situation. For example, Jan, a noncommunicative 17-year-old, admitted having regular sexual activity to the clinic nurse. Jan also stated that she did not wish to get pregnant and she did not want to use birth control. Silence followed. The nurse reflected, ''Anne, a junior in high school and a rather large girl who had always had irregular periods, discovered that she was four and a half months pregnant. She did not want to drop out of school, and did not want to have a baby. She had big plans to go to the junior-senior prom in two months. How do you think she felt? What could have been some reasons that she didn't use a contraceptive? What could she do in this situation? What were some possible choices for her?'' Jan responded that Anne probably did not use a contraceptive because she was afraid her mother would find the equipment if she used a diaphragm or foam, and that Anne had a friend who had gained weight while taking the contraceptive pill. The nurse then talked about the possibility of Anne's finding a private place to hide a diaphragm and jelly and asked Jan to add ideas for places to keep a diaphragm. The nurse then talked about side effects of contraceptive pills and how changing to a pill of lower dosage could relieve side effects. As Jan explored the hypothetical Anne's feelings and options in her predicament, Jan stated, "I want to go on the pill; I was afraid it would make me nervous and fat. Now I know that if there are side effects, it could be changed." With this resolution, the nurse's initial feelings of frustration changed to feelings of success.

The very young, uncommunicative mother who appears uninterested and aloof arouses similar feelings of frustration, defeat, and helplessness. What can the public health nurse do? Recognition of the young adolescent's developmental stage enables the nurse to focus on the *mother's* need. Only if the mother's feelings about herself as a good, worthwhile person can develop, can she have energy to direct to an infant. Only by focusing on the mother's feelings about her situation (Did she really want to keep her baby?) and on her concerns (She has no one to keep the baby while she goes to school) can progress be made. School is the priority work of the young adolescent; therefore, are there resources to help her attain this priority? The young adolescent needs the security of a mothering person to meet her dependency needs. Does she have a mother who can serve as a role model and meet these dependency needs? If not, what can be done to assure a surrogate mother for her?

A crucial factor in working with adolescents is to continually reflect on the adolescent's developmental need and ask whether our expectations are too high. If we are expecting a 14-year-old with an adult body to respond to mothering with adult cognitive sophistication and emotions, we only increase our own frustrations when we attempt to intervene to promote health.

Adolescents' Responses to Health Professionals

The adolescent gets cues for his response from interactions with health professionals, from the news media, and from social conditions and laws. In his work toward achieving his identity, the responses from the significant persons in his milieu affect and direct his response in fulfilling the adolescent role.

STEREOTYPICAL RESPONSES

Anyone who is not a teenager may be viewed by the teenager either as a mere child or too old to understand, to feel human emotions, or to be trusted. Somehow, all adulthood seems to be clumped together and is described as an "ancient" group "who lived in the old days." Obviously, anyone who was an "adolescent in the old days" cannot understand the problems of adolescence as they are today. The preceding discussions have supported the idea that there is some truth in this stereotype.

All adults seem to dress alike and seem to hold to similar values which are assiduously quoted by them as superior to other values—over and over. These look-alike, "square" adults who grew up in the "old days" are sometimes frightened by the adolescent's bluffs, which in turn frightens the adolescent who is seeking a stable role model. The more personally involved the adult, the more personally responsible the adult may feel, and hence the less objective the adult may be able to be. The youth may then see adults as "wishy-washy," hypocritical, and ineffective. Because adults say, "Do as I say and not as I do," withhold information, and keep secrets behind a smug exterior, the youth responds with secretiveness and an appearance of superiority. The youth's turn to intellectualism and asceticism at this stage in life supports his belief in the superiority of his thinking.

There is one occasion, however, when the adolescent does not view his parent as a stereotype of everyone else's father or mother. This is the occasion on which he wishes to go somewhere that the parent considers "off limits." At this time, the parent is the "only" parent who isn't allowing his child to go!

HOSTILITY

An epidemiological survey of 6,709 Australian adolescents 13 to 18 years old assessed their hostility.[5] A "Hostility and Direction of Hostility Questionnaire" with three subscales measuring extrapunitiveness (acting out hostility, criticism of others, and paranoid hostility) and two subscales measuring intropunitiveness (self-criticism and guilt) was used. Total hostility was found to be at a maximum during the period from 13 to 15 years; hostility fell by the seventeenth and eighteenth years. Boys had significantly higher hostility scores at ages 13, 14, and 16 than girls. As age increased, a significant decrease in extrapunitiveness was noted in both sexes. Girls were consistently less extrapunitive than boys. Girls, on the other hand, were more intropunitive than boys over all ages. Intropunitiveness decreased with both boys and girls as age increased, although the decrease was not as great as for extra-punitiveness.

Although this study reflects hostility manifested by Australian adolescents, if there are universal conflicts experienced during the years of storm and stress, a similar response might be found among American youth. If pregnancy indicates acting-out behavior, national statistics suggest a correlation of similar hostile behaviors at similar ages. Fewer pregnancies are observed in American girls under the age of 16—when Australian girls were significantly less hostile than boys—than in the 17- to 18-year range when hostility was similar in both sexes. The Australian study, suggesting the tendency for girls to respond with anxiety or depression during stressful conditions and for boys to respond by more overt antisocial behavior, supported the findings that girls are more intropunitive and boys are more extra-punitive. The fact that the rate of attempted suicide for girls is almost five times that for boys (in Australia) further supports the research findings.

The implications of this important study are that health professionals need to recognize male-female differences in the expression of hostility and that different approaches in dealing with hostility are warranted. In determining at what point hostile behavior is more than just a symptom of adolescence, the total situation must be considered, however. The particular stressor, the age, the social conditions, and the amount of the perceived stress must be weighed against the knowledge of adolescent developmental behavior.[6] Society stands to gain greatly if rebellious or aggressive behavior is given constructive channels for expression.[7]

STRUGGLE FOR INDEPENDENCE

The adolescent in his quest for independence and in his struggle with his parents to assert independence, may transfer this struggle to the nurse, the physician, or the teacher. All represent adult authority figures of whom they wish to be independent. If the health care worker happens to give a teenager a diet with a lot of "don'ts" on it, the adolescent may automatically reject it and eat potato chips and a cola drink for lunch. Inner independence, acquisition of prioritized values, and responsibility for behavior are all prerequisites of choice.[8] The adolescent's choices are not always wise, but he is working on this task. Providing the adolescent with the opportunity to make choices in planning a health regimen facilitates his growth. When a therapeutic action in the youth's best interest is mandated, the therapist needs to be aware that in taking authoritarian action in the client's best interest he is taking away the person's opportunity to choose and to struggle toward his eventual values.[8]

Testing one's independence is a must; role playing always helps the incumbent in a new position to adapt to new roles. If the nurse can view the adolescent as role playing a new adult role and realize that it is even more crucial to share appropriate information and behaviors in a role-modeling manner, perhaps some of the interactions can be viewed as more helpful by both parties.

Hazards for Professionals Working with Adolescents

Laufer[9] cautioned that working exclusively with adolescents can lead to dangers for the professional; among these are an air of omnipotence; an unconscious demand that the adolescent idealize him; a living out via the adolescent's sexual life of one's own difficulties; and the need to be a perfect parent, or savior, with consequent downgrading of the adolescent's parents in order to make oneself look superior.

The person who chooses to work with young people ideally has examined his motives, values, and goals for doing so, and continues his self-analysis following professional encounters with adolescents. Potential traps or shortcomings for the nurse or professional who works with adolescents are reviewed according to the initial tasks of adolescence that were introduced in Chapter 1.

ACCEPTANCE OF AND ACHIEVEMENT OF COMFORT WITH BODY IMAGE

Whether the young person is concerned about severe acne or whether she is concerned about obesity, many feelings may be expressed. The overweight adult who handles frustrations by eating something may have feelings of envy when viewing svelte, firm, shapely bodies, or may even feel hostility because youth has all of the advantages.

Are you as an adult comfortable with your self-image? This does not suggest that anyone or everyone should be complacent with self-image, but the professional who feels sufficiently comfortable will be able to cope good-humoredly with adolescent candidness. A nurse interviewing a high school girl who voiced concern about being overweight commented, "You don't look overweight to me." The young woman immediately replied, "I agree *my* weight problem isn't nearly as large as *yours!*" An ability to laugh and to agree with such astute and accurate observations is important. A defensive response in the above situation would have ended a fruitful interview; as it was, the interview continued with mutual respect for each due to the nurse's sense of humor.

DETERMINATION AND INTERNALIZATION OF SEXUAL IDENTITY AND ROLE

Comfort with his or her sexual identity and sexual role does not exempt the health professional from countertransference or from having conscious and unconscious feelings about the client. If the health professional had problems dealing with her own sexuality during adolescence, the pain currently experienced by the client can exacerbate all of the counselor's early pain. Undue effort to take away or ease the same pain for the adolescent may result. If the adolescent senses, on the other hand, that the health professional becomes upset when she talks about her sexual experiences, she may choose to avoid talking about these experiences, or she may deliberately upset the interviewer by dwelling on them. In situations in which the adolescent experiences problems similar to those of the health professional, therapeutic response is even more difficult.[10]

It is important that each professional analyze her personal feelings about sex and assess her comfort in talking about sexual matters. Young people need factual information; biased or restricted information makes it more difficult for them to resolve their conflicts. Some professionals may feel that adolescents' discussion of or interest in sex leads to sexual behavior; the notion of sex as a taboo topic to be indulged in by adults only may then be unconsciously conveyed. At a time when reproductive capacity has just come into being, curiosity about the body's functioning is at a peak, and it is an absolute right of the individual to know and understand about the body's functioning for biological and emotional or for pleasurable purposes.

A professional's discomfort with the topic of sex may lead an adolescent to withdraw from the topic to protect the professional and thus go unprotected herself. If there is not a climate of acceptance and nonjudgmental sharing of concerns, facts, and feelings, this is an enormous disservice to the young person. Are we open to the most sensitive or intimate question with which an adolescent is faced, or are we unconsciously unapproachable?

An adolescent's behavior may be, at times, seductive, and this requires a mature response to the situation so that the adolescent's self-esteem is not undermined. A nurse practitioner was doing a physical examination on 17-year-old Don. Don stated, ''I'll bet you'd enjoy more than just listening to this muscular chest.'' In a situation of this sort, any number of factors would be operative: Don may have a ''crush'' on the practitioner as often happens among high school students and their teachers; Don may be testing the nurse's ability to handle the situation; he may be testing his masculine appeal to a young woman; he may have experienced rejection from a girl whom he wished to date; or he could have been approached by a male homosexual because of his very attractive body build. The nurse may clarify what Don means by an open-ended statement: ''You have an excellent physique; this could result in a lot of different reactions from others. . . .'' Don, who is probably somewhat anxious and nervous, may blurt out, ''But I can't get a date for the prom,'' or ''This fruit on the beach propositioned me.'' Depending on verbal and nonverbal cues, the nurse may decide to reaffirm that Don is attractive and has masculine appeal or discuss the confused, angry feelings a young man may experience when he sought to impress the girls on the beach and was instead approached by another man. If Don happens to be overtly romantically pursuing the nurse, firm limits may be set without placing Don in a position to feel total rejection: ''It is very gratifying to examine someone whose food and exercise habits are obviously very good. I do not date clients, however.'' According to her own personal style the nurse can convey the idea that Don as a person is attractive and likable, but not for her emotional involvement.

DEVELOPMENT OF A PERSONAL VALUE SYSTEM

The troubled adolescent needs a creative listener as he presents a potpourri of good, bad, or questionable problems. A creative listener *hears what the youth is saying* rather than what her value system condones. Clarifying what the adolescent is saying and what he values involves saying ''Tell me more about what you mean,'' instead of nodding ''I understand this is a difficult decision.'' A breakdown in communication can result in a situation in which neither the adult nor the adolescent is understanding the other; in fact they may be speaking about entirely different matters.

Personal biases can end all communication with the adolescent who is contemplating whether she wishes to relinquish her infant for adoption. If the nurse says, ''You people should not get pregnant until you can afford a family,'' the troubled young person feels totally rejected, becomes angry and defensive, and may refuse further antepartal care.

The adolescent's personal value system suffers many disappointments as he sees adults whom he admires fail to live up to his idealistic expectations. If the nurse's ashtray is overflowing as she talks about the dangers of nicotine, her image as an honest person to rap and exchange ideas with may be destroyed. Similarly, the youth who smokes ''grass'' easily rejects his father's admonitions if the father abuses his family following excessive drinking.

PREPARATION FOR PRODUCTIVE CITIZENSHIP

Often the health professional or the teacher was born in an era when few occupational choices were possible for women: they could be teachers, nurses, or secretaries. Can the adult professional enjoy seeing the wide range of choices available to the young woman today? Does she resent how "easy" the young person's life is, with respect to the schools or the money available, compared with a previous time? Does she appreciate the difficulties of the young person in making a choice when so many are available? The professional who understands some of these differences between generations can communicate more effectively with impatient parents who are demanding that "Susan must get a graduate degree in engineering" or are concerned that she select a major during her first year of college.

If the professional is not comfortable working with adolescents, recognition of this should motivate him to seek a transfer to a different setting or to negotiate for a different function within the same setting. Dissatisfaction or conflicts emerging from interaction with an age group should be faced constructively; how else can a professional encourage constructive action in an adolescent?

ACHIEVEMENT OF INDEPENDENCE FROM PARENTS

Very few persons emerge as adults without some unresolved conflict, either minor or major. Developmentally, adults are in transition throughout life. What is important is that individuals assess and reflect on their interpersonal interactions with others as a part of the personal growth process.

Does the professional feel a need to have a client remain in a dependent relationship with her because of her own unresolved conflict with authority figures? Does the professional enjoy watching the young person assume independence and grow beyond the need for professional interaction? These are the kinds of questions that need to be asked over and over. Does the nurse feel rejected when the adolescent says that he no longer needs the class, or that she no longer needs help with the parenting role?

Can the professional cope with broken appointments? Does she call to determine what is going on and tell the adolescent she missed him—or send a note if she cannot call? The adolescent may be testing his independence.

The seeming ease with which adolescents can cancel appointments or just "not show up" can be very frustrating to the nurse in the busy clinic who has difficulty seeing everyone who needs to be seen, and to the public health nurse who drives ten miles to make a home visit. Although adolescents are busy people involved in many activities, professionals are equally busy and have a responsibility to reach many other clients who have equal needs.

It is important for the professional to interact with the adolescent who has broken the appointment as an adult. As stated above, a courteous call or note to inquire about possible difficulty encountered in keeping the appointment, with emphasis that the client was missed, lets the adolescent know he is important to the professional. Once this information is obtained, if the reason for breaking the appointment is legitimate, or even if it is not, the nurse can set limits for her expectations—e.g., a phone call is expected if an emergency arises, to make it possible to schedule an appointment for another client. The time allotted to the adolescent is available, but not to be wasted. The setting of limits is equally important for the habitually late adolescent. "If you are not here by 15 minutes after the appointed time, you will have to make another appointment, for I will be involved with another client." Honesty is important in dealing with the situation; the youth can see that the limit setting is not punitive or dictatorial but a matter of expediency.

Making a contract or verbal agreement with the adolescent about the time for an appointment and the length of time the appointment is to last is very important. Time may be viewed by him as meted out according to his worth. This connotation should be avoided. When the time limit is specified, the adolescent knows in advance what to expect. It is helpful to remind the adolescent during the appointment that ten minutes remain. This allows the adolescent to assign priorities to his concerns and ask a question that needs to be addressed that has not yet been discussed.

The frequent moves made by families in today's society sometimes make follow-up difficult. A good relationship—one which the adolescent values—is essential to motivate him to share with the professional any projected moves. The lack of continuity from one district in the city to another is evident when the young person moves and is not referred to another professional in the area. The immature youth may use the opportunity of a family's residential move to end the professional-client relationship and may deliberately withhold information so that follow-up by another professional is not possible.

DEVELOPMENT OF AN ADULT IDENTITY

Ideally, the health professional is comfortable with her own identity and her roles so that she is able to respond to individuals in a personalized, sincere manner, rather than in a mechanical fashion. Awareness that all personal interactions reflect to the adolescent something of himself as a person and of how he appears to others facilitates consistent, therapeutic responses. If adolescents are perceived as responsible individuals who can identify and discuss their own concerns and needs, this is reflected by the mode of implementing health care programs. For example, does the teacher decide that a class on grooming is needed because of the sloppy attire she sees and then post a sign announcing that a special class will be held, or does she ask the group if they have any interest in a class in grooming and then talk to individuals to find out if such an interest truly exists? The approach one uses in planning for educational programs, special group sessions, or other activities says something to the adolescent about how the professional feels about his thoughts and concerns in the matter.

The adult is always the outsider in an adolescent group. If this can be remembered, perhaps greater care can be taken to assess the group's wishes, needs, and concerns, and greater care will be taken to interpret the adult's concern or perceived need for a class or group. Adolescents also want specifics: How long will the class last and over what period of time? What do you expect to be the outcome of such an action? What do you expect from the young people? Adolescents are busy individuals with school, various extracurricular lessons, sports, homework assignments, etc., and failing to determine a compatible, specified time will prevent some classes from ever getting started.

Once a class or group session is initiated, the role of the leader continues to have an impact on the adolescent's perception of himself. An authoritarian role projects to the adolescent that he is still a child who needs didactic ''telling'' rather than a blossoming adult who has something very important to contribute to the group discussion and interaction. While adolescents have a strong need to know, at the same time they are often reluctant to bare their ignorance by forthrightly saying ''I don't know.'' The climate must be nonthreatening and all questions must be handled seriously, or else the group will assume an ''all-wise'' attitude and say, ''We know that.''

Communication Problems

Perhaps one of the most frustrating of interviews is a non-interview. The adolescent remains sullen and withdrawn and appears not to listen. If she is in her home environment, she may watch television or listen to the radio during the interview. The professional feels helpless in making ''contact'' with the young person.

Addressing the young person by his name and phrasing questions that cannot be answered by yes or no or a grunt helps. ''Tell me what you enjoy doing during your spare time,'' is sometimes a good opener, since it gives the adolescent an opportunity to talk about something pleasurable and nonthreatening.

Since school is the work of the adolescent just as play is the work of the child, it is important to know something of the youth's feelings and performance in this important facet of his life. Questions such as ''What do you like best about school?'' and ''What do you find the most uninteresting?'' may be useful in helping the adolescent to open up. The statement ''Tell me about your friends and what you do together'' gets at information about his ability to get along with his peers. After a discussion of recreational activities, school, and friends, some rapport may be established and similar statements can be made which seek information about how he gets along with family members—i.e., ''Tell me about your brothers and sisters,'' ''Tell me about your parents.''

To facilitate communication, privacy is important. The adolescent may share little information if people are popping in and out of the room or if there is a lot of traffic past the place where the interviewer and adolescent are seated in an open area.

If the adolescent's behavior continues to be sullen or hostile, it is well to remember that he or she may be very emotionally immature. A question that sounds similar to that of a parent will be responded to as the youth responds to a parent. In any interview, both listening and observing for body communication are important ways of enhancing sensitivity to feelings of depression, rejection, or inadequacy that the adolescent is communicating. Efforts can be made to foster the adolescent's self-esteem by expressing interest and concern. A flat response to the adolescent's flat response will not stimulate any interest.

Role modeling in effective communication may be needed. Demonstrating courtesy, concern, and interest through change of voice tone and body posture, may sometimes help to break the ice. A phony is readily recognized by the perceptive adolescent.

An adolescent may appear at a clinic completely against his will. When this seems to be the case and he refuses to acknowledge all attempts at communication, a statement like "You must be very upset and angry about coming here today completely against your wishes. You may leave any time you wish," might help. The angry adolescent will not communicate anyway, and acknowledging his feelings and giving him a choice shows respect for him as an individual. The statement "You may set an appointment for another day when you feel like talking, if you wish," gives him an opportunity to state his reasons for desiring to leave or for not wishing to come in the first place.

Because of the "normal" turmoil of adolescence, health care professionals may fail to recognize signs of depression that need appropriate professional referral for both the adolescent and his family. Wouters and King[11] emphasized that the adolescent does not necessarily say that he is depressed but may use vaguer terms such as "sad," "low," "blue," "hopeless," "worried," or "discouraged." If four of the following symptoms are present, the adolescent may be considered as having the "depression syndrome": change in eating habits or weight, from loss of appetite to overeating and obesity; insomnia or hypersomnia; loss of energy, fatigue; change in psychomotor behavior ranging from inactivity to constant movement; loss of interest in usual activities, out-of-proportion feelings of self-reproach or guilt; difficulty thinking and concentrating which is reflected in school performance; and preoccupation with death.[11]

Summary

The professional cannot be a miracle worker; however, the professional is the adult in the interactional process who is expected to have a knowledge and an experiential base. The adolescent has certain expectations which in reality are usually reasonable. Conflicts experienced by both the professional and the adolescent may be the result of stereotypic thinking which must be identified and changed.

The helpful professional cannot be all things to all people, and this can be honestly acknowledged. The professional in meeting the adolescent's health needs can strive to be: an objective friend without attempts at familiarity; available without being angry about occasional impositions; empathetic without being overeager; firm in his or her convictions without vacillation or proselytizing; a communicator as a peer, not as a pal; honest without being bluntly cruel; respectful without disdain; and one who keeps confidences confidential.

Because of the inner turmoil the adolescent experiences, the professional must remain vigilant to recognize signs of depression which indicate that additional help is needed.

REFERENCES

1. Davis, K. "The Sociology of Parent-Youth Conflict." In Winder, A. E., and Angus, D. L., eds. *Adolescence: Contemporary Studies*. New York: Van Nostrand Reinhold Co., 1968, 69–79.
2. Anthony, J. "The Reactions of Adults to Adolescents and Their Behavior." In Caplan, G., and Lebovici, S., eds. *Adolescence Psychological Perspectives*. New York: Basic Books, Inc., 1969, 54–78.
3. Woodmansey, A. C. "The Common Factor in Problems of Adolescence." *Brit. J. Med. Psychol.* 42:353–370, 1969.
4. Josselyn, I. M. "Value Problems in the Treatment of Adolescents." *Smith College Studies in Social Work* 42(1):1–14, 1971.
5. Henderson, S., et al. "An Assessment of Hostility in a Population of Adolescents." *Arch. Gen. Psychiat.* 34:706–711, 1977.
6. LeBow, J. A. "Evaluating the Seriousness of Adolescent Adjustment Reactions." *Primary Care* 2(2):281–287, 1975.
7. Gibson, R. "The One With the Elephant (A Further Reflection on Adolescence)." *Brit. Med. J.* 2:1541–1544, 1976.
8. Portnoy, I. "Choice: The Human Prerogative." *Am. J. Psychoanal.* 31:35–38, 1971.
9. Laufer, M. "Prevention Intervention in Adolescence." *Psychoanalyt. Study of Child* 30:511–528, 1975.
10. Rotman, C. B., and Golburgh, S. J. "The Psychotherapist's Feelings About the Adolescent Patient (Countertransference)." *Adolescence* 11(43):335–339, 1976.
11. Wouters, M. L., and King, L. J. "Depression in Adolescents." *Primary Care* 2(3):431–440, 1975.

16

The Health Care System
and the Adolescent

RAMONA T. MERCER, R.N., PH.D.

The presence of an excellent health care facility in a community does not mean that adolescents will take advantage of it. Despite the increased number of family planning clinics with easily available contraceptives, unwanted and unplanned pregnancies continue to occur among teenagers. Despite special schools and special maternity-infant care programs, large numbers of young mothers do not finish high school and do not receive the necessary counseling for planning goals and for their mental health. What brings about a gap between the availability of health services and the utilization of these services by the teenage population? What characteristics of the health care system do the young people find so objectionable that they do not utilize available care?

A national survey of the nature and degree of agreement between youths and their parents in regard to health perceptions and attitudes found that both groups generally ranked symptoms for which one should see a physician in the same order.[1] Adolescents perceive a need for medical care much as their parents do. National Center for Health Statistics data show that almost three fourths of adolescents saw a physician in 1972; 72% of 12- to 19-year-olds visited physicians and 60% made visits to dentists.[2]

This chapter explores some of the characteristics of the health care system and their effect on the adolescent's use of it. The failure of the system to meet the needs of young persons and the system's characteristics that are not congruent with adolescent developmental tasks are discussed.

The Health Care System

The term ''health care system'' is used broadly and incorporates the philosophical stance of a health care providing institution, the rules and regulations that direct the institution's functioning, and the local, state and federal programs that may control it through the withdrawal or contribution of funds. A health care system has certain characteristics that set it apart. It includes a group of professional and nonprofessional persons who are interacting to achieve a purposeful goal. There is a recognizable boundary to the system so that one usually knows what is a part of the system and what is not. For example, a local public health agency is a system made up of the personnel interacting within a specifically identified base (the building). The health care system may be either open or closed, depending upon the organizational structure. In an open system there is a constant interchange between the system and the environment; in a closed system there is no interchange with those outside the system or the environment.

The health care system of some countries is controlled solely by the government so that there is no discrimination in the delivery of health care to all citizens. No such homogeneous picture of a health care system exists in the United States. There are many quite diverse patterns for delivery of care, ranging from urban areas where university hospitals deliver the highest level of care to the most critically ill patients to the rural area where there is no doctor, and a public health nurse or a nurse practitioner meets the local health needs and refers those who are ill to institutions some 100 to 300 miles away from their homes. The adolescent may have access to a special clinic for adolescent health, or he may live in a city in which no institution exists to consider his special needs. Therefore, many of the health care systems are only tolerating the adolescent as a difficult client with whom to deal; their main concern or focus lies elsewhere. This may be the crux of the problem when many adolescents fail to receive necessary health care and counseling.

Eisen observes a posture of avoidance of adolescent health problems in Australia.[3] He postulates that this avoidance filters through to the health care system from professional literature that continues to be colored by suspicion. Although Eisen describes the prevalence of adolescent physical illness as being somewhat less than that of adult illness, he points out a great discrepancy between the delivery of health care to the adolescent and to the adult. Disorders may be overlooked in the adolescent, and the preventive aspects of health care such as obesity control, dental care, and nutrition may be neglected. Drucker[4] suggests that the incidence of serious illness in the 10- to 20-year-old is similar to that in the adult population but that the type of illness is different. The adolescent has fewer cardiovascular illnesses than the adult but a higher incidence of suicide, drug abuse deaths, and injuries.[4]

The terms commonly used in describing problems in the United States health care system: *fragmented, crisis-oriented, inefficient, traditionalistic, physician-oriented, uncoordinated,* and *inappropriately utilized* present greater problems to the adolescent than to the adult, especially if he is poor.[5] The majority of poor adolescents are from ethnic groups such as blacks, Puerto Ricans, Mexican-Americans, and American Indians, who tend to have higher incidences of infectious diseases, orthopedic and visual impairments, mental illness, and untreated dental caries.[5] This group of adolescents is more vulnerable to illness and more often live in areas in which health care is inadequate or absent. What kinds of problems do these and other adolescents face in the health care system?

RIGIDITY OF THE SYSTEM

The system may be viewed by the adolescent as rigid from several perspectives. It may be operating as a closed system; that is, the staff are inflexible, and the rules and regulations are immutable, with no outside input. A closed system does not consider the developmental tasks of the adolescent—his work of achieving independence and assuming responsibility for his welfare, of resolving his concerns with body image, and of building his personal value system. Direct conflict results between an impulsive and rebellious adolescent and an immutable clinic schedule and inflexible staff. The conflict most often is resolved by the adolescent's ignoring the services and reporting the unreasonableness of the clinic to his peers, who follow his advice to stay away from that particular clinic.

Alternatives in health care must be presented to the adolescent along with the merits and shortcomings of each alternative so that the young person himself makes a decision about his care. Direct, didactic instructions to an adolescent whose parents are fearfully submitting to him may simply be ignored, because of the lenient attitudes he has experienced with his acquiescing parents. Or, if the parents are very strict and enforce difficult rules, the rebellious adolescent may defy the health care provider's instructions as he does his parent's.

However, though rigidity of the system must be avoided, clarity and communication must be maintained. The teenager *wants* to know the expectations of the health care provider very clearly. He needs to know the rules governing the keeping of appointments and what his responsibility is when an appointment has to be missed. A certain amount of structure is needed and expected to facilitate the smooth operation of the health care system; information should be provided to the adolescent so that he knows the limitations that have been set.

Rigidity may be viewed from the perspective of automated, or mechanized, assembly-line care. In a rigid family-planning facility there is "one" favored method of contraception. All young persons are coerced into choosing this "one" method. No consideration is given to the individual who has sex sporadically and for whom foam and condoms may be preferable to taking the contraceptive pill. Likewise, no consideration is given to the erratic life style of the individual who will have difficulty remembering to take a pill every day.

Rigidity may be viewed from the perspective of clinic hours. If the clinic operates largely from 9:00 A.M. to 4:00 P.M. the student will have difficulty going to the clinic for counseling and care. Schedules need to be arranged so that a student does not have to miss class or a special function after school in order to receive health care. Availability of services and accessibility of the facility must fit the life-space of the adolescent.

GAPS IN THE SYSTEM

The fragmented care that has developed as a concomitant of increased specialization is especially frightening to an adolescent. Fragmented care may seem as diffuse to the youth as his evolving identity, and therefore quite impersonal and threatening. When he sees several health care providers, each of whom knows very little about him or his problem, he does not become comfortable enough to discuss his concerns. His emotional and social problems are never identified and dealt with. A longtime relationship with one person facilitates identifying and helping the adolescent to recognize any psychosocial problems with which he may be faced. When health care workers do not recognize his problems, the adolescent may feel that no one cares; he may become depressed and/or act out through antisocial behavior, or he may harm himself, as in a suicide attempt.

The adolescent's needs for health education may go completely unnoticed in a system in which he deals with multiple persons and there is no continuity with one person. He may need sexual or contraceptive counseling; he may need knowledge about drugs—tobacco, alcohol, and other street chemicals. Factual knowledge is necessary before the individual can make wise decisions about practices that may affect his health over a lifetime.

The fact that a clinic holds special classes for nutrition, contraceptive counseling, avoiding venereal disease, etc., does not mean that adolescents will attend them, especially when adolescents are not segregated from older adults. Adolescents are reluctant to ask questions when in a group of older adults who may be viewed as near their parents' age. Teenagers also show a certain immaturity in not wanting to expose their lack of knowledge. Adults in such classes also tend to respond to adolescents on an adult-to-child basis rather than as adult-to-adult.

Fragmented care also results in multiple examinations. The young person whose body image is in flux is highly sensitive and modest about exposure to others. For the female, multiple pelvic examinations are particularly devastating. Especially frightening is the university hospital scene in which a resident and two interns enter, examine the young female, talk to each other about the internal organs they are palpating (or baseball), and ignore her. The adult is offended and threatened by this rude behavior; the adolescent doubly so.

AVAILABILITY OF THE HEALTH CARE SYSTEM

Health care systems are less accessible to the poor adolescent. In the city, his welfare status points him to the city hospital emergency room or to a busy waiting room in the clinic. There the care may be rushed and impersonal, and the gaps in care that were identified earlier are all operative—his emotional and social needs go unidentified; consequently, he does not receive social counseling with regard to alternatives in health care and educational or job opportunities.

Further, many young people are concerned about permanent records and who has access to them. They are afraid that their parents will learn that they were treated for gonorrhea.

The rural adolescent, especially the poor native Indian or Mexican-American, often lives in remote areas where resources are sorely limited. Neither funds nor personnel for teen contraceptive clinics or teen medical examination clinics are usually available. If the one available family physician treats him, he fears that the entire community will know that he was afflicted or ill. Many ethnic groups believe that some illnesses are caused by careless or unclean behavior or promiscuousness.

To become ill when one is not guilty of any of these stigmatizing behaviors has an even more frightening impact on the adolescent, who may prefer to suffer rather than appear to be guilty of the wrong behavior.

The problem of the distribution of health care services is one that will probably have to be solved at state and national levels. Attempts are made to channel health care providers into isolated areas by exempting repayment of scholarship funds if the health professional agrees to work for two years or more (depending on the amount of the scholarship) in a medically deprived area upon graduation.

Since health services are based on social models, practices, and norms which reflect the norms of middle- and upper-class providers, the poor adolescent's health needs often suffer most. Private physicians are the major source of ambulatory health care for the total population, including the poor; public clinics provide the second major source of care for the poor.[6] The poor adolescent may lack money for transportation to reach a clinic, as well as funds to see a private physician. The poor usually have less scientific knowledge about health care and tend to seek advice and treatment from friends, family, or others before seeking professional help.[6] When health care is sought, their lack of knowledge about health, their difficulties in communication, and the dissimilarities between their social backgrounds and those of the health professionals make it difficult for them to obtain satisfactory counseling and help.[6] The formal bureaucracy of public organizations creates additional blocks that prevent the poor from receiving adequate care.[6] As a consequence, the poor very often receive health care only on a crisis basis.[7]

Cobliner[8] surveyed 2,485 students aged 13 to 18 in 10 schools in a borough of New York City by questionnaire; 71% stated that they would go to see a physician for advice on health care, 28% specified an older person, and 1% did not answer. Students were queried about the kinds of special arrangements for health care they would use; 36% stated that they would visit the outpatient clinic of a municipal hospital, 59% would visit the outpatient clinic after hours, 61% would visit a teenage clinic at convenient hours, and 22% indicated that they would visit a cruising medical trailer. When asked which health care facility they would utilize for sex and drug problems, 12% indicated an outpatient clinic in a hospital, 4% an outpatient clinic in a hospital after hours, 34% a teenage clinic, 40% a private physician, 6% would not seek help, and 4% gave no answer. These data show the reluctance of the teenager to use the outpatient clinic of the municipal hospital for sex or drug problems. Questions relating to the privacy and autonomy that adolescents desire in visits to a teenage clinic showed that 61% preferred to go alone, 10% would go with a friend, 28% would go with an older person, and 1% gave no answer. Cobliner suggests that the optimum setting for prevention of adolescent pregnancy is a special teenage clinic that would be open after hours and would allow the young person to go with a friend.

Utilization of private physicians by adolescents means either that they have funds to pay for care, or that their parents are aware of their visit. A survey by Rosenbloom and Ongley[9] of private practice data in 1972 showed that pediatricians saw only 5.5% of 13- to 21-year-olds. Pediatricians, however, reported no visits for venereal disease during that year. Half of the visits to private physicians for venereal disease were with generalists and one fourth were with obstetricians/gynecologists. This survey also noted that although the 13- to 21-year old group made up 16.8% of the population, this age group made only 10.7% of all private physician contacts; the numbers of contacts for the year varied by region—i.e., only 4.3% for 13- to 21-year-olds in the South.

Much planning and coordination for a comprehensive health care program that includes mental health counseling as well as treatment and prevention of infectious diseases is necessary if all adolescents are to have access to basic health care. Currently, mental health facilities are overcrowded, and local residents and property owners fight the placement of larger and better facilities, or even halfway houses, for adolescents in their neighborhoods.

Millar[10] notes that special problems arising from the teenager's life style require new approaches, especially in ambulatory health care, for services. These particularly include addictive problems, emotional disorders, suicidal states, and sexual health problems such as venereal disease, contraception, and unwanted pregnancy. Millar cites various innovative services already in operation that merit more extensive development.[10] Age-specific services staffed by professionals with special preparation in adolescent growth, development, and attitudes are necessary. Millar cautions that if confidentiality is not assured many will not seek help with sensitive sex- or drug-related problems. For young people in communes or other styles of group living, a very nontraditional facility is needed—one that is free and located in their immediate environment. Mobile medical vans have been utilized successfully in some cities. Telephone hotlines provide objective listeners for distraught young persons. They are particularly helpful for suicide prevention and V.D. information. Using teenagers in conjunction with regular staff members in health care centers has proven helpful in many situations.[10] Peer counselors communicate more effectively in situations in which an older person may be distrusted or unsuccessful.

LEGAL RESPONSIBILITIES OF THE HEALTH CARE SYSTEM

Pediatricians include among their reasons for not seeing more adolescents economic factors, limited training in adolescent care, inflation, increased third-party payments with accompanying paper work, and increasing malpractice insurance rates.[11] The lack of specificity governing the adolescent's constitutional rights as opposed to parental rights when parents are responsible for the youth's behavior until the age of 21, may increase the physician's reluctance to increase his adolescent caseload.

In a survey of 63 pediatricians, adolescent behavioral problems were reported frequently: 68% saw communication problems between the young persons and their parents; 45% saw school problems; 40% saw acting-out behaviors; 33% saw peer problems; 22% saw depression; and no one reported seeing psychosis.[11] Because of the high percentage of communication problems observed between parents and child, any health care worker must validate the accusations of either party before taking action. For example, the adolescent's acting-out behavior of running away or joining a religious group may be extremely embarrassing or in some cases terrifying to the parent (when the group is known to be dangerous), but it is not grounds for committing the young person to a mental institution. Likewise, the youth's report of abuse may not be accurate grounds for seeking foster home placement.

The rights of minors over 15 are recognized more clearly, by virtue of the fact that no legal suits have been won by parents with respect to their minor children's seeking and receiving medical care on their own. The young person's right to freedom of religious thought can thus be protected by the First Amendment, in cases in which parents seek to institutionalize minor youths whom they have removed from religious cults for deprogramming.[12] As was pointed out earlier, the adolescent who has the right to consent to treatment has the right to refuse treatment.[12]

Disclosure of confidential material presents further problems for health care providers. Confidentiality is expected in any psychotherapeutic relationship except situations in which the client may do harm to himself or to others. This means that the decision for disclosure of confidences rests with professional judgment.[12] In some situations, institutions clearly state their stand on confidentiality to both parties involved so that adolescents may opt not to have treatment under those circumstances. For example, case workers and psychiatrists in the program of the Association for Jewish Children of Philadelphia tell the adolescents and their parents that they will share confidences with the agency administration or a court of law, if the divulged information has the potential to contribute to the individual's growth and development or mental health.[13] Each party then knows at the outset that any information may be used in the best interest of the developing young person.

In dealing with adolescents, health care providers cannot assume that parents always have the young person's best interest in mind. The difficulties and conflicts associated with this period of turmoil detract heavily from the objectivity of either party's perspective.

Potential Strengths and Assets of Health Care Systems

Although there are areas of weakness in the health care systems, there are strengths and assets upon which communities should build in these systems. As was just pointed out, the loss of objectivity in parent-adolescent conflict can result in embarrassment for both parties. The health care system can reflect and reinforce objectivity in matters of mental and physical health. The health care system may represent security for some individuals who have not even a modicum of anything that can be depended upon at home, e.g., no regular hours for meals, parental absence from home at all hours, and no regulations or rules for functioning in the home.

The health care institution can also pursue an advocacy role. It can provide concrete help and guidance, and should make this known to the community, so that the adolescent can receive the supportive help he needs.

PARENT-ADOLESCENT CONFLICT

Whether the adolescent is an early, middle, or late adolescent can indicate the degree of parental involvement needed for proper treatment of the young person's difficulty. The younger adolescent who is rebelling against simple household chores or requirements for body cleanliness or who has withdrawn from communication probably needs counseling both alone and with his parents. He most likely has not achieved the level of thinking or autonomy necessary to negotiate meaningfully, and his parents may be reinforcing a pattern of indecision and conflict.

The middle adolescent who is learning to solve problems, can be helped to begin to look at situations from the perspectives of others. In some situations, he can be helped considerably in learning to make responsible decisions for his welfare and value system and to interact appropriately with family members on an individual basis. In situations of obvious scapegoating or parental stress—i.e., in such circumstances as divorce, marital instability, etc.—unless parents receive help, it is difficult for the adolescent to resolve his problems.

The older adolescent usually can, with help, develop the ego strength needed to deal with stresses, unless he is psychotic. Some of the older adolescent's upsetting, acting-out behavior may be a last fling or a direct confrontation with his parent's authority before he moves to operating his own value system. His value system often is more like his parents' than not.

Knowledge of the parents' pattern of interaction is, however, very important in any situation. A comparative study of Jewish adolescents who needed treatment in a residential treatment center and well adolescents who were living at home with their parents indicated that the interaction pattern of a submissive father and a domineering mother often led to certain neurotic illnesses requiring placement in a residential treatment center.[14] Fathers of the institutionalized young persons studied seemed to have weak personalities despite a high level of educational achievement; they married women with higher levels of education. This study also found interesting male-female differences. There were no differences in ease of verbal communication between institutionalized and noninstitutionalized females. Males who were institutionalized, however, were less verbal than those who lived at home. The cultural attitudes of the ill young persons were weaker than those found in the well. All adolescents communicated more with their mothers than with their fathers. For communicating important and unpleasant feelings males chose their parents over their peers, whereas females chose a best friend. The best friend role seems very special to females. Because of the tendency toward best friends or very small cliques, group work was difficult in the residential treatment centers for females. It never lasted for any length of time, whereas males were more easily involved in group activities.

COMMUNITY RESOURCES

Because the tasks of adolescence are so closely intertwined and so little is known about the impact of one task on the other, health care systems need the collaborative support of community resources in providing optimal adolescent health care. Some community resources are schools, employment agencies and businesses, individual and organized housing agencies, day-care centers, and political leaders.

The school may contribute to various health education programs. School personnel may need consultation regarding specialized instructional content, especially if a teacher is unprepared to discuss the physiology of reproduction as applied to contraception. Health care providers may volunteer or may contribute to educational programs on a consultative basis. An exchange between a professional who is comfortable discussing reproduction and sexuality can contribute much to an adolescent's acceptance and achievement of comfort with body image and comfort with sexual role. An embarrassed, uncomfortable teacher will add to the adolescent's embarrassment with a new body.

Through dialogue with teachers, general developmental and behavioral problems of adolescents may be shared in order to help the teacher to become more tolerant of the adolescent's testing of authority in his working toward independence.

Selection of and preparation for a vocation or profession is an essential task for the adolescent, one that is prerequisite to his achieving independence from his parents. Employment agencies and businessmen in the community can be encouraged to provide more summertime jobs for young people who are experimenting with future occupational roles. The involvement of businessmen in appropriate high school courses can add to the adolescent's interest in professional and career roles. For example, if in civics class a lawyer or judge attends class and shares some of his knowledge of the legal process, a young person will gain a clearer picture of adult roles and may perhaps be motivated toward seeking these roles, as he learns about the legal system.

For adolescent parents who seek housing apart from parents or older adolescents who wish to live in an apartment before finally seeking total independence, renters may be approached by a social worker or public health nurse and encouraged to rent to young tenants. Communication between rental agencies, parents, and adolescents may facilitate understanding of the young adult's need for separate housing.

Day-care centers for young parents who are attending school or who are working are important if these young people are to become prepared to achieve a quality level of life and a positive self-identity. Day-care centers may be part of a health care system. Professionally staffed day-care centers provide an opportunity for positive role modeling in adult-child relationships by the health care professionals. Much informal counseling occurs between the professional and parent on an important day-to-day basis.

Last, but perhaps the most powerful and influential assets, are the political leaders in the community. The political leaders are chosen by you, the reader. Those in political office invite information about the special needs and health problems in a community, including those of adolescents. Meeting a community's high priority needs results in votes on election day.

The young people of today are our leaders of tomorrow. Their optimal health and functioning in tomorrow's roles depend on intervention and manifested concern about their health today. Does this age group not merit our empathic concern and enthusiastic action and support?

REFERENCES

1. Oliver, L. I. "The Association of Health Attitudes and Perceptions of Youths 12–17 Years of Age with Those of Their Parents: United States, 1966–1970." Rockville, Md.: U.S. Dept. Health, Education, and Welfare, Pub. No. (HRA) 77–1643, 1977.

2. Millar, H. E. C. "Approaches to Adolescent Health Care in the 1970s." Rockville, Md.: U.S. Dept. Health, Education, and Welfare, Pub. No. (HSA) 76–5014, 1975.
3. Eisen, P. "The Challenge of Adolescent Medicine: The Adolescent in Society." *Austral. Paediat. J.* 13:1–6, 1977.
4. Drucker, D.: "Hidden Values and Health Care." *Med. Care* 12(3): 266–273, 1974.
5. Fielding, J. E., and Nelson, S. H. "Health Care for the Economically Disadvantaged Adolescent." *Ped. Clin. N. Am.* 20(4):975–988, 1973.
6. Herman, M. W. "The Poor: Their Medical Needs and the Health Services Available to Them." *Ann. Am. Acad. Polit. Social Sci.* 399:12–21, 1972.
7. Leveson, I. "The Challenge of Health Services for the Poor." *Ann. Am. Acad. Polit. Social Sci.* 399:22–29, 1972.
8. Cobliner, W. G. "Preferred Preventive Health Care Facilities: A Survey Among Urban Adolescents." *Bull. N.Y. Acad. Med.* 49(10):922–930, 1973.
9. Rosenbloom, A. L., and Ongley, J. P. "Provision of Private Physician Services to Children and Adolescents." *Am. J. Dis. of Children* 128:504–507, 1974.
10. Millar, H. E. C. "New Approaches to the Delivery of Health Care to Adolescents." *Proceedings of the First International Symposium on Adolescent Medicine Helsinki, August 4 to 8, 1974. Acta Paediat. Scand.,* Supplement No. 256, 39–45, 1975.
11. McAnarney, E. R., and McAveney, W. J. "The Adolescent and the Pediatrician: Their Future Together." *Clin. Pediat.* 16(2):169–172, 1977.
12. Holder, A. R. *Legal Issues in Pediatrics and Adolescent Medicine.* New York: John Wiley & Sons, Inc., 1977.
13. Taylor, J. L., et al. *A Group Home for Adolescent Girls: Practice and Research.* New York: Child Welfare League of America, Inc., 1976.
14. Appelberg, E. "Verbal Accessibility of Adolescents." In Feiner, H. A., ed. *The Uprooted: The Collected Papers of Esther Appelberg.* New York: The Child Welfare League of America, Inc., 1977, 57–65.

Index

413